THE HEALING ECHO

DISCOVERING HOMEOPATHIC CELL SALT REMEDIES

VINTON McCABE

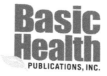

Basic Health
PUBLICATIONS, INC.

The information contained in this book is based upon the research and personal and professional experiences of the author. It is not intended as a substitute for consulting with your physician or other healthcare provider. Any attempt to diagnose and treat an illness should be done under the direction of a healthcare professional.

The publisher does not advocate the use of any particular healthcare protocol but believes the information in this book should be available to the public. The publisher and author are not responsible for any adverse effects or consequences resulting from the use of the suggestions, preparations, or procedures discussed in this book. Should the reader have any questions concerning the appropriateness of any procedures or preparation mentioned, the author and the publisher strongly suggest consulting a professional healthcare advisor.

Basic Health Publications, Inc.
www.basichealthpub.com

Library of Congress Cataloging-in-Publication Data

McCabe, Vinton.
    The healing echo : discovering homeopathic cell salt remedies /
Vinton McCabe.

    p. cm.
    Includes bibliographical references and index.
    ISBN 978-1-59120-073-4 (Pbk.)
    ISBN 978-1-68162-633-8 (Hardback)

    1. Medicine, Biochemic. 2. Salts—Therapeutic use. I. Title.

                                          2008031642
    RZ412.M33   2009
    615.8'8—dc22

Editor: Karen Anspach
Typesetting/Book design: Gary A. Rosenberg
Cover design: Mike Stromberg

Contents

"The Cure of the part should not be attempted without treatment of the whole. No attempt should be made to cure the body without the soul, and, if the head and body are to be healthy, you must begin by curing the mind . . . This is the great error of our day in the treatment of the human body, that physicians first separate the soul from the body."

—PLATO

"No thought without phosphorus!"

—JACOB MOLESCHOTT

Author's Note

I would like to thank Wenda Brewster O'Reilly for her kind permission to quote from her excellent translation of Samuel Hahnemann's *The Organon of the Medical Art* (Redmond, Washington: Birdcage Press, 1996) in these pages. As she has in the past, Wenda has once more allowed me the use of what is, in my opinion, the finest translation of the seminal book on the theory and practice of homeopathic medicine ever to have seen print in the English language. Without it, this book would be a lesser thing.

For that reason, and because she has also suggested that there might, for me, be a life after homeopathy, this book is dedicated to her.

It is also for Norman, who bought a pig in a poke.

Healing From Within

This book belongs to a group of three. And these three books are, by and large, based upon the work of three men. First and foremost of the three is Samuel Hahnemann, whose work is the foundation upon which the other two men, Edward Bach and W. H. Schuessler, built. Hahnemann was a German physician who radicalized the practice of medicine by coining two simple words. And by asserting a simple phrase.

The first word was *allopathy*,* a term that he gave to what he called the "old school" of medicine, the form of medicine that treats symptoms by working in opposition them—by suppressing them until they seem to disappear. This is the form of medicine that still dominates throughout the Western world, what many of us think of when we think of the concept of medicine.

The second term was *homeopathy*.** That was what he called his "new" form of medicine, although it was based in philosophies and practices that could be traced all the way back to Hippocrates.

The simple phrase, the three words that explained his whole approach to medicine and to healing, reads as follows: "Like cures like."

In his lifetime, Hahnemann didn't exactly set the world on fire with his practice of "new medicine." But he had many successes and began a movement that had its followers in its day and still has many thousands of adherents across the globe today. It remains as controversial today as it was two hundred years ago, however, and as likely to inspire intense debate.

Just go to at least two different gatherings of homeopaths anywhere in the world and you'll see what I mean. First, you'll see many of the same people at both. This is because the homeopathic community is rather small, at least in this country. But after you get over the small-town aspect of the gatherings, you'll see the second aspect—pas-

* From two Greek words, *allos*, meaning "different," and *pathos*, meaning "suffering." Allopathy, therefore, literally means "different suffering."

** From two Greek words as well. Homeopathy is taken from *homios*, meaning "similar," and *pathos*, meaning "suffering." Homeopathy literally means "similar suffering.

sion. It is certainly true in this country, if not across the world, that those who explore homeopathy, those who have experienced the true philosophy of homeopathy and its wise practice, most often become rather intense in their interest. They will cross state lines in minivans to hear a lecture on the use of snake venoms as homeopathic remedies. They will put up with bad hotel buffets and even worse ballrooms, taking notes on their laptops as they sit cross-legged on the hideous wall-to-wall carpet.

This passion is also shown in the manner in which homeopaths argue with each other. Put a dozen homeopaths in a room together and you will likely get a dozen different takes on just what homeopathy is and how it should be practiced—especially how it should be practiced. On that subject, homeopaths can come to blows.

Those who feel that homeopathy is utter nonsense at best and quackery at worst are equally dogged in their activities. From angry medical doctors who hold tight to their materialist viewpoint to ex-magicians who have nothing better to do, those who wish to debunk homeopathy never rest in their vigilance and are always willing to give the media a quote.

So suffice it to say, homeopathy has in the past and continues to cause a quiet revolution in medical thought. It has infiltrated the practice of allopathy in the treatment of diseases like chronic allergies. And it continues to wax and wane in popularity as each new generation thinks that it is the first to discover once more what has to be called the one true "holistic" medicine.

Hahnemann lived, worked, and died roughly two hundred years ago. He left behind a written text of his work, called *The Organon of Medicine*. This book has made his philosophy available to any and all.

Among those who uncovered homeopathy and dusted it off once more, while they themselves worked in the field of allopathic medicine, were Edward Bach and W.H. Schuessler.

Bach was a British physician and Schuessler a German doctor. They lived and worked at about the same time, Bach in England and Schuessler in Germany, in the latter part of the nineteenth and early twentieth centuries. Each became interested in finding a more natural form of medicine offering the possibility of a gentler form of healing. Both ultimately became passionately interested specifically in homeopathy, since each, as a practicing physician, could see its potential for healing.

Both studied homeopathy and, to one degree or another, incorporated it into their daily practice of medicine. Over time, both began to separate themselves, if not from homeopathy, at least from Hahnemann. Indeed, in later years, Schuessler would even sometimes deny having studied Hahnemann's writing or ever being influenced by him.

Over time, each man contributed to what we call the homeopathic materia medica, the pharmacy of medicines from which homeopathic treatments are taken. Schuessler's cell salt remedies, also known as tissue salts and sometimes collectively called "biochemical" remedies, were the basis of his particular offshoot of homeopathy, but they are still very much a part of the homeopathic materia medica today. Bach also contributed to the materia medica with his powerful bowel nosodes, which still are valuable tools in treating those with chronic digestive and allergic complaints, although his most famous medicines, the Bach flower remedies, are often considered to be quasi-homeopathic at best.

What each man did was take the complex and, perhaps, top-heavy practice of homeopathy and simplify it. Bach especially sought a form of homeopathic treatment that would be simple enough for laypersons to use to self-medicate and to help those they loved. Schuessler, on the other hand, sought a practice of medicine that could be formatted easily into what might be considered a spa setting, one in which the patient's total experience of healing could be measured and controlled.

Where Hahnemann had insisted upon the treatment of the whole man—body, mind and spirit—in his practice of medicine, Schuessler's methods of simplification moved the patient's physical complaints to the foreground of treatment. And along with the use of the cell salt remedies (a specific group of homeopathic remedies often used in combination, always in low potency) Schuessler also controlled the patient's food intake and exercise in his overall approach.

In exploring his overall system of treatment, he developed a sort of paint-by-number form of homeopathy that was simple enough for self-treatment and yet potent enough to bring curative results.

Even as Schuessler got more controlling, Bach became ever looser in his thought process, especially as he moved from being a practicing allopath to a brilliant student of homeopathy and then on to whatever you decide to call what he did at the end of his life (I think of it, as I do of Schuessler's protocols, as an offshoot of homeopathy, but not homeopathy itself). Instead of dwelling on the aches and pains of the body, seeing the body more and more as a mechanism, a material thing, as Schuessler did, Bach came to more or less ignore the body and treat only the emotions and the spirit, with the belief that, as the mind cleared, the body would follow and become well. Therefore, the Bach flower remedies are given solely on the basis of mood, or emotional state.

The work of these three men, therefore, can give us a unique and, I think, rather total understanding of the full spectrum of the philosophies and practices of everything that can collectively be considered homeopathy. On the one hand, we have Bach, with his loose system that works with simplicity and ease, based almost completely on the symptoms of the mind and spirit. On the other hand we have Schuessler, whose system is equally easy to understand and incorporate into our lives, based almost completely on the patient's physical complaints.

In the center is Samuel Hahnemann, who sought healing for the whole being, body, mind, and spirit, and who himself was a man of tremendous passion, overwhelming will and ego and, of course, unquenchable spirit. Because of the nature of the man himself and his quest to find a method of healing for the whole patient, we have the practice that we today would call "classical" homeopathy.*

As an inquiry into the work of these three men, and what their discoveries have meant in my own life, the three books I offer, *The Healing Enigma*, *The Healing Bouquet*, and *The Healing Echo*, are meant to be read as one, as the life's work of each of these men is intertwined, just as their treatments are interconnected. These texts on the Bach flower remedies, cell salts, and the original homeopathic remedies may be read in any order. Each may also stand totally alone.

The Healing Echo

The book that you are holding tells the story of a unique system of healing treatments. It is unique in that the remedies Schuessler used were all taken from substances that are naturally present in the human body itself. Because of this, each of the twelve remedies is totally benign. Schuessler's treatments are nourishing to your system and to your health. They bring balance to our bodies; a balance of nutrition, form, and function that can lead to a state of total health.

As I searched for a title for this book, one that would fit with the titles of my other books, I kept returning to the idea of an echo. Just as an echo is the sound of your own voice, returned to you changed and magnified from an external source, so too are Schuessler's remedies echoes. Schuessler takes our own substances, the building blocks of our own bodies, and changes them, polishes them into a new state of being. In doing so, he magnifies their actions. He then returns them to us as healing substances.

Schuessler's cell salts (so named because they contain the materials that are the building blocks of the cells that comprise the human body)** are, like the Bach flower remedies, a simple, safe, and surprisingly effective means of self-treatment. Unlike Bach's remedies, however, they were not created for that purpose. But in that they, like

---

* Classical homeopaths would, of course, object to this term, as what is called "classical" today is, in all actuality, homeopathy as Hahnemann defined it, in both philosophy and practice. What we call "modern" homeopathy today tends to be a bastardization of the Hahnemannian philosophy and practice and is, therefore, at least to the classical homeopath, something other than homeopathy. Related to it perhaps, but not truly homeopathy. Effective perhaps, but still just not *true* homeopathy.

** The cell salts are also known as "tissue salts" for the same reason. Schuessler's entire philosophy of treatment is sometimes referred to as "biochemics" or "Biochemic Medicine." For the purposes of this text, they will be referred to only as cell salts.

Bach's method of treatment, represent a simplification of homeopathy, they are well within the easy grasp of every person who is seeking a means by which they can encourage good health.

While the cell salts can be useful in acute situations, the very fact that they are very low potency homeopathic remedies makes them especially useful in cases of chronic illness. They can be helpful for cases that involve functional illnesses, like indigestion, in which no pathology is apparent, but in spite of the fact that no specific disease state can be found, the patient still feels that his health is compromised and, as a result, his enjoyment of life is limited.

Since Schuessler's system contains only twelve remedies and these remedies are, by and large, used in the same level of potency for all cases (some in 6X, others in 12X), the use of the cell salts is about as simple as it gets, while still staying within the realm of what might be called a form of homeopathic treatment.

In these pages, I give a history of the Schuessler system of treatment and explain how Schuessler's and Hahnemann's work is similar and yet not the same. In the following sections I provide information about each of the twelve remedies, as well as a way to group the remedies and identify the need for a specific remedy in any patient. The next portion of the book describes the correct use of the remedies, and the last section details specific uses of the remedies in common household ailments.

In these pages, therefore, is all that anyone needs to know in order to use Schuessler's cell salts for self-treatment or the treatment of those they love in cases of simple, household illness.

Perhaps more important, these pages also explore the philosophy by which these remedies are used, a sort of "allopathic homeopathy" which at once simplifies the task of homeopathic treatment and undermines it. Do with that what you will.

Taken alone, *The Healing Echo* gives an understanding and overview of that off-shoot of homeopathy known as biochemics. Taken together, the three books give the full range of homeopathic thought, from the one extreme of Schuessler's cell salts, in which the invisible nature of the patient—his mind, spirit and emotions—is largely ignored, to the other extreme of Bach's flower remedies, in which the physical nature of the patient is seen as unimportant to treatment and only his invisible nature is explored. In the center stands Samuel Hahnemann, whose pioneering work insists that, if we are to be made well, we must be treated as whole beings, indivisible in body, mind, and spirit. To understand the work of these three men and the philosophy and practice that are the foundation of their modes of treatment is to understand the full range of homeopathic thought. And that is a valuable thing indeed.

PART ONE

Schuessler's Cell Salts

"A disturbance of the molecular motion of one of the inorganic materials in a tissue causes a sickness, for the cure of which it suffices that a minimal dose of the same inorganic substance be furnished, since the molecules of the material thus used as a remedy fill the breach in the chain of molecules of the cell-salts or tissue-salts under consideration."

—W. H. SCHUESSLER
IN *THE BIOCHEMICAL TREATMENT OF DISEASE*

CHAPTER ONE

The History of the Cell Salts: Hahnemann, Schuessler, and Cells

Wilhelm Heinrich Schuessler (1821–1898) was born on August 21, 1821 in Zwischenalm, within the Grand Duchy of Oldenburg in Germany. At this time Samuel Hahnemann (1755–1843), the father of homeopathic medicine, was sixty-six years of age and well known throughout all Europe, and especially in Germany,* for his revolutionary methods in the practice of medicine.

Schuessler was born into a family that was prosperous enough that they could afford to educate their son. He, like Samuel Hahnemann before him, showed an early talent for foreign languages, ultimately becoming proficient in Latin, Greek, French, English, Spanish, and Italian, in addition to his native German.

Early in his life, Schuessler decided that he wished to follow in the footsteps of Hahnemann, whom he admired both for his medical technique and for his passionate dedication to his process of discovery, and become a homeopathic physician. His brother, upon hearing of Wilhelm's interest in medicine, agreed to pay for his brother's full education with the proviso that he promise to see his educational process through and actually become a licensed homeopath. Wilhelm made full use of his brother's funds to this end and studied medicine at universities in Berlin, Paris, Giessen, and Prague. In 1857, at the age of thirty-six, he passed his final examination at the Collegium Medicum of Oldenburg and received his license to practice. He established his practice in homeopathy right there in Oldenburg, Germany.

Schuessler and Homeopathy

Wilhelm Schuessler learned the basic tenants of homeopathy as he was taught them, directly from the writings of Samuel Hahnemann. Chief among them were the principles of uniquity, wholeness, expression of symptoms, and vitalism.

---

* Homeopathy was not yet known in the United States, however. A German doctor, Heinrich Detwiller had brought homeopathy to the United States in 1817 when he emigrated to Allentown, Pennsylvania, but his practice was largely confined to Allentown's large German-American population. It was not until 1833, when Constantine Hering, the so-called "father of U.S. homeopathy" arrived in Philadelphia that the homeopathic movement within America began.

The concept of *uniquity* is important to homeopathy. It states, quite simply, that each patient is a unique being. The traditional, "old school" of medicine, which Hahnemann would name allopathy, stresses that all patients are similar beings and, therefore, what successfully treats one patient's disease will likely also treat all others who share that disease. The idea that each patient is unique in the universe is revolutionary in terms of medical treatment. For the allopath, the disease diagnosis is very important, in that once a disease state can be correctly identified (which, as any of us who have visited more than one doctor in search of a diagnosis knows, is not an easy thing in and of itself), the method or methods used in the treatment for that disease have also been identified. If a particular school of medical practitioners can come to the conclusion that all patients suffering the same disease are more similar than they are dissimilar, then treatment becomes fairly simple: a particular medicine or group of medicines is identified through trial and error as being effective in combating that disease state, and the doctor simply fiddles with the medicines and adjusts their dosage until the desired results are achieved.

If, however, a physician comes to the conclusion, as Hahnemann did, that each patient is unique and has a system that reacts uniquely both to those stresses that cause disease and to those medicines that cure it, then treatment becomes more complex. Whether or not a patient receives a particular disease diagnosis is more or less irrelevant, in that the diagnosis itself can suggest no specific treatment if the patient is seen as unique. The medicine that might be curative to this patient might be ineffective or even damaging to that one over there.

With the idea of uniquity, Hahnemann demanded that those who would call themselves homeopaths start each and every case from scratch. That they never make assumptions as to what remedy or remedies might be curative to that patient during case taking, but, instead, use all their skill, their insight and their powers of communication (both giving and receiving information) when working with their patient.

The idea of uniquity takes away from homeopathy the idea that there is a remedy for backaches, a remedy for colds, a remedy for cancer. Instead, this concept demands that each homeopath approach each patient as if they were the first of his or her race that the homeopath has ever encountered. They must start from the beginning with each case taking, each patient, always seeking information and using that information in the selection of the most appropriate remedy for the case.

Therefore, the allopath, who seeks a disease diagnosis—an umbrella term that identifies not only the cluster of symptoms the patient is experiencing, but also predetermines the outcome of the case, whether it is treated or not—then has only to grapple with a small group of drugs that the pharmaceutical firms have assured him are effective in treatment and safe to use. The homeopath, on the other hand, must always begin by considering the patient's *drug diagnosis*.

For the homeopath, the disease diagnosis is almost completely useless. Certainly, the nature of the complaint is important in determining the severity of the symptoms and their possible outcome, but the disease diagnosis does not in any way suggest to the homeopath what remedy might be useful in treating the patient who is in that particular disease state.

Instead, the process of homeopathic treatment is always the same: one of matching the full range of symptoms that the patient is suffering against the full sphere of action of a homeopathic remedy. In finding the best possible match, the homeopath must consider the uniquity of his patient, and he must also consider the patient in a state of *wholeness*.

Like Hippocrates before him, Hahnemann saw his patient as a whole being—one who is joined in body, mind, spirit, and emotions. And only by taking into account the whole being can the patient be healed of all disease.

The allopath makes the mistake of trying to create an artificial separation of the various aspects of the patient's state of being. For the allopath, the patient who is experiencing a deep feeling of fear while suffering from his disease is no different from the patient who, with that same disease, instead feels anger. For the homeopath, these are two very different patients, who very likely will require two very different remedies. This is because the homeopath is as interested in the patient's emotional state as he is in his patient's physical state. Both must be considered in the selection of a remedy.

It is the patient's reaction to the stressors, toxins, traumas, or other causes of disease that will determine the remedy that is needed to put things right. As I used to say to my students, for the homeopath it is less important to identify the model of the bus that hit the patient than it is to identify how the patient reacted to being hit by that bus. If you ask me, allopaths spend a great deal of their time trying to find out the license plate number of the bus, while homeopaths are busy trying to ascertain the patient's actual injuries, both visible and tangible and invisible and intangible.

The patient's *reaction* to the cause of disease is all-important in selecting an appropriate remedy for that patient*. The location of symptoms, the duration of the symptoms, the sensation of the symptoms—these are all very important. Also very

---

* It may actually be considered more important than the actual cause of the disease itself. Again, we don't need to spend a whole lot of time trying to get the license plate of the bus. Something, whether it is bacteria or virus, exhaustion or physical trauma, has weakened the patient, quickly or slowly, into a state that we call disease. The homeopath puts his or her effort into trying to understand the patient in their discomfort, understanding what specific changes have taken place on all levels of being, visible and invisible, in that transition from healthy to diseased, and then into trying to find the remedy that can reverse that trend back to health.

important are what the homeopath calls the *modalities* of the symptoms, those things that make the symptoms better or worse—which can range from time of day, heat or cold, sleeping or not, touching or not, and on and on. The homeopath will likely seek to understand the modalities not only of each symptom, what things make that symptom feel better or worse, but also the modalities of the patient as a whole. Does he feel better in general from eating or from fasting? What foods or drinks does he crave, or does the idea of eating and drinking revolt him? Does he want to be alone, or wish for company? Again, the list goes on and on, and includes both the physical aspects of the patient's life in general and his specific symptoms and his emotional and spiritual being as well.

As Hahnemann developed his healing art, only by understanding the patient as a unique and whole being can that patient be made truly well. And this goal can be achieved only by helping that patient express his or her symptoms—to let them go completely, and never by suppressing them as the allopaths do.

The concept of *expression* is central to homeopathic practice. Again, going back to the teachings of Hippocrates, when a patient has a set of symptoms that are troubling him, there are only two ways of approaching the symptoms. You can either work in opposition to them or with them.

In making the decision to work either way, you are making a judgment about the symptoms themselves and the reasons for their presence.

The allopathic practitioner who works in opposition to the symptoms that the patient is experiencing does so because he sees the symptoms as invaders. And because he assumes, correctly or incorrectly, that if these symptoms are somehow magically removed, the patient will, in their absence, be in a state of health.

Working from this philosophy, the doctor who treats allopathically gives the patient a medicine that, in a healthy person, would create a pattern of symptoms that are opposite to those the patient is experiencing. In other words, for the patient with a runny nose, you give a medicine whose action is to dry up the sinuses.

By working in opposition, the doctor blocks the patient's experience of his or her disease, blocks the discomfort of the symptoms associated with the disease, without touching the disease state itself. Think about it: does a sleeping pill "cure" insomnia; will it keep you from having trouble sleeping again the next night? Does a cold medicine actually "cure" the cold, or does it only keep the patient more comfortable while they still have their cold?

By working in opposition to the patient's symptoms, the allopath suppresses the symptoms while actually doing nothing to bring about a restoration of health or to prevent another occurrence of the same or similar diseases in the future. In fact, it can be argued that, by suppressing symptoms deeper into the patient's being, the allopath's treatment actually weakens the patient's overall state of being and encourages future illness, because the suppressed symptoms will move to the surface again at some future point.

The doctor who treats suppressively does so because he makes several assumptions. First, that the symptoms themselves are bad things, things that are to be struggled against as vigorously as possible. Second, that the patient's own immune system, if allowed enough time, will ultimately bring an end to the disease.* And third, that the absence of symptoms can be equated to a state of overall health.

Homeopaths would disagree with two of these assumptions, the first and the third, and more vigorously with the third. The second assumption would lead a homeopath to comment that the patients of allopaths are more often cured in spite of their treatments than they are by them.

In homeopathic medicine, the goal of any treatment is not, as it is in allopathic medicine, the eradication of the symptoms of disease. Instead, the goal of homeopathic treatment is always to improve the patient's overall state of health. It is not enough for the homeopath to remove a patient's headache. The homeopath seeks a treatment that, instead, will also help prevent the patient from having another headache in the future. He does this by working with the patient's symptoms and not against them.

The homeopath believes that the symptoms are not invaders. Instead, they are a part of the patient's being. They represent his or her reaction to a particular stressor or toxin or mechanical injury. In other words, the bruise on your arm is not a spontaneous thing; it is your body's reaction to the fact that the arm received an injury. Therefore, the bruise is not a bad thing; it is, instead, a very positive thing—it is the sign that your body's immune function is behaving as it should and that your body is healing itself. The homeopath will see all symptoms, no matter how painful they might be, as a sign that

> In homeopathic medicine, the goal of any treatment is not, as it is in allopathic medicine, the eradication of the symptoms of disease. Instead, the goal of homeopathic treatment is always to improve the patient's overall state of health. It is not enough for the homeopath to remove a patient's headache. The homeopath seeks a treatment that, instead, will also help prevent the patient from having another headache in the future. He does this by working with the patient's symptoms and not against them.

---

*This is what makes me most frustrated with allopathy—the fact that, in most cases, it actually does nothing whatsoever to cure a patient. Suppressive treatments always ultimately count on the body's own defenses to bring about a cure, no matter what our television advertising might tell us.

the body is trying to heal itself, bring itself into balance. Therefore, those symptoms should be noted, understood in their entirety, and worked with, not against.

The question is, therefore, how does the homeopath work with the patient's symptoms? He does so by giving the patient a medicine that, in a healthy person, would create the same symptoms the patient is already suffering. So he would give a patient with insomnia a remedy that would keep a healthy patient up all night long. And he would give a patient with a cold a remedy that is proven to give a healthy person a runny nose, sore throat, and sneezing.

The very word *homeopathy* reflects this method of treatment. The term was coined by Samuel Hahnemann, who took it from two Greek words, "homios" and "pathos," which together mean "similar suffering." Thus, the core homeopathic philosophy is "like cures like."*

The homeopath makes the assumption that, as the body knows what it is doing in healing itself, it is the role of the doctor to help that process by actually encouraging it. Therefore, the doctor seeks to find that single homeopathic remedy that most closely resembles the patient's own symptoms in their totality. (Homeopaths also believe that all medicines have a sphere of action on all levels of being—body, mind, and spirit— and, as a result, use only one remedy at a time, as we shall see in the next chapter.) The patient is given that remedy in the belief that, as the remedy acts, the patient's symptoms will be released through the process of expression, and, once released, they will be gone from his or her body permanently, leaving the patient in a state of increased health and less likely to suffer from the same disease again.

Often, especially in the treatment of patients with acute conditions, the patient's symptoms will worsen temporarily before they dramatically improve. This is known in homeopathic medicine as an *aggravation*. It should last for no more than a few hours. An aggravation is a sign that the patient's system is expressing symptoms very quickly and that the artificial disease state created by the homeopathic remedy is deeply in tune with the patient's own natural disease state. It may also be a sign that the potency of the remedy was too high, in which case the treatment may have to be blunted for the sake of the patient's comfort, but aggravations, although uncomfortable, are not dangerous.

While the idea of giving a patient a remedy made from coffee to a patient who is suffering from insomnia may fly in the face of logic to a culture that is steeped in allopathic philosophy, the core idea of working in concert with a patient's own immune system to restore that patient to a state of health cannot help but have some appeal.

The line between working against and working with a patient's symptoms is the

---

* In the same way, the word allopathy, also coined by Hahnemann, reveals its core philosophy. It is also taken from two Greek words, "allos" and again "pathos," which together mean "opposite (or, more precisely, "dissimilar") suffering."

line that divides allopathy and homeopathy. Further, it is the line between the suppression of symptoms and their expression. Homeopaths warn that suppressive treatments come with a cost—that the allopath makes a foolish assumption when he believes that the apparent lack of symptoms equals a state of health. Symptoms, the homeopath knows, disappear in two ways. They can either be suppressed or expressed. The patient who receives either form of treatment may look the same in a day or two after that treatment—hale and hearty. It is over time that the differences are seen, however. The patient who receives allopathic treatment has had his or her symptoms suppressed into invisibility. But, having been pushed down, they will return to the surface, either as the same disease state or another, deeper disorder. On the other hand, the patient who receives a treatment that allows his or her body to fully express and expel his or her symptoms has no symptoms to recall, as they have been released from the body. Therefore, they are stronger for their treatment and less prone to future diseases.

Finally, there is the concept of *vitalism*.

In some ways, vitalism is the most important aspect of homeopathic theory, and yet, homeopathy is not the only form of medicine that might be called vitalistic—acupuncture, for instance, shares the concepts of vitalism with homeopathy, as do other forms of holistic treatment. However, homeopathy is without a doubt the most completely vitalistic of all forms of treatment, holistic or otherwise.

The concept of vitalism itself dates back long before the time of Samuel Hahnemann. In fact, it predates the known history of medicine. It can be traced back at least as far as the ancient Egyptian culture.

Before he began to map the interior organs of the human body, ancient man saw himself as a whole being, rather than as a biological mechanism, and life as a force, not the product of an active metabolism. This animating energy, which was said to be shared by all living things, was known by several different names, from French philosopher Henri-Louis Bergson's (1859–1941) *"elan vital"* (which translates as the poetic "momentum of life"), to the Greek *dynamis*, a term for a more explosive force from which the English word dynamite is derived, to Hahnemann's own term for it, *lebenskraft*, about which he writes in his *Organon of the Medical Art*, in the ninth aphorism: "In the healthy human state, the spirit-like force that enlivens the material organism in admirable, harmonious, vital operation, as regards both feelings and functions, so that our indwelling, rational spirit can freely avail itself of this living, healthy instrument for the higher purposes of our existence."

Hahnemann's comments do much to reveal his notion of vital force. First, that it is dynamic, which is to say it is a thing of pure energy. And second, that the vital force is capable of impacting not only our physical selves, but our intellectual and emotional selves as well, in that he assures us that the balanced vital force creates harmony "as regards both feelings and functions." Therefore, vital force touches upon all aspects of our lives, the visible and the invisible, the tangible and the intangible. Its balance allows for a sense of freedom and well-being. Its blockage or its imbalance leads to a sense of restriction and illness.

For Hahnemann, vital force was all-important in the lives of his patients. In aphorism ten, he writes: "The material organism, thought of without life force, is capable of no sensibility, no activity, no self-preservation." Thus, the vital force is that which animates us, allows us to function as individual whole beings, and, importantly, allows for "self-preservation," which is to say, allows us to heal when injured.

The footnote to this statement sums up Hahnemann's thought: "Without Life Force, the material organism is dead and is only subject to the power of the physical external world. It decays and is again resolved into its chemical constituents."

As I have written before, we are, each of us, a combination of that which is visible and that which is invisible. We are a combination of things that are tangible and intangible. While we most certainly are comprised of muscles, bones, blood, and fat, while we have arms, legs, eyes, and ears, we are also creatures of intellect and emotion, and, most important, of spirit. While our physical selves can be easily reduced to component parts, to chemical compounds, our spiritual selves transcend that which can be mapped, studied, or surgically removed. In other words, there is more to our minds than just our physical brains.

The vitalist tradition upholds a belief in a life force that both animates and balances, that inhabits the flesh and yet is unique in itself.

While modern science—which could rightly be called "materialistic" modern science, as we shall see—tends to consider the human to be something of a meat machine, a thing made up of organic mechanical parts that can be swapped in and out like the parts of an old Volkswagen, those who uphold the vitalist tradition insist there is something more to human existence than a chemical combustion that triggers a period of animation that is called "life."

That tradition goes further and deeper when its proponents insist that not only is our invisible nature independent from the body's mechanical or chemical reactions, but also that it actually is dominant over the physical self. For Hahnemann and other vitalists, illness begins in the invisible, intangible level of being and only manifests in the physical when the vital force becomes weakened or blocked. In this way, homeopathic belief runs parallel to acupuncture, in which a blockage of chi leads to physical illness.

This idea becomes a guiding principle in medical treatments in any form of therapy that upholds the vitalistic viewpoint. Homeopaths and acupuncturists alike, among others, believe that if the nature of a disease, whatever its symptoms, is to be found within the vital force, then its cure must also take place within the vital force. The practitioner who spends time dealing only with specific symptoms, treating and, in many cases, suppressing them with material treatments, will accomplish little more than palliation of symptoms at best. Only treatments that encourage the re-energizing of the vital force are capable of being catalysts to true healing.

It is therefore part of the vitalist tradition to look at the patient as not only a blend of the visible and invisible, tangible and intangible, but also as a whole being. The symptom that manifests in one specific area of the body indicates illness within the being as a whole. The physician who trains his beady little eyes only on that one part of the body that actually feels the pain, ignoring the rest of the patient's body, mind, and spirit, does his patient a great disservice.

In developing and refining his practice of what would come to be called homeopathy, Samuel Hahnemann brought with him the vitalist tradition and made it intrinsic to his new medical art. Thus, while the remedies themselves and the process of potentizing and succussing in a systematic manner was something new, the concept of vitalism was the "something old" that Hahnemann brought into the marriage of old and new traditions. But without the principle of vitalism, there can be no homeopathy as Hahnemann developed it. The recognition of the vital force and of what Hahnemann called the "*wesen*"* are central to both the philosophy and practice of homeopathy.

These were the building blocks of Schuessler's medical training. These and the other aspects of homeopathy study: case taking and management, and a thorough understanding of the remedies themselves as gathered in Hahnemann's own materia medica.

From all accounts, Schuessler was a good homeopath, a competent practitioner with a thriving practice. Had there not been on the horizon a radical shift in medical thinking from vitalism to materialism, a shift provoked by advances in cell theory,

---

* In her excellent translation of *The Organon of the Medical Art*, Wenda Brewster O'Reilly, Ph.D., gives the following definition of *wesen*: "Wesen is a mult-faceted term which can mean any of the following: essence, substance, creature, living thing, nature or entity. There is no single English word that adequately translates *Wesen*. In almost every instance in the *Organon*, Hahnemann uses the term to refer to that entity which is the essential unchanging essence of something: its being, its quintessence. A wesen is not an abstraction; it is a dynamic, self-subsisting presence even though that presence is not material and has no mass. A wesen is also not a property; it permeates the whole of something and is indivisible from it. The romantic philosophers of the nineteenth century (such as Coleridge) used the word 'genius' in the same way that Hahnemann, Goethe, and other German thinkers used the word 'wesen.'" On the deepest level, therefore, the physician, in seeking to understand both the patient and the true nature of the patient's illness, seeks to comprehend the *wesen*. This was central to Hahnemann's belief system and stood as his goal as a practitioner.

Schuessler might well have continued in the practice of homeopathy for the rest of his life. Instead, he took what he had learned of Hahnemann's method and made something else—something that reflected his early training in homeopathy, something that was and remains homeopathic and yet not homeopathic. Something that he would come to call *biochemics* in the days ahead, when he would also insist he had never heard of a man named Hahnemann.

Cell Theory

Cell theory, also known as "cell doctrine," was finally coming into its full flower in 1847 with the publication of Rudolph Virchow's (1821–1902) *Archiv fur Pathologische Anatomie und Physiologie*, also known simply as "Virchow's Archives." The concepts that informed Virchow's work (which could perhaps be most clearly summed up by his 1845 comment, "life is essentially cell activity"), as well as that of Jacob Moleschott (1822–1893), Theodor Schwann (1810–1882), and Matthias Schleiden (1804–1881), among others, dated back to Robert Hooke (1635–1703), who, in 1663, looked at a piece of cork in an early microscope and announced to the Royal Society of London that his bit of cork was not really a solid, but was made up of tiny structures that he called "cells."* He wrote, "These pores or cells, were not very deep, but consisted of a great many little boxes, separated out of one continued long pore, by certain diaphragms."**

Hooke continued with his research into cell structure and published his classic and, I think, wonderfully named book, *Micrographia*, in 1665.

It is hard for us today to realize the importance of Hooke's observations and understand just how revolutionary and controversial they were in their day. Hooke was so controversial in his time and in the years after his death that no less than Sir Isaac Newton—a great rival of Hooke's, who considered Hooke to be a difficult man, a miser, a hypochondriac, and, unforgivably, a rival in the scientific community who had at one point actually suggested that Newton had plagiarized his wave theory from Hooke's *Micrographia*—insisted upon the removal of Hooke's portrait from the walls of the

---

* Hooke called these structures "cells" because, on seeing them in that bit of cork, they reminded him of the rooms, called "cellula" that monks lived in in monasteries. He thought this way because, along with being a scientist, Hooke was also an architect, who was among those who contributed to the rebuilding of London after the Great Fire in 1666. Among his greatest contributions as an architect is the Royal Greenwich Observatory. He also worked on the designs for the Bethlehem Royal Hospital, the world's first psychiatric hospital, from whose name the word "bedlam" is taken.

** Somewhat ironically, while Hooke was correct in noticing that living tissue is made up of small component parts, for which the word "cells" is as good as any other, what Hooke saw through his microscope were not actually living cells, as cork is a dead substance. What Hooke saw were the cell walls left within the cork, walls that no longer contained any cytoplasm.

Royal Society of London. (The result of this was that, interestingly, while we have clear images of the cells that Hooke saw through the lens of his microscope, thanks to the loss of the portrait, we have no clear image of what the man himself looked like.) Newton went so far as to try to have all of Hooke's papers burned at the time of his death, an attempt that was thwarted by the other members of the Society. Hooke, himself a renaissance man, who contributed not only to medicine and biology, but also to physics, mathematics, astronomy, and architecture, remains something of a mystery to us today. His personal life is unknown, he amassed a great fortune but died without an heir, having never married, and his face today is veiled by history.

It would take nearly 150 years for the concept of cells as the building blocks of living tissue to be fully recognized by the scientific community.

Throughout that next century and a half, research continued into the question of cells—whether or not they really existed and, if they did, what their nature might be. Anton van Leeuwenhoek (1632–1723) developed his own single lens microscope and became the first man to actually see bacteria and protozoa. He reported his findings to the same Royal Society of London in 1673. His work was more generally accepted than Hooke's had been, and he was made a full member of the Royal Society and, no doubt, granted a portrait.

But it wasn't until 1805 that a German scientist and teacher, Lorenz Oken (1779–1851) became the leader of a German movement called *Naturphilosophie* and took the principles of philosopher Immanuel Kant (1724–1804) and applied them to "nature studies" or biology. (He had been born Lorenz Ockenfuss, but shortened his name for simplicity's sake as his scientific star began to rise.)

While Oken became one of the most influential philosophers and educators of his day, his contribution to cell theory can be simply stated with his words, "All living organisms originate from and consist of cells." With this one observation, Oken both originated and defined cell theory.

In 1833, a British naturalist named Robert Brown (1773–1858), who had taken a four-year trip to the "colonies of Australia," next stunned the scientific community with a new discovery. On his return from Down Under, he studied the species he had gathered on this trip. And noticed again and again that the cells he viewed had what he referred to as "an opaque spot" on them. Again and again, he saw the same spot, cell after cell. While others before him, Leeuwenhoek chief among them, had seen the same spot, it was Brown who named it, giving every cell its *nucleus*.

By this point in time, microscopes had developed enough and were more common as scientific tools, and the idea that all living beings were composed of small structures called cells was common knowledge.

This new viewpoint, the ultimate discovery of the cell as the building block of all living things, animals and plants, did much more than just instruct us as to the nature and function of our bodies. It changed the way in which those bodies came to be seen, and created a schism in medical thought that still exists today. In other words, something as small as a cell, with its nucleus, its walls, its very simple function and structure, would loom quite large in the debate between holistic and mechanistic medicine.

But first we have to get from Brown's opaque spots to the cell theory.

It all began when M. J. Schleiden, who was a professor of botany at the University of Jena at the time, built upon Brown's observations of the existence of the nucleus and brought the information to popular attention. While he acknowledged that his own research was indebted to Brown, it was Schleiden who recognized the fact that the nucleus was of vital importance to the life and function of the cell.

He shared this information with his friend and colleague Theodor Schwann, a professor of physiology at the University of Lovain.

As the story goes, the two men were enjoying a dinner together during the year 1837. Since they were academics in the related fields of botany and physiology, the conversation turned, as it likely would, to the subjects of their studies, and Schleiden shared the exciting new discoveries about cells and their nuclei with his friend. Hearing Schleiden's description of the nuclei of plant cells, Schwann instantly thought of similar structures he had seen while studying animal cells under his own microscope. Connecting the dots, the two men came to understand that cells of the same structure existed in both plant and animal tissue.

For Schwann, this discovery ultimately led to the publication of his book *Accordance in the Structure and Growth of Plants and Animals* in 1847. This work not only formed the basis of the study of cell theory, but also brought Schwann no small amount of personal fame.*

Perhaps more important, this discovery led Schwann to break with the vitalist philosophy which was central to both the study and practice of medicine at that time. In its place Schwann became part of a new movement, one that had been shaped by the Dutch physiologist and philosopher Jacob Moleschott.

In 1852, Moleschott published a collection of his lectures that he called *The*

---

* Schwann's fame seems to have come at the cost of his friendship with Matthias Schleiden. In 1839, when Schwann first published a treatise of his findings on the nature of cells, he did so without acknowledging Schleiden's contributions to his work. He did, however, summarize his findings in three conclusions: first, that the cell is the unit of structure and organization for all living things; second, that cells are both individual things and part of an organized whole; and third, that cells are created through a process of spontaneous generation. As they say, two out of three ain't bad. Schwann was, of course, wrong about that third conclusion, as Virchow would prove in 1855.

Circuit of Life. With the publication of this work, Moleschott fully espoused his new philosophy, which he named *materialism*.

Simply put, materialism suggested that all aspects of organic life could be reduced to physical and/or chemical causes. That not only physical processes such as digestion and respiration were mechanical acts, but also that thought and emotions were based in chemical reactions.

The schism between the vitalists, who obviously objected to this radical new theory, and the materialists erupted in 1854, when a zoologist named Karl Vogt (1817–1895) publicly clashed with anatomist and physiologist Rudolf Wagner (1805–1864). Wagner, to Vogt's thinking, gave equal credence to Biblical history and scientific thought. Wagner admitted to his Christian faith and, in doing so, lost the support of many in the academic community, handing the victory to Vogt and his fellow materialists.

Fully radicalized and triumphant, Vogt most famously concluded that human thoughts "stand in the same relation to the brain like bile to the liver and urine to the kidneys." This, understandably, alienated the vitalists and the church alike. But Moleschott stood up for his colleague, declaring, "No thought without phosphorus," a comment that reduced human thought to a chemical reaction.

It is important to note that the emergence of materialism as the dominant philosophy of "scientific" medicine was as much a social and political action as it was a scientific revolution. German institutes of learning were under the control of the government, which had developed an official philosophy that guided and controlled scientific study and largely suppressed any subject or mode of inquiry that the state did not deem appropriate. This controlling philosophy largely left it up to the church to determine what topics made for appropriate study and exploration. Thus, the scientists who shaped the radical new philosophy of materialism were as much rebelling against the church and state as they were evolving the cause of science. With the emergence of materialism, the rules governing scientific inquiry swung as far from the old system as the academic pendulum would allow.

The new breed of scientist, embodied in the public imagination by Jacob Moleschott and Karl Vogt, in very short order, turned away from vitalism, which they saw as part of the Old Order and akin to metaphysics.

This is not to say that all the proponents of cell theory were materialists. No less than Rudolph Virchow, who could appropriately be considered the Father of Cell Theory, stayed true to his vitalist roots, although he agreed that it was important to avoid the metaphysical while exploring the physical and the chemical.

In 1855, Rudolph Virchow built upon exciting cell theory with yet another statement. He announced: *"Omnis cellula e celula,"* which translates as "All cells come from cells." In other words, cells come from pre-existing cells and only from pre-existing cells, giving rise to the possibility that disease might be caused by new cells coming from diseased or damaged cells and health might be the product of new healthy cells growing from older, equally healthy cells. Virchow's statement would come to be known as "biogenic law" and would largely shape the thinking of scientists and physicians alike for generations to come.

Perhaps Virchow's most important statement on the subject would come in his 1858 work *Cellular Pathology*, in which he wrote, "Every form of suffering is only based on a disorder in the cells. Only the cell can become sick—the cell, the smallest functioning unit of the human body."

This brief statement would have a profound impact upon W. H. Schuessler, who had followed the development both of cell theory and of materialism with some interest.

Schuessler and Biochemics

Even as Schuessler was setting up his homeopathic practice, he was closely following the development of cell theory. Thus, he was struck by the conclusion that Moleschott reached in his book *Kreislaug des Lebens* (*The Circuit of Life*), in which Moleschott wrote, "The structure and vitality of organs are conditioned by the necessary amounts of inorganic constituents." In other words, in order to be healthy, cells need to be nourished. And, as Virchow had already concluded that the life of the body was dependent upon the life of its cells, it could therefore be concluded that the health of the whole body was to a great part dependent upon the proper nourishment of its cells.

In the years between 1857, when he was finally licensed to practice medicine, and 1872, when he published his first major work, *An Abridged Homeopathic Therapeutics*, Schuessler practiced homeopathic medicine, studied cell theory, and, over time, developed a new system that blended aspects of both and yet paid allegiance to neither.

> From Moleschott and the materialists, Schuessler took the idea that through the use of specific inorganic substances, given in specific doses, the cells of the body could be nourished to the extent that general health and vitality could be attained and maintained. From Hahnemann he took the idea of potentizing raw substances into homeopathic remedies, in this case the cell salts that were the products of his research and practice, which he prescribed in low dilutions.

From Moleschott and the materialists, he took the idea that through the use of specific inorganic substances, given in specific doses, the cells of the body could be nourished to the extent that general health and vitality could be attained and maintained. From Hahnemann he took the idea of potentizing raw substances into homeopathic remedies, in this case the cell salts that were the products of his research and practice, which he prescribed in low dilutions.*

All of this, by 1872, led Schuessler to announce the creation of a new and unique form of medical treatment, which he called biochemics. As a form of medical treatment it borrowed much from the work of other scientists, researchers and practitioners, often without acknowledgement. As a philosophy of treatment it stood on its own, in a gray area between homeopathy and allopathy, and between vitalism and materialism.

---

* It should be noted that there was a great struggle among homeopaths during this time in history. Some quarters held the belief that homeopathic remedies are most effective if given in high dilutions, which is to say in potentizations well beyond the point where molecules of the original substance still remain in the remedy. Others—Charles Julius Hempel (1811–1879) and Richard Hughes (1836–1932) chief among them—believed that remedies given at such levels of dilution worked only as placebos, and that homeopathic remedies only truly worked in low dilutions. Schuessler agreed with this latter group and made use of his new remedies only in very low dilutions. Biochemical or cell salt remedies are still used this way today, although all twelve cell salts are also used in higher dilutions as part of the traditional homeopathic materia medica. It should be also noted that the same homeopaths who grouped around the concept of low potency also tended to group around the concept of materialism, and tended to be practitioners—one hesitates to call them homeopaths—who used their remedies in the direct treatment of diseases or in treatment of specific organs of the body.

CHAPTER TWO

The Dynamics of the Cell Salts: Homeopathy, Biochemics, and Deficiency

I f you were looking at a Venn diagram illustrating the relationship between cell salts and homeopathic remedies, you would be looking at a large circle representing the pharmacy of homeopathic remedies with a much smaller circle completely contained within it. That smaller circle would illustrate the cell salts, because all cell salts are homeopathic remedies, but by no means are all homeopathic remedies cell salts. There are literally thousands of homeopathic remedies, taken from animal, vegetable, and mineral sources, but there are only a dozen cell salt remedies, all of which are taken from the chemical compounds that are the building blocks of our bodies.

And if you were looking at a picture of Samuel Hahnemann, the Father of Homeopathy, and W.H. Schuessler, the Creator of Biochemics, you would likely be looking at a portrait of two men standing at the same podium, with their backs turned toward each other.

Hahnemann and Homeopathy

Samuel Hahnemann was an allopathic doctor in the early part of his medical career. But he became increasingly alarmed about the sheer toxicity of the medicines that he used in treating his patients. He began to suspect that more patients died from their medicine than from their illnesses.

It was the resulting deep dissatisfaction that Hahnemann felt for the medical status quo of his day that led to the development of homeopathy, a radical new system of medical treatment that was really based in two very simple concepts.

The first was dilution. If arsenic—a part of the traditional medical pharmacy in Hahnemann's day—was toxic in its pure, material form, then, Hahnemann reasoned, it might be less toxic in a diluted form. He began experimenting with dilution, working toward a systematic method of dilution that could render a given medicine benign in its action while still maintaining its medicinal effect.

In learning to dilute his medicines, not just slightly but ultimately to the point at which all the molecules of the original substance were washed away, leaving only the energy signature (vital force, if you will) of the substance in the potentized* remedy, Hahnemann established the manner in which his remedies would be created. But he had yet to work through the other aspect of his new system of therapeutics: the philosophy governing the manner in which those remedies would be used.

For that, Hahnemann looked backward in medical history to principles predating the Roman system of medicine that remains the root of allopathic medicine. Before the Roman physician Galen began dissecting corpses and came to the conclusion that the human body resembled a machine structured from organic parts, the Greek physician Hippocrates considered the human being to be a whole entity, comprised of body, mind, and spirit. In Hippocrates' school of medicine, a patient was as likely to be prescribed a cathartic experience or a change in locale as he or she was to be prescribed an herbal medicine.

Hahnemann went back to the dawn of Western medicine and studied medical treatments that Hippocrates set in place on the Isle of Cos off the coast of Greece. From these, he learned a simple truth—that medicine, in reality, comes down to how any given doctor thinks about pain. About any or all symptoms that can be equated with illness. According to Hippocrates, when you have a patient who is displaying symptoms that involve discomfort, there are only two things you can do, if you choose to do anything at all in terms of medical treatment.

First, you can look at that pain as a bad thing, as an invader that needs to be removed. This concept leads to a system of medicine in which pain is to be controlled, suppressed, pushed down for the sake of the patient's comfort. If the pain cannot be controlled the reason for it should be identified through a system of medical tests and then removed. If symptoms are a bad thing, an invasive thing, then they must be vigorously worked *against* to the greatest degree possible, short of actually killing the patient. In this scenario the patient is seen as the victim of his or her disease, as invaded territory. And all disease states—all sets of invasive symptoms—are seen as more or less the same. When you focus on restoring health by eliminating disease (which carries with it the assumption that "underneath" the diseased patient is one who is well, if you can just peel away the disease), then you have to also assume that all disease states are similar enough and all patients are similar enough that a successful treatment for one patient with a given disease will also work for all other patients with a diagnosis of the same disease. If you cannot learn to more or less equate all patients who share a given disease state, then you cannot practice this form of medicine.

It was Hahnemann's on-the-job experience with this system of medical treatment that ultimately led him to reject it. That sent him toward the alternative viewpoint,

* For more information on potentization, see Chapter Three.

Hippocrates' alternate option for medical treatment. The option in which you have to accept the fact that pain is, in fact, a good thing.

In doing this, you make a different assumption: that the pain is not invasive, but is, instead, native to the patient. That symptoms of all sorts are reactive in nature. That some catalyst or some number of catalysts, deep down within the patient, have created a response that is uncomfortable. That the symptoms are not caused by the presence of a stressor of, say, a virus, but, instead, are caused by the patient's individual reaction to the presence of that stressor. This scenario suggests that the patient's being is attempting to restore balance in the face of some sort of change, some sort of perceived attack, and that pain has resulted as a part of that response.

Pain, therefore, however uncomfortable it might be, is a good thing, a sign that the patient is strong enough to try to work back to balance. A sign that the patient's vital force, or immune system—however you want to look at it, whatever you want to call it—is trying to right itself. This treatment system suggests that symptoms should not be resisted or worked against, but, instead, respected as part of what doctors used to call "The wisdom of the body." This system of medicine suggests that the appropriate thing to do is to work *with* symptoms instead of trying to remove them, as the symptoms are, in and of themselves, the being's attempt to work through some stress, or its response to some catalyst. Of course, as with any treatment, it is helpful if you can come to recognize and eliminate the source of the illness. (Hahnemann was always using the example of the patient with rheumatism who lived in a damp basement. Until he got out of that damned basement he would never have full relief from his rheumatism, and all treatments given would basically be bandaids.)

But the concept of working with a given patient's symptoms leads to a way of working in which the doctor can make no assumptions about the patient or his or her symptoms, other than to seek to understand them and, in understanding them, help the patient release them. This means that each *patient* must be treated, not his or her disease, as the so-called disease in not an attacker from outside the body but a response from within. It also carries with it the implication that any treatment given must seek to support and strengthen the patient so he can work through the illness and heal himself.

Therefore, in treating, you are going to have to select a remedy carefully, basing it on the specific symptoms the patient is experiencing. You must gather this information in the greatest detail possible, and then you are going to have to give a medicine that works in quite the opposite manner from the way you have gathered the information. The remedy must not be specific to a particular symptom at all, as allopathic drugs tend to be, but must, instead, be as general as possible in its action. It must support the patient as a whole being, trusting that, in doing so, you give the patient's vital force the support it needs to remove those specific symptoms, no matter how many of them there may be. The case taking must be detailed, but the remedy must be wide and deep in its action. This is just another way in which homeopathy stands in opposition to allopathy. In allopathy the diagnosis is much more general, with the name of the disease being enough to suggest a course of treatment, and the medicines are very targeted toward specific symptoms.

This leads to another assumption, which is that, ultimately, giving a set of symptoms a name for the sake of diagnosis of the disease is rather pointless. If each patient is an individual, then his or her individuality overwhelms the fact that a patient is suffering from a set of symptoms that have a name. The naming of diseases is only of value if the focus of the treatment is on the disease and not on the patient. If you focus the treatment on the patient and his or her specific response to the stressor in terms of the specifics of the symptoms involved, then the fact that two patients both have colds is really rather meaningless.

The doctor who treats the cold will use the diagnosis, "You have a head cold," as a map to the territory of treatment. They will continue, "When you have a head cold, you must drink fluids, take bed rest, and eat light foods." The disease diagnosis controls the method of treatment.

If, however, you place the emphasis of the treatment on the patient with the cold, then you have to get specific about the treatment in terms of the individual's personal experience of the cold symptoms and his or her reaction to it. The patient who has a sore throat on the right side of the throat may well need a different remedy from the patient who has a sore throat that manifests on the left side. In the same way, the patient with a cold who is angry and chilly may need a different remedy from the patient who is rather happily watching TV and eating potato chips during his cold.

In other words, if the patient is central to the treatment, then each case must be taken on its own terms and a unique treatment must be found, not for the disease, but for the patient. That means there is no such thing as a cold medicine, or a treatment for backache, arthritis, or anything else that can be named. There can be only treatments for individual patients, whose grouping of symptoms can be named or unnamed as you like, as the name in no way implies a course of treatment. This simple change of emphasis from treating the disease to treating the patient with the disease makes for a profound difference in the way medicine has to be practiced.

For one thing, it makes the practice of medicine a good deal harder.

Hahnemann developed his system of therapeutic treatment based on two assumptions—that diluted medicines were safer medicines, and that the most effective and safest medical treatments were those that worked with a given patient's symptoms and not against them. This enabled the patient to heal himself by supporting the patient's remaining vital force, that which had not been suppressed by the illness or by medical treatment. Hahnemann developed a new pharmacy of medicines and encoded a new practice of medicine that was solidly based in principles dating back to Hippocrates, the Father of Medicine himself.

But, in removing the concept of a disease diagnosis as the guiding force in the selection of the course of treatment and medicines, Hahnemann made his practice of medicine much more complex. In insisting that the needs of the individual patient were the overriding concern and in developing a pharmacy of medicines that today number in the thousands in terms of the sheer number of remedies, each available in dozens of potencies—any or all of which are potential medicines for any given case— he created a system of treatment that makes the selection of the best possible remedy in the best possible potency something of a Holy Grail. He called this—the right remedy given in the right potency and in the exact right number of doses—the *simillimum*. This is the remedy that will always lead to a cure. This is the buried treasure that every homeopath digs for through his or her pages of notes concerning the case taking of the patient's mental, emotional, and physical symptoms.

But the most powerful and impressive aspect of Hahnemann's methods was the single statement that summed up this entire train of thought. That statement, "Like cures like," would become known as the Law of Similars, and would become the rallying cry in a medical revolution. Those three simple words stand for all that had come before— the years of work that had taken Hahnemann from the moment of his disillusionment with the system of medicine as he had learned it to the eureka moment when he not only realized that another way of working was needed, but also fully realized just what that new mode of treatment was and how and why it worked.

Think for a moment what that means: Like cures like. It means that if you seek to treat a patient with certain set of symptoms using a medicine (or, worse, a number of medicines) whose action it is to work against the patient's symptoms, then all you can do at best is cover up those symptoms, suppress them. That the only thing that can cure a given set of symptoms is a medicine that can create the same set of symptoms. That if you give a patient with a set of symptoms a medicine that can be shown to create those same symptoms in a well person, then that medicine will be curative to the person already experiencing those symptoms. If you can give the patient that medicine in the right dose, just slightly stronger than the disease state, then the patient's vital force will rise up in opposition to the medicine's action and move him or her away from the symptoms created by the remedy, away from the symptoms of the disease and back toward health.

This is the concept of similarity. It is the heart of the homeopathic process. Of both the philosophy and the practice of homeopathy.

The paths to homeopathy were two trains of thought that started from two very simple ideas: that diluted remedies might be safer than those that were not diluted, and that, if working against symptoms did not seem to bring about a true restoration of health, then perhaps working with the symptoms would. These two paths came together as Hahnemann blended the philosophy and practice of homeopathic medicine. They merged together in the concept of similarity, and homeopathy as it is known today was born.

This, in thumbnail form, is the system of medicine that is called homeopathy, as it was developed and practiced by Samuel Hahnemann, and as W.H. Schuessler learned it and initially practiced it himself.

Schuessler and the Biochemic Method

As Schuessler became more and more involved with cell theory and the materialistic viewpoint that was replacing the theory of vitalism in the scientific community, however, he began to move away from homeopathy as well, and from the homeopathic/vitalistic viewpoint of health and healing.

Instead, like others who shared his conclusions on the importance of cell health to the health of the whole body, he came to conclude that diseases occurred only in those patients whose bodies did not maintain a balanced and normal cell metabolism. In other words, the health of the cells was not just important, but it was important to the point that it determined the health of the body as a whole.

This is certainly a valid enough point, as far as it goes.

In order to function correctly, the individual cells have to be fed. Among those things that nourish the cells, allowing them not only to function independently but also as a unit, the human body needs "essential minerals," those materials that the body cannot manufacture. These are nutritional substances that must be taken into the body in food. Among these minerals are calcium, sodium, magnesium, potassium, phosphorus, sulfur, chloride, iron, and zinc, all of which are essential to the smooth functioning of the body and its individual cells. These minerals appear in the human body as chemical compounds, such as sodium chloride, which contains the essential minerals sodium and chloride. In the same way, these minerals form and reform in any number of chemical combinations within the body. Some are constantly present and always needed in the healthy functioning of the body, while others are only present sometimes and are of lesser import.

The human body maintains an intricate balance among these minerals in order to function properly. Sodium and potassium, for example, carry on an elaborate dance within the human system called the "sodium-potassium pump" (also called the "Na+/K+ pump"), a process present in every cell of the body, but especially important to nerve and muscle cells. Through the process of active transport, three ions of sodium move to the outside of a cell for every two ions of potassium that move into it. When the process remains in balance, a state of health is maintained. When the process goes out of balance and the sodium-potassium pump is disrupted, the cells are starved of glucose and amino acids. The fluid balance of the body is disrupted, and illness results. The body no longer functions as it should, just from the disruption of the nutritional process of the cells.

While Schuessler, using the technology of his day, could not have been able to track the sodium-potassium pump, he concluded through clinical research that illness results if the cells are not properly nourished and if the balance of minerals needed by those cells was not maintained. Taking it a step further, he concluded that all illness had its basis in the cells and in a disruption of the balance among what he identified as the twelve essential tissue or cell salts in the body. They were those minerals—"cell" or "tissue" salts as he referred to them—that were always present in the human body and most necessary to its function. Even Schuessler had to admit the number of cell salts present in the body at any given time in various and sundry chemical compounds was far more than twelve. But these, he concluded, were the most important of the cell salts. Further, he concluded that these twelve were the cell salts that were always present and always required to maintain the health of the body, a fact that he verified by studying the minerals present in the ashes of the human body after it was burned.

> Schuessler concluded through clinical research that illness results if the cells are not properly nourished and if the balance of minerals needed by those cells was not maintained. Taking it a step further, he concluded that all illness had its basis in the cells and in a disruption of the balance among what he identified as the twelve essential tissue or cell salts in the body. They were those minerals—"cell" or "tissue" salts as he referred to them— that were always present in the human body and most necessary to its function.

These conclusions led Schuessler to adopt a nutritional approach to medicine. He believed that if the balance among the cell salts could be restored, then the cell's metabolism could be restored as well and health and vitality would result.

Then the issue became just how—in what form—the minerals could be supplied to the depleted cells. They would have to be readily and easily assimilated in order to nourish the cells that were weakened from having been starved of these essential minerals.

This led Schuessler partway back down the path to his homeopathic past. He began to create these essential minerals, these cell salts, in potentized form of homeo-pathic remedies, using the same methods of dilution that Hahnemann set forth in the creation of homeopathic remedies. In doing this, he created* what were in essence homeopathic remedies, in their physical form at least, although he did not intend to use them in accordance with the Law of Similars, as Hahnemann did.

Instead, Schuessler worked by the theory of *deficiency*.

The idea of deficiency is that, if we can ascertain exactly which mineral salt or salts the body's cells are starving for, and if we can give the body those salts in a manner in which it can absorb and digest them, then the cells will be nourished and the balance needed for function, form, and good health will result.

By giving the cell salts in the form of low-potency homeopathic remedies, Schuessler not only supplied the body with the salts it needed, but administered them in a form that stimulated the body to absorb and utilize them in the optimal amounts needed to maintain balance and health. Thus, the action of the salts was at once nutri-tional and homeopathic, and the remedies were at once homeopathic and allopathic. Homeopathic because they were created as homeopathic remedies. Allopathic because they are not used in accordance with the Law of Similars, as all homeopathic remedies are, but, instead, under the guiding principle of deficiency, which is an allopathic the-ory because it implies that the material substance of the mineral salts is responsible for health and not the balance of energy, of vital force.

The cell salts are, therefore, a strange balance between allopathy and homeopathy or, better put, a balance between homeopathy and nutritional medicine. Unlike home-opathic remedies, which have no direct action on the human body, the cell salts, because of their low dilution, have a physiological action on the human body. They are, at once, substance and energy.

Schuessler came to call his system of therapeutics the biochemic method, taking it from the Greek word *bios*, which means "life." With his method, he sought to develop a simple system whereby all the ills of mankind could be removed by simply shifting the fundamental parts of the body, the cells, into a state of nutritional health and func-tional balance. In doing this, he developed a system that utilized homeopathic reme-dies in a new way (some may say in a "bastardized" way and refer to Schuessler as what Hahnemann himself would have called a "mongrel homeopath") that achieved some

---

* In the majority of cases, Schuessler did indeed create his cell salts, in that he was the first to make the specific chemical compound into a potentized remedy. It needs to be noted that for some others he simply borrowed remedies that Hahnemann had already created from chemical compounds. Among these are two of the most important and most used of the homeopathic remedies, Natrum Muriaticum and Silicea, which Schuessler borrowed for his biochemic system of treatment, adapting their use and potency to his own methods.

sort of a balancing point between that which we can think of as nutritional and that which must be considered medicine.

Indeed, since Schuessler's time, the cell salts have many times been used as if they were not homeopathic medicines at all, but were, instead, a form of multiple vitamin, the purpose of which is to nourish the body rather than to restore the vital force.

Homeopathy and Cell Salts

Suffice it to say that biochemics and homeopathic medicine are not the same, although they share a method by which the remedies are created. They do not work in the same way and the principles that guide the treatments are different. And yet the two systems are linked, and undeniably have much in common. (They do, after all, share the twelve remedies that make up the entirety of the biochemic pharmacy and a minute part of the homeopathic pharmacy.)

This biochemic balance between homeopathy and allopathy makes the biochemic method the subject of suspicion by both camps. Like a Republican who is too liberal, or a Democrat who is too conservative, the cell salts are often scorned equally by both camps. The allopaths scorn them because this nutritional system, which has some undeniable truth to it, also uses potentized remedies. This marks it as a form of holistic medicine and makes it the target of quackbusters everywhere. The homeopaths scorn the cell salts because Schuessler denounced not only homeopathy but also Hahnemann himself, and, in his later years, insisted that he had not gotten any of his ideas for his biochemic method from his misspent youth as a homeopath.

The result is that the cell salts have been relegated to a small medical niche and are not well known. In health food stores, where the cell salts can usually be found next to the homeopathic remedies, they are given a very small amount of shelf space. Most who know of them at all today know them only as a group of low-potency remedies, and not as the full therapeutic system that they are.

This is a pity, really, because in home use the cell salts are a simplified form of homeopathic medicine and an alternative to over-the-counter allopathic medicines for the treatment of common illnesses. They are far less toxic than over-the-counter medications. They are safe, easy to use, inexpensive, and, unlike homeopathic remedies, finite in number and potency. The cell salts

> The cell salts are ideal for those who are seeking relatively simple, safe, and effective treatments for common household ailments. With only twelve remedies to learn instead of the hundreds or thousands used in homeopathic medicine, it is actually possible to learn by heart those symptoms—skin color, tongue color, skin temperature, quality, and other such indicators—and recognize the need for a specific remedy quickly and easily.

are ideal for those who are seeking relatively simple, safe, and effective treatments for common household ailments. With only twelve remedies to learn instead of the hundreds or thousands used in homeopathic medicine, it is actually possible to learn by heart those symptoms—skin color, tongue color, skin temperature, quality, and other such indicators—and recognize the need for a specific remedy quickly and easily. In cases of simple chronic conditions, such as indigestion, they can be nothing short of miraculous and offer an alternative to costly and far more toxic allopathic treatments. In acute ailments, they can be very helpful and often yield results that seem miraculous (to the parent whose child has suddenly stopped screaming in the middle of the night because his teething pains have been soothed, for example).

They are a means of treatment in which the caregiver and the patient alike need not fear side effects or toxic results. In which both can rest assured that the cure will serve only to strengthen the patient.

For these reasons they are worthy of consideration, of study, and of a place in the family medical kit, if not exactly in the homeopathic kit. I do not suggest that the cell salts are superior to other homeopathic remedies, simply different from them (although I would, in many, many cases say that they are in every way superior to their allopathic alternatives). Most certainly they have value as a system of treatment—a system whose unique status as a synthesis between that which is homeopathic and that which is nutritional sets it apart from homeopathy and allopathy and, because of its unique status, makes it part of each. I have at times over the years found the cell salts to be a good stepping stone for those who are interested in learning about homeopathy but not particularly interested in leaving all things allopathic behind. In the same way, I have found the cell salts to be very useful for those who are in the beginning stages of learning homeopathy. They can be used just like other homeopathic remedies, should the caregiver choose to use them in this manner. They can be a doorway into homeopathy or considered an end in themselves, a fully realized form of holistic medication. Either way, the cells salts have value, as we shall see.

PART TWO

Nutritional Homeopathy

"The Human body is composed of two kinds of matter—organic and inorganic. The former greatly preponderates, but it does not follow that it is more essential to life than the latter; indeed, the organic could not perform its proper function without the inorganic. These are not mere theories but scientifically proven facts. It has been discovered that the human body will survive for a shorter period of time from the deprivations of inorganic (mineral) salts than of the other (organic) constituents of the diet."

—J.B. CHAPMAN, MD
IN *DR SCHUESSLER'S BIOCHEMISTRY*

CHAPTER THREE

An Introduction
to the Cell Salts

The Cell Salts—just like the Bach flower remedies—beg the question: "But is it homeopathic?" Anyone considering using them has to wonder about their true nature, whether or not they should be considered to be homeopathic remedies. And, again, as with the Bach Remedies, the answer to the question has to be yes—and no.

Just as the floral essences* represent the perfect balance between homeopathic remedies and herbal medicine—remedies that are in the state of "zero dilution," prepared as if they were going to be potentized into homeopathic remedies but then left unpotentized, floating in a limbo between substance (herbal medicine, which is, by its nature, allopathic) and energy (potentized homeopathic remedies), the cell salts represent a balance between homeopathic and nutritional (perhaps what would best be termed "naturopathic") approaches to medicine.

> The cell salts represent a balance between homeopathic and nutritional (perhaps what would best be termed "naturopathic") approaches to medicine.

When Schuessler took the inorganic compounds that he used in the creation of the cell salts he developed (or borrowed from the homeopathic pharmacy), he ultimately decided to prepare them in the manner of homeopathic remedies and then made an important decision about just how his remedies would be potentized. He decided to potentize them only to a specific low level, where they were left, as Bach's

---

* I keep mentioning the flower essences not just because I wrote about them in a companion volume to this book called *The Healing Bouquet*, but also because, for me, these two offshoots of homeopathy represent the two extremes to which homeopathic thought can be taken. If you think of it in terms of a government, Hahnemannian homeopathy represents the centrist stance, the flower remedies (in that they largely ignore physical symptoms and deal with emotional states, with the belief that, if emotional issues are cleared away, physical issues will surely follow) take the role of the far left and the cell salts (which focus very much on the physical body—indeed, upon the cells of the body, the smallest aspect of the human form—and the symptoms of that body, almost to the exclusion of the mind and emotions) represent the far right. In looking at these three philosophies of medicine, it is possible to identify the full sweep of all that can be called, to some degree, "homeopathic."

were, in a limbo between material medicine (that which is used in allopathic treatments) and energy medicine (that which is common to such treatments as homeopathic medicine and acupuncture, among other therapies). Because of this, the Schuessler cell salts are undeniably homeopathic in that they are created in the same manner as all other homeopathic remedies, and yet they are not truly to be considered homeopathic, in that they are used in a manner that stands in sharp contrast with homeopathic philosophy.* As has already been noted, the concept of deficiency is in no way homeopathic. Indeed, Schuessler himself at the end of his life insisted that his treatments had nothing whatsoever to do with Hahnemann's. While this most certainly is not true—it stretches the imagination beyond the breaking point to suggest that Schuessler could have studied medicine in Germany when he did without hearing of the work of the great and controversial Samuel Hahnemann and that he, Schuessler, just somehow stumbled onto the same concept of potentization and used it to create remedies from the same source materials as Hahnemann—it does seem that Schuessler came to the conclusion that, in giving his approach to treatment a new name—biochemics—he was somehow re-inventing the homeopathic wheel.

However, the value of the cell salts does not lie in their origin, or even in the moral nature of the man who created them. It lies within the remedies themselves. Whether they are an admitted offshoot of homeopathy or not, they are undeniably linked with homeopathic medicines both in source materials and in the process by which they are created. In the same way that the flower remedies are a balancing point between homeopathy and herbal medicines, the cell salts are a perfect balance between homeopathic medicines and nutritional supplements. This gives them great potential. Since they are remedies that have been potentized to a low level, the original compounds from which they were taken have not been diluted to the point that all original substance has fallen away. As a result, they are capable of acting nutritionally as well as medicinally. It is important that they have been potentized slightly, only to a degree at which substance and energy combine. This allows the needed cell salt (in which the body has been found to be deficient) to nurture the body, while the vital force of the substance, released in the process of potentization, stimulates the body to heal itself. The cell salts therefore represent a more directed, more powerful form of nutritional supplementation: one that is completely safe, because they are taken from source materials that nat-

* James Tyler Kent (1849–1916), an American homeopath and eclectic physician (naturopath), who was a major influence on the development of homeopathy in the United States, drove this point home, when he insisted that homeopathic remedies must be homeopathic in two ways—in the way in which they are created and in the way in which they are used. The fact that the cell salts are potentized in the homeopathic manner suggests that they are homeopathic remedies. It therefore depends upon the way in which they are used by various individuals to determine whether or not they may truly be called homeopathic remedies in both aspects of that definition.

urally occur in the human body and are required for the processes that are the source of good health, and one that is more powerful than supplements taken in material form. Because of this dual aspect of the cell salts, I have given this system of treatment a new name that reflects both their function and their potential. I think of it as "nutritional homeopathy."

To better understand the meaning of the term, it's important, at this point, to consider the method by which all forms of homeopathic remedies are made.

Potentization

Potentization is a two-step process for homeopathic remedies. It consists of dilution, a term that is rather self-explanatory, and succussion, which means "shaking," as the remedies are, once they are in a state of dilution, shaken systematically in a process that ends with an impact. In Hahnemann's day, succussion involved the rapid up and down motion of the right forearm, while the diluted remedy, sealed in a glass container, was gripped in the right hand and slammed against a leather-bound book, with a Bible often being the book of choice. The succussion took place through ten stages of shaking and slamming to sufficiently stir the dilution to the next stage of potency.

Even the process of dilution was systematic in Hahnemann's process of potentization. When he began working with his remedies, he started with a general notion that medicines that were toxic in their material state might be less so if they were simply diluted. He developed a scale of dilution of one part medicinal to nine parts water (or alcohol, if the substance was insoluble in water). This dilution would then be succussed, as described above, and one part of the resulting potency—called 1X if it was the first level of potentizing, with a dilution in tenths—would be mixed again with nine parts water (no need for the use of alcohol, as the remedy was now in a state of dilution) to create a 2X, and so on, ad infinitum. This "X" scale of remedies was the basis from which Hahnemann worked in the development of his remedies, always exploring what changes each new level of dilution brought about.

Over the years, Hahnemann developed another system of dilutions and another scale of remedies, the "C" scale, "C" representing the Roman numeral for one hundred. This potency scale involved taking one part of medicinal substance and diluting it with 99 parts water before succussing. Like the "X" scale, the "C" scale continued onward from there, until the 999th dilution, at which point the next dilution was called a 1M, "M" being the Roman numeral for one thousand. (Hahnemann, making his own remedies by hand in his laboratory, considered the 30C potency, which we now consider a nice low potency, to be a very high potency, as it took thirty full stages of dilution and succussion, hours of labor, and dozens of glass vials to reach. He conjectured, however, about the effects of much higher potencies—potencies in regular use today, now that remedies are machine-made in factories.)

As Hahnemann worked with medicinal substances in order to polish them into homeopathic remedies, he had to develop a method by which he could potentize remedies made from substances—mineral compounds, mostly—that were not soluble in either water or alcohol. For these substances, like calcium carbonate, from which Hahnemann created the remedy Calcarea Carbonica, he developed the process known as *trituration*.

In trituration, one part of the medicinal substance is blended with nine parts of milk sugar and the mixture is ground in a mortar and pestle. This grinding of solid substance—nine parts milk sugar and one part medicine—takes place for the first three levels of dilution until the 3X potency is reached. At this point, all mixtures are soluble and are mixed with water and succussed from the 3X potency onward.

This process of trituration is vital to the cell salts since the majority of them are made from chemical compounds that are insoluble in water or alcohol. As a result, most companies now make all cell salts through this process, whether the substances are (like sodium chloride, or common table salt) soluble in water or not. Some feel that the process of trituration always results in a more potent remedy when making remedies from mineral sources, no matter their solubility. But whether created through dilution or through trituration, all homeopathic remedies become homeopathic in the same way: via some form of systematic dilution and succussion, in the process known as potentization.

Avogadro's Number

The concept of Avogadro's number is important to understanding the idea of nutritional homeopathy.

Amadeo Avogadro (1776–1856) was a physicist working in Turin, Italy who, in 1811, published his findings concerning the number of molecules, atoms, and other particles that were to be found in a single mole of any substance. (A mole is a unit of mass equal to the substance's molecular weight. For example, a gram mole of the carbon-12 isotope would be twelve grams.) Just the fact that Avogadro could calculate this number was astounding. The fact that the number of molecules was found to be a constant seemed the stuff of science fiction, at least what would have been science fiction in nineteenth century Italy.

The identification of what came to be known as Avogadro's number is important to homeopathy because it allows us to calculate the exact point in dilution at which not one single molecule of the original substance remains in the remedy, no matter from what substance that remedy was derived. That level of dilution is found at the 23X or at 12C, meaning that remedies 24X and above, or 13C and above, no longer have any original substance left in them. Only the traces of vital force, or the "energy signatures" of the original substances remain.

This remains a central mystery of homeopathic medicine. Just as Hahnemann found two hundred years ago, we today also find that the medicinal action of a remedy becomes stronger, not weaker, once it passes Avogadro's number in terms of dilution. Common sense might suggest that the more diluted a substance becomes, the less potent it is, but homeopathic clinical experience suggests otherwise. Two hundred years of clinical use suggests that, as homeopathic remedies become more diluted, they become both less *toxic* (and certainly most if not all material or allopathic medicines are toxic to one degree or another) and more *powerful* at the same time.

This is particularly important to the cell salts, because Schuessler chose to always use them in potencies of 12X or under—potencies that are well below Avogadro's limit. Remedies created in these potencies include not only the energy signature of a given substance, but the substance itself as well. The selection of this low level of potency was not an act of laziness on Schuessler's part. It does not reflect either a lack of muscle strength in his right arm or his lack of belief in the power of the Bible. Instead, it is a clear indicator that, with this system of therapeutics that he named biochemics, he was not seeking to reinvent medicine, as Hahnemann had sought to do, but, instead, to reinvent homeopathy—to simplify it and to ground it within the substance of the body itself.

Nutritional Homeopathy

If we can accept any aspect of the concept of deficiency—even if we accept it only as a nutritional given that, for better or worse, we all need the same nutrients in our diet in order for our bodies to function—then it stands to reason that we might well be on to something if we can somehow use the idea of potentization and apply it to our nutritional needs as opposed to our medical requirements.

So, it is safe to say that, in his development of biochemics, Schuessler was on to something. He started from ashes. Literally. He started with the ash that remains when the human body is burned. He looked at that ash and at its component parts, searching among them to identify the building blocks, the chemical compounds that give the structure and function to the human body. In the end, Schuessler identified twelve compounds and used these (or, at least, used the compounds that Hahnemann or some other homeopath had already beaten him to) as the basis of his system of treatment.

It was important to Schuessler that these substances be "native" to the human system because of his belief in the concept of deficiency. Since he believed that the health of the body as a whole was determined by the health of each individual cell of the body, it was of great importance to him that each of those cells had all the nutrients it required to form, grow, and function.

When choosing the substances that could be identified as being a part of all human bodies, Schuessler also chose remedies that were totally benign—that were actually more than simply benign. Not only did they have no degree of toxicity, they also were nurturing substances, compounds that gave cells elasticity and strength that encouraged their formation, their growth, and even their removal when individual cells died.

In identifying his twelve remedies, Schuessler created a simple system of treatment that could inspire the body to find a new balance, a new state of health beyond that which it had while still in the state of deficiency he saw as the source of disease. In limiting his potency to 12X and under, he made sure that the remedies still contained their nutrient substances. But in limiting the number of his remedies to just twelve, he made the mistake of limiting his entire system of treatment.

Before we go further, it is important to note that Schuessler was limited in his research—as Hahnemann was before him—by the technology of his day. Therefore, he was reduced to literally sifting through the ashes in a way he would not have been today. Indeed, he found, no doubt to his chagrin, that one of this remedies, Calcarea Sulphurica, did not actually occur naturally in human systems, and therefore technically did not belong among the biochemical remedies.*

In limiting his remedies to an even dozen, Schuessler perhaps fell prey to the desire to make things nice and tidy, to have a system about which nice books like this one could be written.

But he attempted to fit any number of square pegs into round holes by doing so. There is that whole issue of Calcarea Sulphurica, and ending up with only eleven remedies. And there is the somewhat odd nature of the remedy Silicea, our little orphan remedy that is not made from a chemical compound as the others all are, but instead from silica itself. And the greatest issue of all, the fact that these few remedies in no way represent all the building blocks of the body. By omitting the other components, Schuessler's system fails to be as far-ranging as it could be.

So, do the eleven or twelve remedies—depending upon whether or not you want to give Schuessler the final say on the number—represent everything that could be thought of as a "cell salt," as a compound that occurs naturally in the human system? Most certainly not. Which means that, as good as the system is, as much potential as it has as a method of healing, it is not complete.

If we could embrace this idea of "nutritional homeopathy," of creating a full pharmacopeia—a body, if you will—of remedies based upon the building blocks of life itself, upon those things not only wanted in the human system but actually required in order for it to function and function well, what an interesting and potentially wonderful system of therapeutics we might have. Calcarea Sulphurica is a perfect example of what I

---

* In his last years, Schuessler dropped Calcarea Sulphurica from use and had only eleven remedies. He split Calc Sulph's actions among other remedies, in some sort of a pretense that it was never really needed to begin with.

mean. If, instead of simply trying to sweep the remedy under the rug when he discovered that Calc Sulph did not appear as a compound in all human bodies, he had enlarged his circle of remedies, using all that contained the basic building blocks of life in various compounds—different variants, if you will, of the original eleven remedies—then he might have created a fully realized system of mineral-based nutritional remedies. Instead, he made his circle smaller. In doing so, he made it less effective for the treatment of the many ailments of mankind. As it is, we have an awfully good beginning with the twelve remedies that are commonly used, each utterly safe and surprisingly effective for the treatment of myriad diseases, both acute and chronic and functional and pathological.

Whatever Schuessler's flaws—whatever wounds to the ego he had experienced that led him to announce that his biochemical remedies had nothing whatsoever to do with homeopathic remedies, whatever need for completion that led him limit his system to just twelve (or, worse, eleven) remedies, when there were so many others that could have been considered while still staying true to the ashes—Schuessler has given us something really quite unique. Something that stands on its own, though it should perhaps be considered an offshoot of homeopathy (as the Bach remedies must also be considered). Schuessler both made use of some standard therapeutics and developed some of his own—the majority of his cell salts were either of his own devising or remedies that had been more or less cast off until he researched their use. In the end, he not only developed his own system but contributed to the homeopathic pharmacy as well, as the materia medica now contains all the remedies that he contributed, each of which is available today in the form of cell salts as well as in the more fully potentized homeopathic form.

Cell Salts Today

The cell salts offer an excellent version of homeopathic medicine for home use. Just as the Bach flower remedies belong in every home—Rescue Remedy at the very least—I believe that every home should have a full kit of the dozen cell salts in the basic 6X potency, and that that kit should be used for the ordinary crises that arise in the home, usually in the middle of the night. (Calcarea Sulphurica has proven itself to be an effective remedy and it is unique in its actions, so I can't help but believe that it deserves to stay put, as its removal would create a therapeutic gap in our home kit. Therefore, I have included Calc Sulph in these pages and given it the status of a cell salt, even though I don't have any of it naturally occurring in my liver.) Used correctly and appropriately (more on this in Part Three of this book), I also believe that they can be an excellent introduction to homeopathy in general, to case taking and management, and to the nature of the homeopathic "cure."

But let's be clear. The cell salts are to classical homeopathy what a crockpot is to a microwave. The healing they inspire is gentle and steady, if a little bit slow. But when efficacy and safety are desired in medical treatment, the small group of homeopathic remedies known as cell salts should always be considered. The cell salts are of particular value in cases of chronic conditions where the homeopathic remedies of higher potency will give a more active and dramatic response. They are excellent in cases requiring pain management and are sometimes superior to everything else in cases involving allergy and skin conditions of all sorts. Most important, they are completely safe for home use. It would not only be far safer but also far more effective for a given patient to take a cell salt, or even a combination of cell salts, for a cold than it would for that patient to take any of the over-the-counter medications available at the local drug store. This is true largely because they are homeopathic remedies by nature. They are *not* allopathic drugs, which only suppress the symptoms of the ailment without actually treating it in any way,

> The cell salts offer an excellent version of homeopathic medicine for home use. Just as the Bach flower remedies belong in every home—Rescue Remedy at the very least—I believe that every home should have a full kit of the dozen cell salts in the basic 6X potency, and that that kit should be used for the ordinary crises that arise in the home, usually in the middle of the night.

and actually manage to weaken the body's healing response in doing so. Instead, they work, as all homeopathics do, by helping the body to express its symptoms, and in expressing them release them from the body completely, leaving a system that is cleansed and stronger than before. And more, the cell salts can be so very effective in the home because they are simple to use—far simpler to use and to learn than the thousands of homeopathic remedies that can be cumbersome, to say the least, for the student who is just beginning a study of homeopathy.

So while I do not share Schuessler's belief that his system of biochemical remedies are revolutionary or that they represent a panacea for all who suffer, I do see them as an excellent variant on classical homeopathy—one that has a place in the home as a means whereby acute conditions can receive appropriate and safe treatment. That is perhaps the most that could be hoped for, given the boundaries that Schuessler himself placed upon his biochemical treatments in terms of potency and the small circle of included remedies. But if you look at it another way—that these simple, safe, and easy-to-use remedies bring relief to those who suffer from pain and illness, and, in doing so, work to strengthen the patient's system to help prevent the next occurrence of illness—they are pretty impressive things, these little cell salts.

CHAPTER FOUR

Considering the Source

The best way to understand the nature of the cell salts, all of which are compound remedies* (which is to say that they are taken from more than one substance and then potentized into a homeopathic state), is to look at the substances used in the creation of the remedies and at the specific actions these component parts of the cell salts have once they are made into remedies. In other words, phosphorus, whether it is combined with potassium into Kali Phos or with sodium into Natrum Phos, will still carry with it the same "message" and will still resonate with a specific type of patient and/or a specific set of symptoms.

Therefore, in looking briefly at the component parts of the cell salt remedies, we can better understand the full working of each of the remedies and the ways in which they may most effectively be used.

Familial Relationships

The easiest way that I know of to think about the cell salt remedies is as if they were the children of specific marriages between parents. Each remedy will share some aspects

---

* Let me be clear in explaining the difference between compound remedies, which are an appropriate part of the homeopathic pharmacy, and combination remedies, which are not. Compound remedies are combined while they are still substances. This combination of materials is then diluted and succussed through the stages needed to make them into fully potentized remedies. The resulting remedy is then fully proved in its medicinal effects using healthy human subjects. Combination remedies, on the other hand, are made up of two or more homeopathic remedies—already fully potentized and proven as individual remedies—that have been combined together with that hope that, jointly, they will have a more powerful medicinal effect than each would have if used alone. The problem with combination remedies is that they fly in the face of Hahnemann's own so-called law of cure, simplex, which tells us that we should use only one remedy at a time. Those using combination remedies are guilty of what Hahnemann called polypharmacy, or the use of more than one remedy at a time. This is problematic because Hahnemann felt that every medicine—homeopathic or allopathic—produces more than one change in the human system. When more than one remedy is used at a given time, it is impossible to know what remedy is creating what series of results. Combination remedies can result in muddled if not incurable cases, especially when they are used for a long period of time.

with each of its parent remedies. Natrum Muriaticum will have some of the attributes common to Natrums and some attributes that it gets from the Muriaticum side of the family. In the same way, each of the compounds will "inherit" a mix of traits, divided between the two parent remedies.

And each of those parent remedies belongs to a family of remedies. Natrum Muriaticum is kin to the cell salts Natrum Phosphoricum and Natrum Sulphuricum, as well as to a host of other homeopathic remedies, including Natrum Carbonicum and Natrum Nitricum, among others, that Schuessler did not select for inclusion among the cells salts, but that are still related remedies with myriad shared symptoms.

So before we look at the individual remedies and their actions, I think it is important to first "meet the families," to illustrate the ways in which the variations of the compounds into which the same substances are blended and reblended can yield remedies that are at once related and quite unique in their actions. This will, I think, offer a

> The best way to understand the nature of the cell salts, all of which are compound remedies, is to look at the substances used in the creation of the remedies and at the specific actions these component parts of the cell salts have once they are made into remedies.

better understanding of the individual cell salts and a means by which we can consider the cell salts among the other remedies of the homeopathic pharmacy.

The Calcium/Calcarea Family

Just as calcium is used by the body to give it structure, all Calcarea remedies relate to this notion of structure, of how things are built and how things are done. Each, therefore, will play out the riddle of structure (or lack of same) in their symptoms.

In the emotional sphere, this sense of structure will play out most commonly in the role of work in the patient's life. These are people with low self-esteem, people who feel that they will soon be found out to be frauds at the things they do for a living. They seek safe harbors in work, tend to rise to the middle of the pack and cling there. In these roles, they give structure to businesses of all sorts. Often, they cling to a single approach, a single way of solving a problem, and cannot adapt to the idea of multiple solutions or new ways of working. Change comes very hard to the Calcarea patient.

Calcareas, typically, are either driven to work very hard or totally averse to work. They tend to be detail-driven and rather passive. Calcarea types avoid conflict, confrontation, and all tasks they find unpleasant. They can be sluggish in their thoughts, unclear in their motivations. They are very clear about one thing, however: they care deeply what others think of them. This can turn some Calcarea patients into "pleasers" who will go to any lengths to please others, even at great cost to themselves.

Calcareas tend to be very loyal and cling to people and relationships as they do to the procedures and methods that they use in problem solving. While they may have a pronounced fear of people and tend to avoid crowds and, especially, strangers, they do not want to be left alone and will cling to those they love, especially to family members.

While they are loyal, Calcarea types, rather ironically, tend to be lacking in empathy for others. While they are themselves very sensitive, hyperaware of their own emotional needs and their overriding need to be seen as pleasant, successful, and, above all else, competent, they are rather immune to the needs of others, and can even manage not to notice suffering that is right in front of their eyes.

Emotionally, Calcareas are most known for their stubbornness. These are, perhaps, our most stubborn patients. (This stubborn streak is also displayed on the physical level. Calcareas can be notoriously chronic in their complaints—they can be very hard to cure, even when they present mild and comparatively simple physical complaints).

The other key indicator of the type is depression. Calcarea is known for an emotional sense of weight that mirrors their physical reality. They are given to depressions, both mild and severe, that can be as stubborn as they are. These depressions are commonly accompanied by an ongoing sense of anxiety, as if something bad were about to happen.

Physically, the remedies taken from the substance calcium are, rather ironically, known for their tendency toward flab. The Calcarea remedies are most commonly known for what is called the three F's: fair, fat, and flabby. These are patients with underdeveloped muscles who gain weight very easily. They have large appetites, often for the most indigestible things, even for things that are not food: they may eat chalk, mud, paste, or other inedible materials. They are known for having a slow digestion—all the remedies within the Calcarea family will display multiple symptoms associated with indigestion—and a slow metabolism. Hypothyroidism is common, as is the condition known as Syndrome X, or metabolic syndrome, which combines overweight with a sluggish metabolism, a tendency toward hypertension, and an inability to metabolize sugar. Calcareas tend to be heavy, dyspeptic, and averse to exercise in any form, perhaps because of their tendency toward emotional inertia and their sense of emotional weight.

Other common ailments include issues with blood and bleeding. Women needing the calcium-based remedies tend to have menses that are too long, in which there is a great deal of blood flow, or that arrive prematurely. They also tend toward ailments of the bones and teeth. Children needing one or more of these remedies often will have slow or delayed development with weak or malformed bones and/or teeth. They are slow to walk, late in learning to talk, and delayed in other ways. Calcareas are also commonly given to allergies of all sorts, especially to food allergies. They are given to rashes of all sorts, and, although commonly chilly patients, they sweat. They are worse when the weather is cold and/or damp, although they also tend to be better in open air, even when the weather is cold.

Cell salts belonging to this group:

- Calcarea Fluorica
- Calcarea Phosphorica
- Calcarea Sulphurica

Other homeopathic remedies in this group include:

- Calcarea Arsenica
- Calcarea Carbonica
- Calcarea Caustica
- Calcarea Iodata
- Calcarea Muriatica
- Calcarea Silicata

The Chloride/Muriaticum/Muriatica Family

The chloride group shares the emotional complaint of neediness, of want of recognition, want of nurturing. This is played out in various ways by the various remedies contained in the group. Natrum Muriaticum, for example, combines the need for loving attention with an unwillingness to accept this sort of behavior from anyone—especially from those they most care for. (As Natrum Muriaticum plays out the ongoing drama of denying itself the very thing that it most needs and wants, it displays the chloride-based tendency to be in a state of simultaneous desire and denial. No other group of remedies displays modalities in which a given patient is, at the same moment, both improved and aggravated by a single catalyst. The Natrum Muriaticum type, like the Magnesia Muriatica, is at once made better and made worse by being near the sea. They are improved emotionally when they are near water and yearn to be near water when they are not, and yet their physical symptoms are made worse when they visit the seashore or bathe in seawater.

These are remedies of specific fears. The Kali Muriaticum patient, for example, fears that he will starve to death. All are solitary people who prefer to be alone, especially during times of stress.

This is the underlying stress of the chloride-based remedies. Each presents himself as being quite capable of taking care of himself on his own, yet each yearns to be taken care of. Each also fears that he will not be nurtured, that he will go unfed, on one level or another.

On a physical level, the Muriaticum/Muriatica type tends to have swelling, physical enlargement of organs (Magnesia Muriatica, for instance, is a remedy for enlargement of the liver), and/or bloating. These are remedies that share a tendency toward dyspepsia, especially chronic dyspepsia, and for chronic complaints in general. Discharges tend to be clear to white in color and watery to thick and, especially, frothy or foamy. They tend to be somewhat chilly types for whom motion is an important component linked with pain. In some cases, as with Natrum Mur, the patient will want to stay still when in pain. In others, such as with the cardiac pains associated with Magnesia Muriatica, the patient will have to move around to find relief. Look for the Muriaticum patient to have a strong preference when it comes to motion and to insist that he be allowed to do exactly what he needs to in order to find relief.

Look to the lips for an indication of the need for a remedy from this group. Most will have chapped lips or lips that are cracked down the middle.

Cell salts belonging to this group:

- Kali Muriaticum
- Natrum Muriaticum

Other homeopathic remedies in this group include:

- Calcarea Muriatica
- Magnesia Muriatica

The Fluoride/Fluorica/Fluorata/Fluoratum Family

The effect of adding fluoride into the mix in a compound remedy can seem subtle, as there is no apparent link among these remedies. This is only enhanced by the fact that these remain rather little known remedies and are likely much underused.

Emotionally, however, each shares a rather unique attribute—a mixture of heat and coldness. Each remedy in this group plays out a variation on this theme. These are warm-blooded, and, on first glance, warm people, emotionally open and available. Only as they reveal themselves more clearly does the coldness within show itself.

The fluorides are cold people, people who tend not to make real connections with others, and tend not to want connection beyond the sexual. They can be highly manipulative types, using their exterior warmth to charm others into giving in to them.

The fluorides tend to be attracted to excess; certainly to sexual excess, but also to excess in terms of possessions and life experiences. They wear tee shirts, literally or figuratively, that read, "I'll try anything twice."

And while I do not want to go so far as to say that an entire group of remedies is made up of patients who are liars, it is certainly fact that they tend not to find themselves hampered in any real way by a need to tell the truth. Truth, for them, is a circumstantial thing at best. As charm is their primary tool of manipulation, you will find that, as part of that charm, they tend to tell people what they want to hear, whether or not it is actually true.

The best known remedy of the group is the cell salt Calcarea Fluorica, whose native coldness is blunted somewhat by the presence of calcium. Calcium's tendency toward insecurity and desire for stability and order counters much of the worst of fluoride's excess. However, even this remedy displays the fear that is most common to the group—the fear of poverty. All fluorides are interconnected by this fear (as it represents the undoing of excess) and by their driving desire to make as much money as possible, by any means possible in some cases. Perhaps it is this driving need for money that gives fluoride its core coldness, even ruthlessness.

These are remedies that are, as a result, highly concerned with how others perceive them, how they look, and, specifically, how successful they appear. They will tend to be concerned with what cars they drive, what clothes they wear, and other aspects of status.

On a physical level, look for the patients needing these remedies to suffer from myriad conditions of the teeth and bones and joints. Cataracts are common, as are all conditions in which the elastic tissues of the body become stretched and lax.

Cell salt belonging to this group:

- Calcarea Fluorica

Other homeopathic remedies in this group include:

- Baryta Fluorata
- Magnesia Fluorica
- Kali Fluoratum
- Natrum Fluoratum

The Iron/Ferrum Family

As iron is an important component of the blood, all the remedies in this group will share symptoms relating to blood. Look for the various remedy types to share the sensation of a rush of blood and look for them to share a tendency toward anemia (what television commercials used to refer to as "iron poor blood"). As iron itself is a great conductor of heat, all the remedies in this group in which Ferrum is compounded with a "hot" remedy type will have the tendency toward heat and inflammation, most notably Ferrum Phosphoricum, in which the iron component carries the heat of the phosphorus type in periods of fever. This attribute of conducting heat does not mean that the Ferrum types are hot-blooded. Quite the opposite, in fact, most Ferrums are chilly patients.

In their emotional symptoms, the Ferrum types display the clichéd "wills of iron." They tend to be extremely stable emotionally, and extremely determined. They will move forward with their own ideas, their own plans, despite what others may do, say, or think. They are not concerned with how they are judged by others, but are far more concerned with their own results.

Although their wills are strong, their bodies are, more often than not, weak. They do not like to be crossed and tend to become quite irritated and angry when others disagree with them. They tend to view any disagreement as an obstacle and any obstacle as reason for anger. Their anger, however, weakens them, exhausts them. The Ferrum types tend toward emotional and physical exhaustion.

On the other hand, no other group of remedies has such a high "say/do" ratio. If they say that they will do something, they actually do it. These are persons who persevere, despite opposition, despite exhaustion, despite saying things like, "I don't care if it kills me." They actually will do what they set out to do.

Ferrum types can be very strict. They can be very demanding. And yet they seek support. They need support. The Ferrum type who has no support—mental, emotional, or physical—will tend to fall into physical illness from overwork and emotional stress or into a maze of compulsive behaviors.

On a physical level there is, first and foremost, the keynote of the sensation of a rush of blood, most commonly to the face. When roused, especially when angered, the Ferrum type becomes red-faced. They blush when embarrassed, flush when they become irritated.

This is a nervous type as well, a type known for palpitations of the heart, throbbing sensations in the pit of the stomach, and throbbing pains running throughout the body. Ferrum types are restless and tend to keep in some form of motion at all times. They will move their hands and feet even when lying down, will toss and turn while sleeping.

As depleted types, they cannot bear too much of anything: too much emotional pressure, too many physical demands, too many changes in their environment. Just as they seek support emotionally, they will seek it physically as well. They seek balance, order, and calm. They believe in balance in all things, order at all times, and seek moderation in all aspects of life.

This is the group that can be most linked to congestion. Their pains, especially their headaches, have a quality of congestion about them. Their pains carry this sensation of congestion, linked with a throbbing sensation.

It is keynote of the group that the aches and pains associated with its remedies come on during periods of rest and are better from simple, calm movements.

Cell salt belonging to this group:

• Ferrum Phosphoricum

Other homeopathic remedies in this group include:

• Ferrum Arsenicosum
• Ferrum Bromatum
• Ferrum Cyanatum
• Ferrum Iodatum

• Ferrum Metallicum
• Ferrum Muriaticum
• Ferrum Sulphuricum

The Magnesium/Magnesia Family

There is a dichotomy to the Magnesia type, almost a split personality. It is as if the pain—the severe pain or the pain to which the patient reacts as if it were far more severe than it is—was the physicalization of their internal, emotional conflict. The issue at the core of the type is aggression. Magnesia types at one and the same time fear and hate aggression (to the point that they may all but retreat from the world) and are themselves aggressive in their mannerisms and behaviors. This ongoing issue of fight-or-flight can tear them apart—right down the middle, apparently, as their many aches and pains tend to cluster on the right side of their bodies. Therefore, in the many different remedies that make up the Magnesia family, there are many different shades of aggression and many different aspects of pain. These are our remedies for those who suffer from pain. These are remedies that relate to patients who are always chilly, who actively seek warmth. Who actively seek peace in the same way, on the emotional level. Those belonging to this cluster of remedies are in an ongoing battle with pain—mental, emotional, and physical pain. These are patients whose pains shift, evolve, but never leave. These are erratic, sensitive types who dedicate themselves not only to solving their own issues with pain, but the world's as well. They are sensitive to the issue of pain—their own, their neighbor's, their world's. Where other remedy groups relate to those who turn inward (Calcarea, Fluorica, and to some extent, Natrum and Muriaticum) and have little or no concern for others who suffer as well, the Magnesia family of remedies contains those who, in their pain, open their eyes to the pain of others and dedicate their lives to trying to solve the issue of pain on a universal level. The Magnesia type learns from his or her own suffering, grows from it, and at times can revel in his or her own pain and find deep meaning in it, if not deep satisfaction. Pain can come to define their lives in the short term, but in the long term, Magnesia types learn to find meaning in the pain that helps them find a greater meaning in life.

Magnesia types are chilly physically and rather warm and open emotionally. They are natural vegetarians in many cases, and dislike meat, either the smell of it or the cruelty of eating it. They like raw foods and dislike cooked things and, especially, fatty foods. They are allergic to dairy and should avoid it completely. They may have other allergies and sensitivities as well, because their systems are in the same state of fight-or-flight as the rest of them and therefore are very sensitive to any form of challenge. This is a remedy group in which asthma, especially allergic asthma, is very common. This is a group in which the symptoms shift from place to place, moment by moment. It is also a group in which symptoms recur periodically. In which patients have the same pain monthly, weekly, seasonally, annually. They are given to warts and tumors of all sorts, especially to malignant tumors.

Like the Ferrums, the Magnesias can become depleted rather easily, and like the Ferrums, they tend to become involved in political movements, charities, and political issues to which they dedicate much time and energy. Like the Ferrums, the Magnesias tend to mean it when they say that they will do it and to follow through on their promises (quite unlike the Fluoricas).

Cell salt belonging to this group:

• Magnesia Phosphorica

Other homeopathic remedies in this group include:

- Magnesia Bromatum
- Magnesia Carbonica
- Magnesia Fluorica

- Magnesia Iodatum
- Magnesia Muriatica
- Magnesia Sulphurica

The Phoshorus/Phosphoricum/Phosphorica Family

This group is one in which the emotional symptoms outweigh the physical when it comes to identifying a need for a specific remedy, and, most often, in terms of the patient's own experience of his life in general and his health specifically. Like the article in *The New York Times* some years ago about scientists who noticed that the particles that make up matter behave differently when they know they are being watched, the Phosphorus type will experience not only life in general, but also the specific symptoms of his disease, quite differently when he has other people near. When he is not only being watched, but being offered the lifeline of human contact. No other group of remedies has the need for human contact on so deep and profound a level as the Phosphorus group. And no other group has the sensitivity that the members of the Phosphorus group of remedies have, especially in terms of sensitivity to other living things—to people, to animals, to all that are in their immediate environment. Where Magnesia types will feel the pain of the whole world, Phosphorus types will tend to feel the pain of those with whom they are in contact. This is perhaps because Magnesia types exist on the frequency level of pain, while Phosphorus types exist on the frequency level of connection. They are masters of doing in reality what the Fluorides can only feign—being completely open emotionally and completely vulnerable in their state of openness.

If anything, Phosphorus types have difficulty learning to build walls and create boundaries. They tend, particularly when they are ill, to not understand that appropriate boundaries actually exist and need to be honored. At times, Phosphorus types can seem as if they are clouds: that they exist without a solid form, that they can surround, choke, and envelop everything around them.

In terms of the cell salts, this group is most represented. With the sole exception of the remedy Phosphorus itself, all of the remedies that are created in combination with the substance phosphorus are included in this group. And as the remedy Phosphorus represents such a sensitive and open state of being, the substance phosphorus seems to stand back from and enhance the attributes of others that are added to it rather than blunt them as some other substances (Natrum and Kali in particular) tend to do. Therefore, the sensitivity and emotional availability of the Phosphorus type gets played out very differently in the different phosphorus-based compounds.

Natrum Phosphoricum, for instance, takes the natural openness of phosphorus and shuts it down within the engine of retention and denial that is Natrum Muriaticum.

The result is that the Natrum Phosphoricum yearns for emotional connection but retreats from it, with no small internal conflict. The result is a secretive, mysterious person, one that others often mistrust, simply because he or she does not seem to be authentic or forthcoming. These are patients who are often underestimated or unfairly judged by others.

The Calcarea Phosphorica has a hard task in blending Phosphorus' natural openness with Calcarea's tendency toward low self-esteem. The result is a needy person, a clingy person who tends to place his or her need for recognition and approval above personal dignity or independence. This makes for a patient who can be somewhat suffocative of others, who fears changes, especially changes in relationships, above all else.

The Magnesia Phosphorica walks an even more problematic path in life. Magnesia offers a mindset in which pain is the connector to the world, the means by which the world can be understood. Phosphorus offers an innate tendency to connect with others at all costs and a desire to reach out (which can manifest in constant motion and travel, coupled with a sense of rootlessness and a deep feeling of being constantly homesick), even to overwhelm others with contact. The result is a patient who is so sensitive on both the emotional and physical level that they have to be careful every moment of their lives, careful where they step, both physically and emotionally. The Mag Phos type can be an emotional roller coaster: open, honest, and level-headed one moment and a bipolar agent of chaos the next. Note that Mag Phos types, perhaps more than any other type, can become fixated on the notion of home and what home means in terms of joy and connection. Calcareas tend to fixate on what home can mean in terms of security. They will feel lonely, even in a crowded room, if they do not find the "other" with whom they can connect emotionally. In physical pain, they tend to become vibrantly sensitive to the touch they so desperately desire, and to move into an emotional state of "Nobody understands me," or "Nobody knows the trouble I've seen."

Kali Phosphoricum, for me at least, is the most interesting type, as it is a blend of Kali, which is all about discipline and duty, and Phosphorus, whose whole message is one of connection and relationship. This makes the Kali Phos a patient who is as obsessed about relationships, about making the connection, as any other Phosphorus type, but who finds the whole process rather wearying, rather depressing. This is a type who goes through the motions of availability and openness common to the Phosphorus type, but who finds no real joy in them.

Ferrum Phosphoricum blends the iron will of Ferrum with the need for communication that is native to phosphorus and produces a patient who demands attention. Who kicks, screams and turns bright red in the face to get your attention. These patients will not stop until they have the attention they crave.

The core remedy of this group, Phosphorus, displays the traits that will be parceled out in various combinations as it is blended with other minerals in the creation of individual cell salts. Phosphorus is the remedy type that exists for the purpose of emotional connection. It is also the remedy of hemorrhages, of bright-red blood—that symptom will run through all the phosphorus-based remedies. Here again, Ferrum Phos is a good example, as it blends the blood issues of iron and phosphorus. The result is a patient who has the flush and congestion of Ferrum combined with the tendency toward hemorrhages with bright-red blood common to Phosphorus. (Phosphorus was even used in homeopathic hospitals as a remedy after surgery to stop bleeding. A keynote symptom of the type is the tendency to bleed a great deal from even a small cut, and for that blood to be bright red.)

Other common physical symptoms include a sensation of burning accompanying all pains, and a frequent feeling of chill accompanying the burning pain. (Sulphur will often be both hot and burning, while Phosphorus can feel either heat or chill, or a combination of both, while having burning pains.) There is a quality of suddenness and unpredictability and a sensation of heat in the symptoms associated with Phosphorus. Even if the patient is quite chilly, they will experience a flow of heat along with the burning in the affected parts.

Sensitivity, emotional availability, hemorrhages, shifting and/or erratic pains, the need for attention and that bright-red blood—these are the keynotes of Phosphorus.

Cell salts belonging to this group:

- Calcarea Phosphorica
- Ferrum Phosphoricum
- Kali Phosphoricum
- Magnesia Phosphorica
- Natrum Phosphoricum

Other homeopathic remedy in this group:
- Phosphorus

The Potassium/Kali Family

This is one of our largest groups of remedies, with twenty remedies listed in the homeopathic materia medica. This is also the most diverse group, which may reflect the ubiquity of the source material potassium or its ability to work in combination with a great number of other materials in the formation of homeopathic remedies. Either way, the Kali group, while the largest, is used much less often than the other groups (notably the Natrum group, the Sulphur group and, particularly, the Phosphorus group) and quite possibly goes underused.

On an emotional level, those belonging to this group may be considered, in turn, fussy, crabby, old-fashioned, duty-bound, dull, stupid, and, surprisingly, rash and impulsive at odd moments in their lives. Kalis are rather plodding types, both emotionally and physically. It can be said that they sleepwalk through life, a fact that is only underscored by their tendency toward chronic insomnia and unrefreshing sleep. They yearn for a good night's sleep like others yearn for money or fame. They walk through life exhausted, wanting a nap.

Like Ferrum types, Kali types are dedicated to getting the job done. But they lack the fireworks of Ferrum types, the tendency toward flashes of anger and the appeal of high drama. Instead, they get to their goal step by unremitting step. They may feel no joy in the work or even in its completion, but they finish the job just the same. The journey they begin is one that they end. Kalis go home with the dates that they brought to the dance.

In moments, however, they yield to impulses, often to violent impulses. These are the bank tellers who rob the bank in a moment of madness. About whom, after the patient suddenly kills his wife, the neighbors all say, "But he always seemed so nice and so quiet." Kalis simmer a long, long time, plodding through and doing their duty, but sometimes they break and act on impulse, almost always with a bad result.

When Ralph Waldo Emerson wrote that "most men live lives of quiet desperation," he was writing about the Kalis of the world. And note that his use of the word "most" indicates the numbers of the type in terms of the world's population.

Physically, they are given to chronic illnesses of all sorts. To rheumatism and arthritis and headaches and PMS. To diseases that involve twitches in the muscles and muscular weakness. They have droopy eyelids, droopy stomachs, flabby arms and legs.

Kali types tend to experience anxiety in their minds and bodies. They suffer from neuralgias, from gout, from pains that involve the sensation of cutting, tearing, or stitching. They have pains that shift from place to place in the body, especially in their joints, without ever ceasing.

Like Calcareas, Kalis tend to be both chilly and sweaty. They sweat all over their bodies (unlike the head and foot sweats that are more common to the Calcarea Carbonica and Silicea types). They are extremely sensitive to cold in any form, especially to drafts.

Kali types have a great hunger and must eat on time. They have a fear of poverty and starvation and demand to be fed. They feel better in every way from eating and especially crave sweets and baked goods. They tend to belch after eating and to feel bloated. However, they tend to like the sensation of bloat, or at least prefer it to the empty sensation in their stomachs that drives them to eat in the first place. Even those Kalis who become quite uncomfortable after eating still generally improve from the act of eating and are happy they did it.

Again like Calcarea, the ailments associated with Kali are most often functional as opposed to pathological. They are slow in coming on and slow and stubborn in going away again. This is a group of remedies for those who are given to chronic complaints and who can prove difficult to cure, partially because of the nature of the illnesses themselves, and partially because the stubborn Kali will often refuse to make any adjustments to his or her diet or lifestyle that could enhance their ability to heal.

Cell salts belonging to this group:

- Kali Muriaticum
- Kali Phosphoricum

- Kali Sulphuricum

Other homeopathic remedies in this group include:

- Kali Aceticum
- Kali Arsenicosum
- Kali Bichromicum
- Kali Bromatum
- Kali Carbonicum
- Kali Chloricum
- Kali Citricum
- Kali Cyanatum
- Kali Ferrocyanatum

- Kali Hypophosphoricum
- Kali Iodatum
- Kali Nitricum
- Kali Oxalicum
- Kali Permanganicum
- Kali Silicicum
- Kali Tartaricum
- Kali Telluricum

The Sodium/Natrum Family

Just as sodium rivals potassium in its importance to the human body and the amount present in the body at all times, the group of remedies built upon sodium rivals the Kalis both in number of remedies and their importance in the homeopathic pharmacy. In fact, the Natrums may be more important as a group than the Kalis, and no single Kali remedy has achieved the importance within the homeopathic materia medica that Natrum Muriaticum has. Indeed, few remedies (Sulphur, Phosphorus, and Silicea among them) rival Natrum Mur when it comes to the sheer sweep of their effectiveness, and no other remedy comes close to Natrum Muriaticum when it comes to the number of patients worldwide that would benefit from its use. Suffice it to say that the Natrums are not only a large group of remedies, but are an important one as well.

Like Silicea, the Natrums act upon digestion and nutrition and are the remedies of pale people. Emotionally, they tend toward depression, even long-term clinical depression. They tend toward sorrow, usually a quiet sorrow or grief that goes unexplored and unexpressed. Natrums do not like to show their emotional hands and instead prefer to wear poker faces. (This can be problematic for those living with this type, as they are expected to know when the Natrum is upset and when he or she is not, while the Natrum displays the same emotionally blank face throughout.) They tend to be rather negative and are utterly pessimistic as they look forward to the future. In fact, Natrums tend to live both in the past (holding on to old hurts and grudges) and in the future (looking ahead to a bleak outcome)—so much so that they often miss what is happening in the present moment.

Although sensitive, perhaps even as sensitive in their way as Phosphorus, Natrums tend to be very closed emotionally and prefer to be left alone, particularly when they are suffering. As Phosphorus reaches out when in pain, Natrums retreat, rejecting attempts to comfort or to tend.

They are sensitive people—physically sensitive to their environment and emotionally sensitive to it as well. They are sensitive to light, especially to glare (they cannot bear bright lights or glare or direct sunlight), and to noise. They are sensitive to music in particular and will respond strongly to it, either with great pleasure or great upset. They cannot bear loud or grating sounds, but have a great love for music that they like, especially for the music of their youth. Natrums are highly nostalgic, although they may not show or admit it.

Natrums tend to be intelligent and tend to have strong powers of concentration. They tend to be detail-oriented and have a tendency toward nearsightedness.

They are often rather chilly people, although they may be warm-blooded as well, but, either way, they cannot abide warmth and cannot stand direct heat, especially the heat of the sun. They prefer cool things, cool air, cool liquids.

Because sodium causes retention, Natrum types can be chronically bloated, and will always feel better after any discharge: better from sweat, from tears, from mucous discharge. They are even better from vomiting or diarrhea. They tend to have chronic toxicity that is a part of their tendency toward retention. They do not sweat enough to remove toxins from their body. In the same way, they can be chronically constipated and given to chronic allergies of all sorts.

In the remedy Natrum Fluoratum, the combination of remedies plays out in a patient who has muscular pains that feel as if he or she has literally been punched. This results in a patient who literally loses the power of speech when in pain.

In Natrum Carbonicum, one of our important homeopathic remedies, sodium combines with carbon to give us a patient in whom all the weaknesses of Natrum are enhanced—a patient who bears permanent effects from sunstroke, a patient with ankles that are so weak he cannot walk at all, a patient who is so sensitive to music that he cannot bear it at all, to the point that he quakes and shakes when hearing a piano, even when it is soothing and beautiful.

Such is the sensitivity of the Natrum type. Often, because they will refuse to show their emotions, they will instead embody them in shaking, quaking, and general weakness. This is a remedy group filled with emotional exhaustion that, over time, translates into physical exhaustion. This is the remedy group of chronic fatigue.

Cell salts belonging to this group:

- Natrum Muriaticum
- Natrum Phosphoricum
- Natrum Sulphuricum

Other homeopathic remedies in this group include:

- Natrum Arsencosinum
- Natrum Cacodylicum
- Natrum Carbonicum
- Natrum Fluoratum
- Natrum Hypochlorosum
- Natrum Iodatum
- Natrum Lacticum
- Natrum Nitricum
- Natrum Nitrosum
- Natrum Salicylicum
- Natrum Selenicum
- Natrum Silicofluoricum
- Natrum Sulphurosum

The Sulfur/Sulphurica/Sulphuricum Family

Sulphur always adds heat, confusion, and a certain excitement as well, to the mix. There is a certain joy that comes with Sulphur, a certain unwillingness to face the reality at hand, no matter how cruel it may be. For this reason, those remedies associated with Sulphur may be said to share the trait of apparently refusing to accept their fate, they may seem to be unwilling to take things seriously. Or they may be unwilling to give the bearer of bad news the full attention that he or she may feel is deserved.

This lack of attention to the reality in front of them is keynote to the Sulphur remedies. They may embody it in the look of boredom you will find on the face of a teenage male, or they may embody it in full-fledged delusions, in which they remove themselves as far from reality as possible.

Either way, the Sulphur imagination tends to work overtime. They may be naturally intelligent types, or inclined toward creative things, or as dumb as a stick, but they are creatures of vast imagination who will escape into their world of imagination more and more completely when they are physically, emotionally, or mentally stressed.

Sulphur types tend to live and work in their own personal time zones and may run chronically late, or come early, or not at all. They tend to be rather sloppy, both in their appearance and in their behavior. They tend not to work out of the same playbook as others. They may be con artists, jerks, and heels, but they are always authentic in a way that the Fluorica is not capable of being. They do not hide their flaws or tricks, but, instead, revel in them. Sulphurs have an innate joy of life that can make them feel invulnerable to harm (which is often the source of their boredom with the reality of life or their illness) and that can make them feel as if the rules that apply to others simply do not apply to them.

Physically they have a tendency toward sweat, toward itch and toward functional disorders. Sulphur is one of the most important building blocks of life. The remedies based upon it are used in all aspects of health and healing and are key players for both acute and chronic conditions. These are important, often-used remedies. They are among our most prescribed remedies (with the exception of Magnesia Sulphurica, which, in my opinion, is greatly underutilized).

Sulphur itself is a remedy that is given when indicated remedies fail to act. It jump-starts the body's ability to heal and awakens the sluggish immune system. In the same way, it awakens the "sleeping" patient who has become sluggish from age, from pain, or from chronic disease. It restores the joy of living. It also is a great remedy for clearing away ailments of very long standing. Often it will not heal the condition in and of itself, but will, instead, begin the process. As I put it, it lights the fuse.

When coupled with a stabilizing influence like Natrum, Sulphur becomes a remedy for deep chronic complaints, for issues like head injuries that have changed the persona of the patient. It restores that which time and injury have worn down and worn away and returns the patient to himself, as if he had been sleeping for a long, long time.

When coupled with magnesium, the result is Magnesia Sulphurica (from Epsom salts), an excellent remedy for females with chronic dysmenorrhea, especially when it is accompanied by migraines. It is similar to Magnesia Phosphorica, in Magnesia's shooting pains and nervous conditions, but it replaces Phosphorus' overall sensitivity and instability with a sense of heat. The Mag Phos pain requires heat, while the Mag Sulph pain cannot bear heat and is only soothed by cold water. It is an excellent alternative to Mag Phos for patients who share that remedy's aches and pains, but who cannot bear heat in any form.

Cell salts belonging to this group

- Calcarea Sulphurica
- Kali Sulphuricum

- Natrum Sulphuricum

Other homeopathic remedies in this group:

- Magnesium Sulphuricum
- Sulphur

CHAPTER FIVE

The Twelve Cell Salt Remedies

In this chapter, I present a simple materia medica of the twelve cell salts. In all cases, the listing begins with an overview of the remedy, its source material, and the process by which it is potentized. This overview gives the essence of the remedy's actions and the symptoms most indicative of the need for the remedy. Next comes a listing of the clinical conditions that most often suggest the need for the remedy.

The mental and emotional symptoms likely to be found in the patient needing the given remedy is then covered. As a group of remedies, the cell salts are most often thought of in terms of physical ailments, but an understanding of the mental and emotional symptoms and the remedies they point to can be vital when selecting an appropriate remedy. Admittedly, these symptoms are often less helpful than the physical symptoms in remedy selection (with the sole exception of Kali Phosphoricum, which is more often selected on the basis of emotional symptoms than anything else). But in that the cell salts represent an offshoot of homeopathy, it is important that the whole of the patient's being—body, mind, and spirit—be taken into account in the process of remedy selection, even if the physical complaints are largely emphasized throughout the process. Therefore, it is important that the emotional and mental state of the patient be taken into account, as the patient who has injured himself and is angry about it is quite likely to need a different remedy than the patient with the same injury who is crying and wants to be comforted.

> It is important that the whole of the patient's being—body, mind, and spirit—be taken into account in the process of remedy selection, even if the physical complaints are largely emphasized throughout the process.

This section is followed by descriptions of the physical symptoms. In all these listings, I begin with the cluster of physical complaints and specific symptoms that most clearly suggest the need for a given remedy. What inflammation is to Ferrum Phosphoricum, cramping pains are to Magnesia Phosphorica—a guiding symptom that indicates the remedy so clearly that it will send your hand moving toward it on the shelf. These are the symptoms that most need to be mastered if one is to learn how to quickly and easily choose the most effective remedy in any given situation.

Next comes an important part of case taking—modalities. Modalities are those behaviors or actions that make a specific symptom or set of symptoms feel better or worse. The pain in the back that is better from simple, slow motion suggests a different remedy than the pain that is better from lying still, just as the pain that is better from applications of heat suggests a very different remedy than the one suggested by improvement from cold applications. Truly understanding modalities means understanding the remedies and understanding how and when to use them.

It is also important to understand the relationships between the cells salts: which ones work well with others in a given situation, and which should not be used either in alternation or combination with a remedy already in use. Individuals will work with the cell salts differently. Some combine two, three, or more at any given time, while others use them singly whenever possible and only use more than one in alternation, placing doses of each individual remedy hours apart. I will discuss the concepts that guide the use of the remedies at some length later in these pages, but it is important to understand the relationships between the remedies that guide their use, because most cases will ultimately involve the use of more than one remedy.

Each cell salt listing closes with a look at potency and dosage. Most of the cell salts are most commonly given in the 6X potency. In some cases, especially in the case of rashes or other skin conditions, lower potencies (3X and under) may be suggested to keep the condition from spreading while it clears. For other cases, especially cases in which emotional symptoms dominate, higher potencies of 9X or 12X may be called for. Every cell salt may be used in any available potency. However, you will learn to use the cell salts most effectively if you learn to match the potency of the remedy to the situation at hand.

The same goes for learning about dosing; learning just how often to use a remedy and when to repeat it and when not to repeat it. Again, this will be dealt with at greater length later in these pages, but each individual listing will give information on how well a remedy works in repetition and how best to figure its appropriate dosage.

A BRIEF MATERIA MEDICA OF THE CELL SALTS

1. CALCAREA FLUORICA

Overview

Calcium fluoride is the chemical compound from which the remedy Calcarea Fluorica is taken. It has a formula of CaF_2. It occurs in nature in the crystalline mineral fluorspar. As it is insoluble in water, the remedy is made through the process of trituration.*

Calcarea Fluorica was first proved as a homeopathic remedy in 1874 by homeopath J.B. Bell, although most of what is known of the remedy and its actions has been taken from Schuessler. In fact, this remedy, although it had become a part of the homeopathic pharmacy after Bell's proving, went almost totally unused until Schuessler included it among his cell salt remedies.

This remedy has a wide range of uses and is unique among the cell salts in two ways. It is an excellent remedy for long-lasting complaints of a chronic nature, especially those, like lumbago and joint pain—especially hip pain—that are seemingly without cause. There is a certain vagueness, even sluggishness, to the ailments that Calcarea Fluorica mends. In the same way, this is an excellent remedy to consider for vague emotional conditions. For mild anxiety and nagging fears, especially fears about money, and about day-to-day things, including the state of one's health. This central issue of vagueness carries over to the patient as a whole. The typical Calcarea Fluorica type is sluggish, has a tendency toward weakness, and a desire to rest. Ironically the aches and pains associated with this remedy are almost universally *worse* for rest, forcing the patient, who wishes to slump on the couch, to get up and keep moving instead.

Perhaps it could be said that this vagueness is carried over to the remedy itself, because Calcarea Fluorica is a cell salt that usually will not work well enough on its own to completely clear a condition, particularly a chronic condition. It works well in concert with other cell salts, particularly with Silicea, with whom it shares both physical and emotional traits, as well as with Calcarea Phosphorica and Natrum Muriaticum.

As Schuessler called Calcarea Fluorica his "bone salt," and as calcium fluoride naturally occurs in tooth enamel, on the surface of bones, and in the skin and blood vessels, it should come as no surprise that the primary use of the salt is in treating conditions of the bones and teeth, and that it also has value in treating those with diseases of the skin and/or blood vessels.

---

* See Chapter Three for information on trituration and the process of potentization for homeopathic remedies.

Conditions that Suggest Calcarea Fluorica

Aneurisms; bone disease and bone pain; cataracts; cold sores; colds, coughs,and espe-cially postnasal drip; flatulence; gout; hardening (induration) of tissue, especially breasts and glands; herpes; hemorrhoids; Hodgkin's disease; joint disease, especially hip disease; liver disease; lumbago; nodes in any part of the body; strains; varicose veins; wrinkles.

Mental and Emotional Symptoms

The Calcarea Fluorica patient typically blends a sense of free-form anxiety with a sense of indecision. The result is that the patient will be somewhat sluggish mentally and emotionally and will often tend to rather fixate on a specific fear—poverty, for instance, even if such a fear is baseless; hypochondria being most common—rather than focus on any given situation at hand. Depressions great and small. The Calcarea Fluorica patient can be very negative, predisposed to believe the worst in any given sit-uation. Calcarea Fluoricas tend to look on the dark side of life.

The Calcarea Fluorica patient is known to have great trouble in communicating his or her ideas to others. He is forgetful, and can often forget what he is saying while still mid-sentence. He will misplace his words in speaking or writing them, switch them around, render-ing communication ineffective.

Calcarea Fluorica patients can appear to be less intelligent than they are, due to their lack of clear ver-bal communication and also to a certain dullness that settles upon them, mentally, emotionally, and physi-cally. They are indecisive, unsure of how to proceed.

Calcarea Fluorica patients can be difficult to treat because their tendency toward vagueness and sluggish-ness makes them something like "dead weight" in the doctor's office. While they do not actively resist treat-ment, they tend to be passively aggressive in their unwillingness to do anything that might help them to break out of their pattern of chronic illness.

> Calcarea Fluorica patients can appear to be less intelligent than they are, due to their lack of clear verbal communication and also to a certain dullness that settles upon them, mentally, emotionally, and physically. They are indecisive, unsure of how to proceed.

And as this is a remedy given more for chronic than for acute ailments, those need-ing it often feel at the mercy of their disease symptoms. They may feel anxious when speaking about or thinking about their illness, or they may display a remarkable apathy concerning their own state of health. Either way, the patient's emotional state will often present itself as a block against treatment, especially when it is presented in the form of a patient who has become weary of life itself.

Physical Symptoms

The same sense of sluggishness and vagueness will be played out in the Calcarea Fluorica's physical complaints as well.

For instance, soft tissues throughout the body will tend toward a lack of elasticity, mirroring the patient's emotional sluggishness. This stands to reason, as calcium fluoride is a chief component of all the elastic soft tissue in the body. Therefore look for complaints that are based in a *lack* of elasticity, in a sluggish response on the part of soft tissue. Fibers are relaxed instead of being supple. This leads to conditions like hemorrhoids and varicose veins, both of which are a direct result of normally elastic tissues becoming lax. Muscles atrophy. Connective tissue fails to support joints. Blood vessels lose their natural elasticity, increasing the risk of aneurism.

Along with these issues, the homeopaths of ages past also note what they call "malnutrition of the bones." Since calcium fluoride is a component of the outer part of the bone and of the teeth, those needing this remedy commonly experience maladies such as sensitive teeth, an uncommonly large number of cavities in their teeth, and weak bones and joints, especially the hip and knee joints. Poor ossification is an indication of the need for this remedy.

The need for Calcarea Fluorica can be linked to a generally poor diet, especially one lacking in calcium. Calc Fluor patients are often overweight. And Calcarea Fluorica is considered to be one of the cell salts that can be used to help patients in need of losing weight, especially those patients whose weight gain was caused by a diet of processed foods and/or foods low in fiber. With weight loss, as with many other conditions, Calc Fluor works best in alternation with other remedies. For weight loss, consider alternating Calcarea Fluorica with Calcarea Phosphorica to achieve better results. (Natrum Phosphoricum is also considered very helpful for weight loss, but is best and most effective for this purpose when used along with Natrum Sulphuricum.) For best results, take Calcarea Fluorica one hour before eating and follow with the Calcarea Phosphorica one hour after the meal.

Overweight patients needing Calc Fluor will often display what it called a "hanging belly," in that the elasticity of their abdominal wall has relaxed and all muscle tone is diminished. These same patients will also exhibit chronic lower back pain, as their abdominal muscles will fail to help support their body weight, putting undue stress on their lower backs. Patients with chronic lumbago or lower back pain, who want nothing more than to lie down on a nice firm mattress as a result of their pain, often respond very well to Calcarea Fluorica given in alternation with the cell salt Natrum Muriaticum, each given two or three times a day in chronic cases, more often in acute cases involving severe pain. Once the pain begins to improve, lessen the dosage to twice a day in alternation (two or three hours apart) until symptoms clear.

The overweight, rather sluggish Calc Fluor patient will also likely suffer from hemorrhoids and/or constipation. In patients suffering from hemorrhoids, Calcarea Fluorica is often enough to bring relief.* (If the hemorrhoids are bleeding, consider alternating Ferrum Phosphoricum with the Calc Fluor. If they are especially irritated or burning, alternate the remedy Kali Sulphurium with the Calc Fluor.) Patients whose symptoms combine constipation with hemorrhoids often find relief in alternating between Calcarea Fluorica and Kali Muriaticum. Taken in alternation, each two to three times a day over a period of days or even weeks, these two remedies will bring relief.

Another aspect of the Calcarea Fluorica picture is linked to diet. Many patients move into the chronic Calc Fluor state by way of a poor diet and lack of exercise, and many of these patients have chronic nasal allergy symptoms, especially postnasal drip, as a result of eating processed foods. As the patient eats foods in an "unnatural" processed form, he or she develops more and more of an allergic reaction to them, often in the form of what seems to be a mild, ongoing cold in the head. The patient may develop an almost constant draining of mucus down the back or his or her throat, or may experience an almost constant mild cough.

A change in diet is, of course, indicated in cases such as these. No pill, homeopathic or not, can be used to substitute for common sense or healthy lifestyle choices. But Calcarea Fluorica can help jumpstart patients on the road back to health by recharging their batteries and giving them the impetus they need to make necessary changes.

It is keynote of the Calcarea Fluorica, by the way, that their mucous discharges have a peculiar and unpleasant smell. The condition, referred to in homeopathic literature as *ozaena*, refers to the fetid smell that comes from such a discharge in cases of chronic nasal drainage.

Calc Fluor types can be rather smelly all the way around. They are flatulent, and smelly. They tend to be belchy and hiccuppy, and smelly. They also tend toward decayed teeth and rather smelly breath (for which the term *ozostomia* is used in classic homeopathic texts). In any cases involving infection, the pus or discharge will also be smelly.

Calc Fluors also tend toward skin symptoms that can be attributed to a lack of elasticity. Cases involving chapped or cracked skin or brittle fingernails suggest Calcarea Fluorica, as do any conditions that involve the thickening or hardening of the skin. Consider Calcarea Fluorica for patients with skin conditions such as scar tissue that has hardened. Also consider it for those with warty growths on the skin, and for cases of ulcers of the skin where the edges of the ulcer are raised and hard. This remedy is also said to be helpful in clearing away birthmarks of all sorts.

---

* Let me note that topical applications of Calcarea Fluorica can be helpful in cases of hemorrhoids. Just dissolve two or three pellets of the remedy in warm water, dip cotton into the water, and apply directly to the hemorrhoids.

It is an important—perhaps the outstanding—use of this remedy that it works effectively against hard swelling of the skin in nearly every part of the body. An example of this is that Calcarea Fluorica is an important remedy in cases of gout that have advanced to the point that hard nodes of uric acid crystals, called *tophi*, have begun to form, particularly if they form on the joints of the patient's fingers or toes. In the same way, Calc Fluor is the chief cell salt to remember for patients with *whitlows*, also called *felons*, which are small, hard inflammations around the area of the fingernail. (A more general term *panaritium* is used to describe any inflammation of finger or toe in the general area of the hard tissue—the nail or bone itself.) No matter what it is called, Calcarea Fluorica is the remedy of choice for these small, hard, painful eruptions.

Any gland in the body that is swollen, and hardened by that swelling, suggests a need for Calcarea Fluorica. It has been given for cases of lumps in breasts, hard knots, or nodes. For any case involving hard swelling of the jawbones, including hard swelling of the cheek as a result of tooth decay. For cases of goiter, in which the gland is hard and swollen. Also consider this remedy for cases of hard swelling of any tissue surrounding joints anywhere in the body. This is, therefore, one of the most helpful remedies for those who suffer from bursitis. It is also the chief remedy for those who suffer from ganglion cysts, especially on the back of the hand or on the wrist.*

Perhaps one of the most invaluable uses of the remedy Calcarea Fluorica is its ability to slow the progression of, or, in some cases, reverse the appearance of cataracts in the eye. This is especially the case for senile cataracts that appear as the patient ages and the lens of the eye stiffens and thickens. In cases of cataract, Calcarea Fluorica is often given in alternation with Silicea in order to reabsorb the opaque areas and restore elasticity to the lens.

Modalities

In general, the symptoms associated with the need for Calcarea Fluorica will be made better by heat and by warm applications to the painful area. Symptoms are also improved by rubbing, and a combination of rubbing and heat will often bring temporary relief. The patient will feel better from drinking warm drinks as well.

The patient will tend to feel better from motion as well, especially from gentle, prolonged motion. The patient will, however, feel worse on first moving—indeed, the first motion may bring a good deal of pain—but as the affected area begins to stretch

---

* Ganglion cysts, a relatively harmless although sometimes painful condition, are also known as "Bible cysts," because the chief home remedy for them has historically been to take a large, heavy book, like a Bible, and smash the cyst until it goes away. Most doctors suggest lancing or even surgically removing the cyst instead.

and warm through motion, relief will result. Pain will return and increase, however, if the affected area is moved too much or too roughly.

The patient will be worse from resting, although he may desire nothing more than to simply lie down. His pain, however, will drive him to move and continually change position when he does attempt to rest.

Calcarea Fluorica patients are highly responsive to changes in weather. They are better in warm, dry weather and much worse in damp weather and during changes from dry to wet.

Relationships

Calcarea Fluorica works best when it is used in alternation with other cell salt remedies. It is perhaps most similar to Silicea in its actions (its action is, after all, to the body's elastic tissues what Silicea's is to the body's connective tissues). They follow each other well and complete each other's actions. Most often, however, particularly in cases of inflammation and the formation of pus, Calcarea Fluorica is given after Silicea to complete the cure.

Calcarea Fluorica is highly compatible with Natrum Muriaticum, Calcarea Phosphorica, and Calcarea Sulphurica, and may be used in alternation with any of these—and with Silicea—for any case in which either of the remedies alone fail to bring about the desired results.

Dosage and Potency

Schuessler most often gave Calcarea Fluorica in 12X potency, although he considered the 3X and 6X to be very effective as well. For cases involving hard growths of any sort, the higher potency should be used. Note that Calcarea Fluorica is also very effective when it is used topically. Two to three pellets of the remedy may be dissolved in water and then applied to the affected area with cotton balls or a clean cloth. As the Calc Fluor patient is often improved by warm applications, the pellets can be dissolved in warm water and liberally applied to the affected area.

Calcarea Fluorica is more often used in chronic conditions and given as a long-term remedy than used in the acute sphere. It may be given in the same manner as other cell salts, with adults taking the remedy two or three times a day and children and seniors usually only twice a day. As always with any form of homeopathic remedy, the doses should be cut back as improvement begins.

Note that, although this remedy can be repeated as needed, it is important to have some patience when using this remedy. Calcarea Fluorica is a cell salt that is fairly slow to work, and it is a rather deep-acting remedy as well. Those giving or taking this remedy would do well to be sure they have given it a chance to work before they give another dose, or switch to—or alternate with—another remedy.

2. CALCAREA PHOSPHORICA

Overview

Calcium phosphate naturally occurs in the human body in the blood plasma and corpuscles, in the teeth and bones, in connective tissue, and in the gastric juices and saliva. It promotes cell growth in both hard and soft tissues and encourages the growth of new blood cells (which makes the remedy Calcarea Phosphorica one of the most important for patients who suffer from anemia) and promotes proper coagulation of the blood. It has a chemical formula of $Ca_3(PO_4)_2$.

The remedy Calcarea Phosphorica was created by Constantine Hering (1800–1880), one of the giants of homeopathic medicine, who was called "The Father of Homeopathy in the United States of America." Hering prepared the chemical compound from which the remedy was made by dropping a controlled amount of diluted phosphoric acid into so-called "lime water" (a highly saturated calcium hydroxide solution that is also called "lime milk") until a white precipitate formed. This precipitated phosphate of calcium was soluble in neither water nor alcohol, so the remedy was created through the process of trituration.

Calcarea Phosphorica is something of a general tonic among the cells salts. It is of particular use among the very young and the very old. In young patients, it ensures the growth of healthy bones and teeth and can be of particular importance in times of rapid growth. In the elderly it again acts as a tonic, especially of the nervous system, and is important in aiding elderly patients during recovery from severe ailments. Calc Phos is also an important tonic for patients who are suffering from any form of wasting disease (most especially those involving the particular symptom of night sweats), or who are in a state of prolonged weakness. It is the first cell salt remedy to think of in cases of anemia. It can be used to assist any patient during the time of recovery from illness or surgery or act as a boost for any patient who feels run down. It is helpful for patients who, in their acute or chronic weakened state, are susceptible to any illnesses that are making the rounds. For children who catch every cold that is being passed around the classroom. For adults who seem prone to illness and slow to recover.

> Calcarea Phosphorica is something of a general tonic among the cells salts. It is of particular use among the very young and the very old. In young patients, it ensures the growth of healthy bones and teeth and can be of particular importance in times of rapid growth. In the elderly it again acts as a tonic, especially of the nervous system, and is important in aiding elderly patients during recovery from severe ailments.

hosphorica can be used in tandem with any other cell salt remedy. ⌐ne practitioners believe that Calc Phos actually will strengthen the activity ⌐very other cell salt and that it should, therefore, be included in the use of any or all of them for all purposes.

If there is one cell salt that is considered to be most general in its action and most beneficial to all patients, it is Calcarea Phosphorica.

Conditions that Suggest Calcarea Phosphorica

Anemia; bedwetting; bone pain; bones slow to grow, weak bones (Rickets); broken bones, fractures of all kinds; colds with sore throat; colic; diabetes; epilepsy; headaches; indigestion; irritable bowel syndrome; joint pain; lumbago, and weakness of the lower back; palpitation; rheumatism; teething delayed; tonsillitis; weakness with exhaustion, trembling and delayed recovery; weight gain and obesity.

Mental and Emotional Symptoms

The patient needing Calcarea Phosphorica displays a certain slowness, a kind of fog-giness. This is the most important cell salt remedy for children who are slow to learn or who display signs of learning disabilities. The remedy also keys to children who, in particular, have difficulties with reading comprehension or who get headaches from reading. When writing, young and old Calc Phos patients will tend to write words more than once, to scramble their order, or to write words other than those they meant to write.

Calc Phos patients, especially elderly patients, tend to have issues with short-term memory loss. They forget things that happened only minutes ago. Forget why they came into a room, what they are looking for, what they just said. They will tend to have clear long-term memory, however.

Calcarea Phosphorica patients tend to be deeply emotional types. They very much want to be left alone. They do not want to be questioned and can become quite angry if they feel challenged. They dread doing whatever they need to do—this, again, is particularly true in the very young and very old. Calcarea Phosphorica children will stubbornly refuse to do their schoolwork and elderly Calc Phos types will refuse to cooperate with those whose job it is to assist or support them.

It is an important keynote of the type that they tend to display a wish to run away. When away from home, they will say again and again they want to go home, but when they are home, they will just as adamantly insist they want to go somewhere else.

Along with Natrum Muriaticum, Calcarea Phosphorica is a remedy for those in grief and those who feel betrayed by a loss of love or a loved one. They tend to brood in their grief. They may also tend toward anxiety, especially anxiety attached to their fears about their health. Look for the Calc Phos' physical symptoms to grow worse when they think or talk about them. In many Calc Phos patients, emotional anxiety will manifest in palpitations. Again, like many Natrum Murs, Calcarea Phosphorica patients are given to sighing—if you pay attention, this single symptom will help guide you to this remedy when combined with other physical, emotional, and mental attributes.

Calcarea Phosphorica is as soothing a remedy for emotional complaints as it is a tonic for physical weakness. It is a remedy that can be used, like Bach's Rescue Remedy, to help patients cope with bad news or with the emotional ramifications of a loss of a loved one. Just as the homeopathic remedy Arnica jumpstarts healing on both the emotional and physical levels, Calcarea Phosphorica can stir a renewed vigor on both planes of being. It can be given to any patient who is in a state of emotional upset.

Physical Symptoms

This is the first cell salt remedy that should be considered for cases of young children who are slow in reaching their milestones in life. Particularly for infants whose fontanelles remain open for too long, are slow to teethe (for cases in which the child displays teething pains and is irritable, alternate Calcarea Phosphorica with Ferrum Phosphoricum and infant and parent alike will rest easier), are delayed in bone development and growth, or have soft or brittle bones. Consider Calcarea Phosphorica for infants who display signs of failure to thrive.

This is also a great remedy to have on hand for children who are given to swollen glands, especially to swollen tonsils, and to chronic sore throats.

The typical child needing Calc Phos is considered "sickly." He or she will likely be thin (playing off the Phosphorus component of the compound remedy, in that the other Calcarea-based remedies tend to be chubby) and delicate in appearance. They tend toward long, thin necks and underdeveloped chests. They are given to earaches and infections as well as to sore throats. They may have chronic middle ear infections and inflammations. The child will complain of a sensation that his ears are "stuffed up" and of aching or tearing pain in his ears. The child may also have difficulty hearing and there may be discharges of thick, dark wax from the ears that is often mixed with blood.

Discharges of blood can be common to the Calc Phos type. Children who would benefit from Calcarea Phosphorica often are given to nose bleeds of bright red blood. They will often have a slight discharge of blood along with mucus when they blow their noses.

The Calc Phos child may have breathing difficulties, mild asthma, a chronic cough that may bring up a mixture of mucus and blood. The child will clear his throat on an ongoing basis and may hack up the mucous discharge. The child will also tend to swallow a great deal, and his throat will be painful for dry swallowing or if he has not swallowed or spoken for period of time. Thus, he will keep swallowing to keep the pain of the sore throat under control. (This applies in both chronic and acute cases—remember this remedy for simple sore throats that are worse for empty swallowing and cause the patient to lose his or her voice, or feel increased pain on first speaking after a period of silence.) The lymph glands in the child's throat will commonly be chronically swollen and tender.

The Calc Phos child often will wet the bed as well. (This is also common in elderly patients who need Calcarea Phosphorica—indeed, many of the symptoms can apply to either end of the spectrum of the very young and the very old.) Even when awake, the patient will have a frequent urge to urinate and will urinate copious amounts.

The child who needs Calcarea Phosphorica will often crave cold things: cold water and soda and, especially, ice cream. But they will upset the child's stomach when he ingests them, and he may vomit them up again when they are warmed in his stomach. This is especially true of ice cream. The Calc Phos type tends to be very sensitive to dairy products and to sugar. The combination of the two in ice cream can lead to intense personality changes within minutes of ingestion. Again, this is a child who is sensitive, over-reactive to many things, and his or her diet must be watched closely.

Food allergies may make it seem as if this child constantly has a cold. He has a nasal voice, a frontal or sinus headache, and a more or less constant dripping from his nose of clear, thick drainage, which will often be mixed with blood. (In acute cases, consider this remedy for all colds in which the discharge from the nose is clear, thick, and mixed with blood.)

To sum up, the Calcarea Phosphorica child tends to be slow in developmental milestones and grows to become a sickly child with a slim and delicate physique, thin and/or brittle bones, and a sensitive or overly sensitive nature. The child will tend to have an inborn weakness in his ears and lungs, will tend to be prone to allergies and upper respiratory infections. Often, the child's ears will act as a barometer of his overall health. When the child's ears turn bright read, it can be a sign of an allergic response or the onset of a respiratory illness. This is often a child who presents a medical puzzle. His physical symptoms can be traced back to a calcium deficiency in his diet, but often he is quite unable to digest dairy products (lactose intolerance is a common feature of the type). Thus his diet is of extreme importance. And the remedy Calcarea Phosphorica can be a godsend to the parents of these children, as it will help them digest and utilize calcium, alleviating the allergy response and providing the mineral to child's teeth, bones, and vitality.

Many of these same conditions will be mirrored in the elder patient who needs Calcarea Phosphorica. Here, too, you will see the bedwetting, the oversensitivity to diet and the subsequent allergic response. You will also see the state of profound respiratory weakness that allows the patient to easily become ill with all the coughs, colds, and flu (influenza) that make the rounds, and for that patient to have a much more difficult time of recovery than he might otherwise have had.

As Calcarea Phosphorica is a great remedy for increasing the absorption and utilization of calcium, it is an excellent remedy for elderly patients who have weakened or brittle bones. Consider it for all patients who have received the diagnosis of osteoporosis. (Since this is a condition more common to women after menopause than it is to men of the same age, let me note here that Calcarea Phosphorica is also an important women's remedy, as we shall see.)

Calcarea Phosphorica is also an excellent remedy for joint pain and rheumatism that comes on with old age. The pain can be located in any joint or bone in the body. Joints feel stiff and painful. Numbness is a common feature as well, as is a sensation of coldness in the achy joints and bones. The pain is worse for any change in the weather. The patient will be, in general, worse in winter. (This again is true of both the young and the old Calcarea Phosphorica, as children needing this remedy will tend to go from one cold to another, as will the elderly, who will add general rheumatic pain to the mix.) The patient is worse from becoming cold or wet, and worse from having to climb stairs. The Calcarea Phosphorica patient's fingers are most likely to be painful, as are his or her hips, lower back, and buttocks. The patient's neck is another point of vulnerability and chronic neck pain and occipital pain are common to the type.

These are patients who tire easily when cold or in pain, who want to lie down and rest, and who are improved by resting, by covering up and getting warm. They feel drafts easily (especially on the back of their head and on their neck), feel worse from feeling them, and do their best to avoid them.

The combination of chill and pain is quite common to the Calcarea Phosphorica type, although it is not unique to it. But the Calc Phos patient can become chilly from being in pain or experience the onset of pain by becoming chilly. The two sensations are inextricably intertwined for the type.

As noted, Calcarea Phosphorica is something of a general tonic remedy. When it is given to aged patients, it can help lower the degree of their rheumatic pain and improve their vitality, their sensitivity to cold, and their tendency toward respiratory illness. It can help with such common ailments associated with age as eyestrain and headaches brought on by trying to read with presbyoptic eyes, as well as with bedwetting, general loss of urinary control, and pain in the region of the kidneys. With short-term memory loss, and the sense of crotchety irritability associated with old age. Further, it can be very helpful for cases of elderly patients who experience bouts of vertigo. To help offset the wear and tear of old age, Calcarea Phosphorica can be given as a nutritional supplement, two or three times a day, in the 3X potency, to increase vitality and decrease the aches and pains associated with old age.

Calcarea Phosphorica is an excellent remedy for many of the milestones of women's lives, from the onset of menstruation to pregnancy and menopause, and for many of the symptoms, osteoporosis included, that have their onset during the menopausal years.

Think of Calcarea Phosphorica for girls who are slow to mature and for whom the onset of menstruation is delayed, or when the menses are irregular, scanty, or come early, late, too often, or too seldom. This is an excellent remedy, especially when paired with Magnesia Phosphorica, for PMS (premenstrual syndrome).

Calcarea Phosphorica is also commonly used during pregnancy, especially in cases of women who have previously exhibited difficulty in carrying the fetus to term.

It is an invaluable remedy during menopause, as it will help the patient with the night sweats, hot flashes, emotional upset, and hormone imbalance associated with that milestone. Further, because it strengthens the overall system, particularly the hard tissue of the bones, and works to forestall bladder-control issues that may arise, it acts as a tonic to assist the patient in a smoother adjustment to the changes in her system.

Among the more general uses of the remedy is as a tonic for the digestive system. It can be very helpful to any patient who feels worse after eating, or whose other symptoms are made worse by eating. It can also be helpful to patients who, in addition to chronic indigestion, suffer from constipation and/or from hemorrhoids that bleed and itch. As Calcarea Phosphorica acts to increase the actions of the other cell salt remedies, patients with severe digestive disorders should alternate Calc Phos with other indicated remedies for complete relief.

In cases involving indigestion, Calcarea Phosphorica acts best when given an hour after eating. In cases of obesity, Calc Phos acts best in alternation with Calcarea Fluorica, with Calc Fluor given one hour before eating and Calc Phos given one hour after. This will not only decrease the appetite through the action of Calc Fluor, but will, through the use of Calc Phos, increase the digestion itself and the ability of the body to absorb nutrients from the food eaten.

Modalities

The modalities for Calcarea Phosphorica patients are pronounced. They are worse from changes in the weather and in temperature. They are worse in damp weather or from becoming wet. They are worse from becoming cold. They are especially worse if they are wet and cold at the same time.

Calcarea Phosphorica patients are worse in winter and better in summer. They are better from dry heat. They are worse from exposure to drafts, to cold air, especially cold, damp air, from snow, especially melting snow, and from any change in the weather, especially changes that stir up the east wind.

They are improved by lying down and resting. They are worse from motion, especially lifting or climbing. Their pain symptoms will become worse if they think about them or talk about them. They are worse from reading, from concentrating, from working, and better from resting.

They crave cold things to eat and drink—ice cream usually tops the list. These cold things disagree with them, as all cold things do, and patients are worse from them. They crave dairy, including milk, which disagrees with them and may cause them to vomit. They also tend to crave smoked meats, bacon, ham, and the like. They crave salty things.

Calcarea Phosphorica patients often have a spell of weakness or vertigo around four in the afternoon, at which time they will be hungry and must eat something.

Relationships

As noted earlier, Calcarea Phosphorica works well with the other cell salt remedies and may be used in tandem or in alternation with any of them. It has a special affinity with Magnesia Phosphorica in female patients, and an affinity with Silicea in patients who are slow developmentally or who display an overall malaise and an inability to completely heal. It also shows a special affinity with Natrum Muriaticum in patients with headaches and/or with rheumatic pains, if either of these is relieved by the patient lying down to rest.

Calc Phos may be given before or after any other cell salt, although it most usually is given after another remedy has begun if that remedy acts with less potency than it should.

Dosage and Potency

Calcarea Phosphorica is a long-lasting remedy. The effects of a single dose may last for up to sixty days. It is, however, a remedy for both acute conditions and chronic ailments.

Calc Phos is most often given in the 3X or 6X potency. Schuessler himself showed a preference for the 6X and felt that Calcarea Phosphorica attained its highest level of functionality at that potency. The 6X potency is also suggested for elderly patients or those with depleted immune systems.

3. CALCAREA SULPHURICA

Overview

The substance calcium sulphate naturally occurs in gypsum, alabaster, selenite, and anhydrite. In its hemihydrate form it is commonly called "plaster of Paris" and has a chemical compound of $CaSO_4 \cdot 0.5H_2O$. While the fine white powder (usually taken from gypsum) is soluble in water, the remedy Calcarea Sulphurica is made through trituration.

Calcarea Sulphurica has undergone several homeopathic provings, beginning with partial provings and tests as far back as 1847. The first complete proving of the remedy was done in the United States by Dr. Clarence Conant in 1873. But the remedy's usage was proven most notably by Constantine Hering. Calcarea Sulphurica is something of an orphan among the cell salt remedies, in that Schuessler removed it from his list of cell salts in the final edition of his *Therapeutics*, leaving only eleven remedies. He split the duties of Calcarea Sulphurica between Natrum Phosphoricum and Silicea. He did this because he came to understand that, unlike his other remedies, Calc Sulph does *not* naturally occur within the tissues of the body. (It had been believed that it occurred naturally in the bile secreted by the liver, but that could not be proven consistently.) But despite Schuessler's curt dismissal of the remedy from his own list, Calc Sulph continues to be included among the dozen cells salts as they are used today. Perhaps this is because most of us like the neatness of the even dozen remedies, but more likely because it does have value as a remedy and works well in concert with the (other) cell salts, whether it is naturally part of the human body or not. Certainly its components, calcium and sulfur are, which renders this a benign remedy even if it is not part of the human system as a compound.

Therefore, I include it here—both because I like an even dozen as much as the next guy, and because it will likely be found in any kit of cell salts, so it is best to have its usage understood.

This is a remedy that can be highly useful in cases involving an infection that has progressed to, or is about to progress to, the development of pus. For any discharge from mucous membranes, ulcers, or abscesses. It should be noted that Calcarea Sulphurica is very similar in its actions to another homeopathic remedy, Hepar Sulphurica, which is not a part of the cell salts subcategory. (Note that sulfur is part of both compounds.) Both Hepar Sulph and Calc Sulph are very useful for cases involving infections, even serious infections. The difference between them in terms of their usage often comes down to a single symptom: The Hepar Sulph patient in his distress cannot bear moving air, is very sensitive to air and to changes in its temperature or motion. The Calc Sulph patient, on the other hand, craves open air, and, even when ill, will want to go out walking in the fresh air, or open a window to get fresh air into his room. (In addition to this, the Hepar Sulph patient will also be very sensitive to being touched and to touch in general, while the Calc Sulph patient will not. They will share a tendency to be very sensitive to changes in weather, however.)

Indications for the need for Calcarea Sulphurica often show up on the patient's skin. Liver spots, eczema, boils, pimples (this is an excellent remedy for those with acne), and rashes of all sorts indicate this remedy. In the same way, gums that bleed easily, sores on the inside of the mouth and lips, and sores on the lips are all indications of the need for Calcarea Sulphurica. It is an important remedy for those with herpes and can be especially helpful during outbreaks if used in alternation with Silicea.

Like the other remedies in the Calcarea group, Calcarea Sulphurica is to be considered for patients with any or all conditions related to hard tissues like bones, to connective tissues, and, especially in this case, to the skin.

Finally, Calcarea Sulphurica is considered to be a strong purifier. Its use can purify the blood. It can act as a natural antibiotic and can clear away infections. It is especially helpful in the early stages of an illness for purifying the system and preventing the onset of disease, from herpes outbreaks to colds and sore throats. The next time you feel a cold coming on, reach for Calcarea Sulphurica. Take the remedy in the 6X potency, every two hours at first (every hour if the illness seems to be taking hold quickly), then less often as the symptoms of the illness subside. Continue to take Calc Sulph two times a day for two days after the symptoms fade away, to ensure that they do not return.

Conditions that Suggest Calcarea Sulphurica

Abscesses; burns; chilblains; colds, coughs, and sore throats; glandular swelling (buboes); hemorrhages; herpes; injuries: cuts, bruises, and wounds; skin conditions: acne, boils, carbuncles, crusty rashes, cysts, eczema, felons, polyps, psoriasis, and ulcers; tonsillitis.

Mental and Emotional Symptoms

The patient needing Calcarea Sulphurica often will fall into a pattern in which the time of day can be used as a measuring rod of his or her emotional state. Calcarea Sulphurica patients tend to be happy and lighthearted in the morning, only to become more and more depressed and difficult as the day progresses. Most often, they tend to begin to feel worse after eating lunch and become increasingly negative as the sun sets and evening comes on. They are emotionally (and physically) better as the sun rises to its peak, and begin to feel worse as it heads down toward the horizon. (The worst time of day for most Calcarea Sulphurica patients is from 9:00 P.M. until 4:00 A.M.)

As his anxiety and irritation increases as the day progresses, the Calc Sulph patient tends to brood and grumble. The Calc Sulph patient can be both contrary and self-contradictory. He or she will feel undervalued and not well cared for. Calc Sulph patients cannot bear to be disagreed with or patronized. They feel pressured by any who do anything but coddle them. They feel hurried in all things, in eating, in sitting up, in answering questions. They may decide that what they want to do is sit silent and brood. And that is exactly what they will do.

Calcarea Sulphurica patients will be restless, especially when confined to bed. They will want to get up, and especially will want to go out of doors into the fresh air, but often lose their desire as they begin to move around, begin to prepare to dress and leave their home. Most often, they will ultimately give up and go back to bed. (The idea of doing work will be the same. Calc Sulph patients will say they want to do some work, will prepare their task, only to abandon it and go back to resting without accomplishing anything.) Theirs is a constant struggle between a perceived desire to go somewhere, do something, and the reality that they feel too weak, too sick, or too depressed to actually do it.

Often they will have a sensation of suffocation and may awaken suddenly as they are falling asleep with the feeling that they are suffocating. Calc Sulphs crave air. They will want the windows open or will want to have a fan going in their room, just to stir the air. They feel they can breathe more easily when air is moving and/or fresh.

It should be noted that, although Calc Sulph patients crave air on an emotional level, they, like other depleted patients, are actually quite vulnerable to their environment and may catch colds often and easily. Consider this remedy for a sudden cold that comes on after a child has been out playing in the fresh air on a cold day, or for illnesses that come on after a patient comes into a warm room from cold weather, or from a draft of cold air or a cold, windy day.

> Think of Calc Sulph first for cuts, wounds, or bruises that do not heal properly. That, instead of forming a healthy scab and then healing, become infected, form pus (yellow) and scabs (yellowish). In home use, this remedy is perhaps most valuable for its ability to clear away and prevent these infections. Think of this remedy for cases of burns or scalds as well, when the affected area of the body fails to heal, but instead forms wounds that produce pus.

Physical Symptoms

Yellow is the color that I associate with Calcarea Sulphurica. The patients needing this remedy will have a thick yellow coat on their tongues. Especially in chronic illness, their skin can become dry and take on a yellowish tinge (and, yes, this is a remedy associated with jaundice). The pus that forms in pimples, ulcers, and wounds is yellow. Even the mucous discharge from their noses during a cold or allergy attack will be yellow.

Think of this remedy first for cuts, wounds, or bruises that do not heal properly. That, instead of forming a healthy scab and then healing, become infected, form pus (yellow) and scabs (yellowish). In home use, Calc Sulph is perhaps most valuable for its ability to clear away and prevent these infections. Think of this remedy for cases of burns or scalds as well, when the affected area of the body fails to heal, but instead forms wounds that produce pus.

It can also be very helpful when the patient is feverish due to infection, most especially when that fever is accompanied by the keynote symptom that the patient, although cold and sensitive to chill, kicks off his or her covers (which will seem contradictory, as the patient, on the whole, may be very chilly or sensitive to cold). As a sulfur-based remedy, it shares the characteristic of having hot and/or burning feet. The soles of the feet, especially, can chronically itch and/or burn, which makes it impossible for the patient to allow his feet to stay under bedcovers for very long.

Another indicator of the need for this remedy is dandruff. Just as the patient's feet will tend to be hot and itchy, especially when he puts them under his bedcovers, his head will tend to be hot and sweaty, especially during sleep. His pillow will be wet in the morning and his covers will have been kicked away during the night. His hair may always seem to be slightly greasy and dirty, no matter how often he washes it.

This is also a remedy that is characterized by swollen glands, especially cases in which glands are chronically swollen.

Also think of this remedy for patients with acne, especially chronic acne of the face, back, and shoulders. Especially if their skin is not only blemished but, like their hair, seems unhealthy, as if it had not been washed for some time.

If all of the above paints a picture of a teenage boy in your mind, you are right: this remedy is often quite helpful during the period of adolescence when young men in particular are smelly, greasy, slovenly, moody, and have bad skin. Further proving my point is the fact that classic texts on homeopathy suggest that those who need this remedy are often given to masturbation, to such a degree that, as James Tyler Kent puts it, "Onanism and sexual excess reduce the economy to a state whereby they feel their constitutional disturbance."* Given as a nutritional supplement during this stage of life— two doses a day in the 6X potency—can make the transition from boy to man easier for all to bear.

An important general symptom of the remedy type, young or old, is that all pains associated with their symptoms will combine a burning sensation with a sensation of numbness. This combination can occur in any part of the body affected by their illness. The numbness, in particular, can be either specific to affected parts or completely generalized.

Like all the other calcium-based remedies, Calcarea Sulphurica is an excellent general remedy for bone and/or joint pain. It can be especially helpful for painful, swollen joints, for gouty joints in the fingers and toes. For patients with pain in their bones day and night, with pulsation and numbness accompanying the pain. For pain in the ribs and chest that descends into the legs. The pain will be aggravated if the patient

* From *Lectures on Homeopathic Materia Medica* by James Tyler Kent (1849–1916), page 348.

stands, aggravated by lifting or bending. Aggravated if the patient becomes overheated through motion.

This is a patient who is sensitive to both cold and heat. Whose ailments can be aggravated if the patient becomes cold or chilled, or exposed to fresh or cold air—which he craves, but to which he is exceedingly vulnerable. And whose symptoms are all made very much worse from warmth, from being wrapped or covered, or by the patient becoming overheated. Thus this is a patient who will try to find some comfortable temperature, some comfortable balance between covering up and uncovering, being in open air and staying warm enough not to take a chill. He will kick off his covers, only to shiver through the night and wake up enough to pull them back on, only to kick them off again in his sleep. This search for a comfortable temperature will be reflected in the patient's temperament as well. He will become more irritable the colder or warmer he becomes, as either end of the spectrum can greatly exacerbate his physical complaints.

The typical Calcarea Sulphurica patient will also tend to sit on one end of the spectrum or the other when it comes to appetite. He will be either very, very hungry or totally lacking in appetite. The Calc Sulph will generally crave the same things that most sulfur-based remedy types crave: salt, sweet, and grease. These patients tend to be very thirsty, especially for cold drinks (they often want drinks that are cold and sweet—sodas and juices primarily). They may eat until nausea sets in, may tend to belch after eating. They are given to heartburn (Calcarea Sulphurica is an excellent remedy for heartburn that comes on from overeating).

Remember Calcarea Sulphurica's role as a purifier. It cleans the skin, the hair, and the nails, giving tissues that have heretofore seemed unclean and sickly a new, vital look and feel. In the same way, it is helpful for patients who are slow in recovery, especially patients who have been given many allopathic medicines that have proved toxic to their systems. Calcarea Sulphurica, given in a 6X potency twice daily for a period of some weeks, helps purify the patient's system and cleanse it of toxins. Like Silicea, Calcarea Sulphurica will allow the patient's body to excrete that which has been trapped and suppressed.

Modalities

The Calcarea Sulphurica patient is better from resting, from lying about. He is worse from standing for any length of time, from walking, especially worse from walking quickly, which overheats the patient into aggravation. The patient is worse from heat in any form, from being wrapped up or covered, although—and this is important—specific symptoms, especially joint pains, may be improved by an application of heat that is applied directly to the affected area and not generally to the whole body. He is worse in a hot, closed room and may feel as if he cannot breathe if he becomes too warm, especially when he is sleeping.

Calcarea Sulph patients are made worse from being touched, either by human hand or by covers, clothing, or such, which can cause increased pain to joints, skin and bone. They are worse from rubbing or being rubbed.

They are improved by fresh air, and from cool air, although they are vulnerable to it and may become ill from being chilled. Chill can begin in the feet, which usually are hot and itchy, and spread upward to the whole body.

They are improved by eating and drinking.

They are improved by sleeping and often feel their best in the morning, with their symptoms improved from rest.

Relationships

Calcarea Sulphurica works best in conjunction with or alternation with Calcarea Phosphorica, which enhances Calc Sulph's actions and works in concert with the patient's vulnerability to chill and inability to heal. It can be used in the same way with Natrum Sulphuricum, another sulfur-based remedy with which it shares an affinity to all things yellow, to improve myriad skin conditions. Calcarea Sulphurica is often used in conjunction with Silicea in the treatment of bone and joint pain.

Dosage and Potency

Schuessler's long clinical history using this remedy before discarding it from his roster of cell salts led him to conclude that it worked best in the 6X and 12X potencies.

Calcarea Sulphurica is considered to be more effective when used for chronic cases than for acute conditions. It may be used safely in repeated doses, although, as with all cell salts, the doses should be lessened as improvement begins.

4. FERRUM PHOSPHORICUM

Overview

The chemical formula for iron phosphate, from which the remedy Ferrum Phosphoricum is made by way of trituration, is $Fe_3(PO_4)_2$. The remedy is taken from the precipitate that forms when iron sulfate is combined with sodium phosphate. The bluish precipitate is then washed, dried, and ground into a powder from which the remedy is made.

Note that there are differences of opinion when it comes to the exact chemical formula, or compound, for the raw material from which the remedy is made. The formula is also stated as $FePO_4 \cdot 12H_2O$.

Schuessler's formula is the one shown above in the first paragraph. He called this compound "white phosphate of iron," and claimed that it was the true form of iron phosphate that occurs naturally in the human system, contrasting it with "ordinary" iron phosphate, which is also know as "ferrous-hydric phosphate."

Schuessler gives us almost all the important clinical information that we have on the remedy and its uses, although its use has extended well beyond the sphere of bio-chemics and it is a well-known and often used part of the general homeopathic phar-macy. Ferrum Phosphoricum is a remedy that is often included in homeopathic home kits, and it is considered an important remedy for many common acute conditions, notably fever and inflammations of all sorts.

As inflammation is, generally speaking, the reaction of the tissues of the body to an envi-ronmental, chemical, or mechanical irritant, the signs of inflammation include heat (fever), redness, swelling, and pain. These symptoms, presented either generally or in specific parts of the body, suggest the need for the remedy Fer-rum Phosphoricum.

Ferrum Phosphoricum is taken from two basic components, iron and phosphorus, both of which are connected with the blood in terms of the actions of homeopathic remedies. It is logi-cal, therefore, that Ferrum Phosphoricum is also an important remedy for patients suf-fering from anemia, from hemorrhages, or from circulatory disorders. As with other phosphorus-based remedies, the patients will tend to hemorrhage easily, so look for bloody discharges. Like other phosphorus types they are given to weakness of the ears (especially the eustachian tubes), the nose, the throat, and the lungs.

This is a chief remedy for patients with neuralgic pain, especially when that pain is right-sided (as is the tendency with iron-based remedies) or more severe on the right side of the body. In addition to the central "burning"sensation of the pain, the pain will also be described as "bruised" or "raw."

More often than not, Ferrum Phosphoricum is a remedy most needed by younger patients, by children and young people, most especially by those in puberty. This is not to say that it cannot sometimes be helpful for older patients, as any or all homeopathic remedies may be required acutely or constitutionally by any individual patient. How-ever, the general pattern of its use will weigh heavily toward younger as opposed to older patients.

There are remedies that are commonly used for patients who are manic in their ill-ness and pain, but this is not one of them. There are, likewise, remedies that are very helpful for patients who become exhausted, almost comatose, in their pain. Again, this is not one of them. I bring this up, not to confuse the portrait of this remedy, but to point out that when it comes to the patient and his or her symptoms, very often Ferrum Phosphoricum suggests itself as the needed remedy by its lack of specificity and, if you will, sheer drama. Thus, this is the remedy to think of for the patient who has a simple fever of perhaps unknown origins, who, although ill, is not critically ill, and in that illness neither thrashes about in his bed nor faints into frightening stillness. Instead, this is a somewhat sensitive, somewhat anxious patient whose pulse will not race but will flow, whose eyes, while perhaps reddened, are not glazed or crazed in their expression. And whose mind—most strangely—will almost seem sharper, clearer as part of the pattern of the symptoms rather than fogged by fear or pain or exhaustion.

Conditions that Suggest Ferrum Phosphoricum

Anemia; cystitis; diabetes; diarrhea; ear infections, especially in children; fevers; headaches; inflammations; injuries; measles; mumps; neuralgia; nosebleeds; rheumatism; upper respiratory conditions: bronchitis, colds, coughs, croup, laryngitis, pneumonia, sore throat, whooping cough.

Mental and Emotional Symptoms

As with the symptoms of fever, it is the generality of the emotional and mental symptoms that often guide us to Ferrum Phos, and not the drama of the symptoms themselves. Ferrum Phos patients will be rather relaxed in their illnesses and not particularly demanding. Very often, they will just want to be taken care of and do nothing whatsoever to impede the caregiver's ability to assist them. They may seem actually indifferent, not only to their illness, but also to their desires. They may want some tea, or something soothing to eat or drink, but they are not demanding. They will tend to want to rest, may or may not want to have conversation, and may or may not become irritable in their pain. They will not, however, become wildly demanding or irritable, nor will they seem as if they are so very ill that they cannot make their needs or distress known. Instead, they will be rather clear-minded, rather self-possessed. In other words, their behavior will usually match their physical health. Those needing this remedy whose chief complaints are rheumatic, for instance, may be more irritable than those whose complaints are laryngitis and a cold. But in all cases, their reaction to their condition is more or less appropriate to that condition, nothing more, nothing less.

Physical Symptoms

Years ago, our television screens were filled with commercials for products whose job it was to combat "iron-poor blood." The customers of these products, women mostly, reported feeling lightheaded, weak, and just plain "run down." The tonics sold on those black and white sets promised to build up the blood and build up the patient in the process, so she could live a happy, active life raising her children, cleaning her house, and cooking (all while wearing a housedress, high heels, and pearls).

While that image of the patient has faded into the past, the use of Ferrum Phosphoricum for those in need of a tonic for "iron-poor blood" has not. This is the chief and most important remedy in the cell salts repertory to combat anemia. And if the cell salts can be considered the perfect balancing point between homeopathy and nutritional supplements, then the idea of taking iron not in a material dose, but, instead, in a potentized, which is to say, diluted form might hold some appeal. It should be noted, however, that anemia can be a serious condition and, like other ailments discussed in these pages, requires the skill of a medical professional to put right. In other words, with cell salts, as with all other homeopathic and semihomeopathic remedies, including Bach Remedies, it is always best to work with your doctor, and not on your own.

In general, however, the need for Ferrum Phosphoricum on a chronic or constitutional level can be indicated by a prolonged feeling of dizziness, exhaustion, and a general feeling of debility. Those needing the remedy will have an almost constant need to lie down and rest. They will find that simple tasks that were no challenge before have become difficult. They will also find that rising up from a sitting or squatting (think: gardening) position leaves them lightheaded.

In constitutional cases, the patients who need Ferrum Phos are usually women. It is, as has been noted, a remedy for those who are anemic. It is also an excellent remedy to consider during pregnancy, especially to combat morning sickness and nausea. It can also be helpful for headaches and rheumatic pains during pregnancy. Indeed, any pregnancy in which the woman is ordered into bed rest indicates the need for this remedy.

Ferrum Phosphoricum is an excellent remedy for those who suffer from headaches (perhaps second only to Natrum Muriaticum among the cell salts). This is the remedy for those who suffer from "blind headaches," who feel a sharp pain in the head, usually running from back to front, or wedged in the occiput and traveling from there up over the skull to the front of the head. The headache may be accompanied by pain in the face as well, by sensations of pressing or throbbing. The headache will be soothed by motion. The patient may shake her head, or bend or stoop forward to find relief from the pain. The top of the patient's head becomes very sensitive during the headache. She cannot bear to have her head or even her hair touched. The top of the head is sensitive to cold air, to touch, even to noise. The pain tends to increase at night. This sensation of pain on the top of the head may be chronically associated with a female patient's monthly cycle.

These headaches will often be accompanied by vomiting (Ferrum Phos is a good general remedy for nausea that leads to vomiting) and by the patient having a red face.

This leads to another indicator of the remedy: the color red. As with all phosphorus-based remedies, the patient will tend to have bloody discharges and the blood will tend to be very red. In the same way, the patient often will display redness—again, bright redness—of affected parts. During a cold or sore throat, the face, the throat, the internal and external ears will all become very bright red. Children with chronic bright red external ears, or whose ears become bright red just as they are becoming sick, show in indication for this and other phosphorus-based remedies.

While the use of the constitutional remedy in adults is most often associated with women, especially pregnant women, the acute use of the remedy is wide-ranging, but its use is most commonly targeted toward young patients.

You will find Ferrum Phosphoricum to be such a valuable remedy for children with chronic or acute ear infections, bronchitis, and nosebleeds, and for sore throats, colds, coughs, croups, measles, and mumps that you will soon decide that it is a very good remedy to have on hand in any household with young or adolescent children. It is particularly helpful for treating fevers in young patients, especially fevers that do not present any notable symptoms: when they are not especially high, dangerous, or sudden. When they are, quite simply, fevers.

Ferrum Phos always works best if it is used as soon as possible after the onset of illness. When the child's ears are just becoming bright red and burning hot. When the sore throat is just beginning. At the onset of the cold. While it can still be an effective remedy at the later or deeper stages of illness (think: pneumonia), it is far more effective for preventing deep or long-lasting illness than it is in correcting it.

Think of Ferrum Phos for cases of whooping cough in which a spell of coughing leads the patient to vomit. When the coughing—whooping or not—is painful. For short, for dry, spasmodic coughs.

This is a restless remedy, meaning that, while these patients will most usually want to rest or lie down, they will have trouble actually sleeping. And as their symptoms will tend to be worse at night, no matter what those symptoms are, they often interfere with their sleep.

Ferrum Phos is the first remedy to think of for cases of chronic nose bleeds in children, especially when the blood is bright red and the child follows the pattern of symptoms and behavior associated with the remedy: worse at night, restless, exhausted, and so on.

This is an excellent remedy to consider for patients of all ages who have pain in the right shoulder, especially rheumatic pain. The affected area may be red and swollen and is sensitive to the touch. The pain may travel down into the right arm or up into the neck, with the patient complaining of a "crick in the neck" on the right side. The patient may experience a loss of strength in the right hand, or may feel that the right hand is numb. It is an excellent remedy for hip pain as well—also right-sided—and for cases of lumbago that are better when the patient moves about and/or walks slowly. Note that in almost all circumstances involving pain, patients will be better from slow, gentle motion and worse from quick movement, overreaching, or stretching. While they may wish to lie down, their pain may dictate that they move about instead.

Modalities

Ferrum Phosphoricum patients will be worse at night, especially from 4:00 A.M. until 6:00 A.M. They will be worse from touch and from quick or sustained motion. They will be worse from cold air, worse from being jarred emotionally or physically. They will be worse from noise and light and excitement, worse from cold drinks and from all but the simplest foods.

Ferrum Phos patients will be better from rest, from peace, from gentle, simple motion, from simple things in general: simple foods, calm surroundings, and from loving caregiving. They will be better, in general, from cold applications to affected areas, especially those areas that are red and/or swollen. They will be better from lying down, better from sleeping, if sleep is possible. They will be better from drinking warm drinks. Ironically, Ferrum Phos patients, who are known for their bloody discharges, feel better from having discharged blood.

Relationships

An oddity among the cell salts, Ferrum Phosphoricum works very well on its own. It has an affinity for the other phosphorus-based cell salts, most notably Calcarea Phosphorica and Kali Phosphoricum, and may be used in combination with or alternating with Natrum Muriaticum or Natrum Phosphoricum in cases involving chronic headaches. But in most cases, especially in acute aliments in young patients, Ferrum Phosphoricum stands alone. Kali Muriaticum may also be used in conjunction with Ferrum Phos in cases of deep respiratory illness like pneumonia or cases of chronic inflammation of tissues. Kali Mur can also be used to follow Ferrum Phos in a case of fever that is not cured by Ferrum Phos alone.

When we extend our reach outside the limits of biochemics to the more general homeopathic pharmacy, Ferrum Phos is often used in conjunction with the homeopathic remedy Aconite. The two remedies have much in common—their use in combating inflammation, the rapid onset of symptoms, the burning, redness, and heat of affected parts. But Aconite carries with it the keynote symptoms of rapid pulse and a manic, fearful patient. This means that, in most cases, a choice must be made whether to give the patient Ferrum Phos or Aconite, and the deciding factors will be the behavior of the patient and the rapidity of his pulse. In some cases, Ferrum Phos may be needed following an initial use of Aconite to clear away the full range of symptoms of the illness—give Kali Mur in the later part of the fever, after the Ferrum Phos has brought about improvement and the fever itself is receding.

Dosage and Potency

Schuessler used Ferrum Phos most often in the range of potencies between 6X and 12X. It is, however, used in a wider range of potencies today. Potencies as low as 1X or 2X are used in cases of anemia, and potencies well beyond the biochemical limit of 12X are commonly used in homeopathic practice. Indeed, most homeopathic kits will include the remedy in a 30C potency that is highly effective in the treatment of indicated childhood illnesses. It is suggested that the remedy never be given in potencies below Schuessler's 12X at nighttime, as these will often cause sleeplessness to occur.

In young patients, Ferrum Phos is most often used as an acute remedy and is very helpful in cases of minor childhood illnesses, from fever to measles to mumps. It can be repeated as needed in acute cases. In adults, especially in adult female patients, it may be used as either an acute or a chronic remedy. In chronic cases, it should be repeated only as needed and as symptoms recur.

5. KALI MURIATICUM

Overview

The remedy Kali Muriaticum is taken from the chemical compound potassium chloride. Its chemical formula is KCl. It is found in nature in the mineral carnallite and in the human body in blood cells (where it is found in nearly as much abundance as its related substance, sodium chloride), muscles, nerve tissues, and, most important, in brain cells. Schuessler insisted that, without the presence of potassium chloride, no new brain cells could be made. Potassium chloride is a building block of the fibrous tissues of the body, especially of the skin. Kali Mur is a remedy that Schuessler himself brought into the homeopathic pharmacy, although Constantine Hering undertook an important proving of the remedy as well.

The remedy Kali Muriaticum tends to play "clean up." It is seldom used as an initial remedy, but is, instead, given after one or more of the other cell salts. It will enhance the work of the initial remedy and complete its action in healing. A perfect example of this is the use of Kali Mur as a follow-up to Ferrum Phosphoricum in cases of inflammation, especially of fever. Ferrum Phos is a remedy that works best in the first stage of an illness, at the onset of symptoms. Kali Mur works best in the second stage of illness, or for cases of illnesses that have been slow in coming on, with symptoms that are slow in developing. Therefore, the two remedies tend to be a perfect team. Give Ferrum Phos at the onset in cases of fever. As the patient's temperature comes down and the associated symptoms such as chills and sore throat begin to fade, follow up with the Kali Mur, which will not only help bring the symptoms to an end, but will stoke the patient's vitality, making recovery time short and the restoration of health assured.

The color white or whitish-gray is suggestive of Kali Mur. Look for the patient's skin, tongue, and discharges to all share this common color. The tongue will tend to have a thick white or gray coat on its base. The Kali Mur is given to dandruff, and that dandruff will be white as well. Discharges are milky white, thick, slimy, and/or lumpy. Even the patient's vomit, should that occur, will contain white, lumpy discharges. Kali Mur is most effectively given at the moment of illness in which the discharges begin to appear. Therefore, it will not be especially helpful at the first dry sneeze of a cold, but will be very helpful later, when the mucous discharge begins, as long as the symptoms of the cold mirror those of the remedy.

> The remedy Kali Muriaticum tends to play "clean up." It is seldom used as an initial remedy, but is, instead, given after one or more of the other cell salts. It will enhance the work of the initial remedy and complete its action in healing.

This is another cell salt, like Calcarea Phosphorica, that can be thought of as a general tonic, so you may have some confusion as to which is best to use. Kali Muriaticum is of greatest value as a tonic for those who have just begun their recovery from an illness, in which case it can help shorten recovery time dramatically. Calc Phos, on the other hand, is the more generalized tonic, and works best for patients who do not display the symptoms of a specific ailment or who are not in a stage of recovery, but, instead, feel depleted and exhausted, apparently for no reason.

"Sluggish" is a good word to use to describe the Kali Mur patient and his or her constitution. There is a "stuckness" about the remedy and those who need it. Think of it as the remedy for patients who are stalled in their recovery from their illness, who can't quite muster the strength to throw off that illness and get back to health and need a push to get better. That push is Kali Muriaticum.

Remember that all the Kali remedies, all the potassium-based remedies, will share a certain "stuckness" one way or another. Potassium-based remedies all relate to a certain slowness, to a sensation of being trapped one way or another, to a need for a good push forward. In Kali Phosphoricum, that "stuckness" will tend to play out as nervous exhaustion and hypersensitivity. In Kali Sulphuricum, it tends to manifest as a sensation of physical weight that pulls the patient down and saps his strength (it may, in many cases, be the real effects of obesity). But in Kali Muriaticum, it plays out as depletion brought on by illness of any sort, from which the patient has not yet recovered. And because of which the patient has never felt truly well since the onset of symptoms, however long ago that might have been. Therefore, think of Kali Mur for the patient who has a cold that drags on and on, and for the patient who had the flu a year ago and who has never felt really well since.

Finally, consider this small but telling keynote symptom that is associated with this remedy: cracking noises. Because this is a remedy taken from one of the body's building blocks, the need for it may be indicated by cracking sounds made by patient's joints. When the fibrous tissues stiffen because of a deficiency of potassium chloride, they tend to make a cracking sound as they are moved. This will be particularly true of the joints in the hands and fingers. The patient may also hear the cracking noise internally: this remedy will be very helpful for those who are suffering from head colds that have a chief complaint of a loud cracking noise every time the nose is blown or the jaw is moved. While the cracking sound associated with the need for Kali Mur may not be of great importance in terms of medical emergencies, it can be very important in helping you select this remedy from the whole group of cell salt remedies and, in doing so, lead you to a successful remedy selection.

Conditions that Suggest Kali Muriaticum

Bronchitis (chronic); chicken pox; colds and coughs; cysts; dandruff; ear aches (especially when they involve the eustachian tube); measles; mumps; nodes; obesity; pain (joint or muscle pain, especially if it is wandering pain with pulsation); rheumatic fever; rheumatism (especially when associated with cracking joints); slow recovery from any illness; sore throats with laryngitis; swollen glands; vaccination (ill effects).

Mental and Emotional Symptoms

Kali Muriaticum patients are, above and beyond all else, hungry patients. No matter what their illness, they will eat.* They will tend to want warm things—food and drinks alike. They may well crave heavy, fatty, or rich foods they cannot digest. They may become nauseous after eating and may even vomit, but they will still want to eat again soon after. Hunger may be a point of mania for them. The patient may become convinced that he or she will starve and must keep eating in order to survive. (Let me note that, in cases of patients who are in a chronic or constitutional Kali Mur state, this mania for eating as a means of survival can and does lead to real issues of obesity. The patient may have moved into the Kali state months or years earlier as a result of a "not well since" sluggish recovery from a past illness. The remedy tends to aid in weight loss in cases such as these, because the issue of "starvation" is removed from the table as it aids in recovery.)

---

* This can be very irritating, I know, but in working with homeopathic medicines, it is best to just accept the fact that every strongly indicated symptom also carries with it its opposite. So you may also find Kali Mur patients who do not want to eat at all, who cannot bear the thought of food, and who will vomit from the thought of food or even from just drinking anything—especially warm drinks. So keep in mind that food is a key issue for the Kali Mur; either they want it all or they want none of it. The patient for whom food is not an issue is likely not to be helped by Kali Mur as much as they might by another, better indicated remedy.

Look for the the Kali Muriaticum patient to not only crave food but to crave foods that sick people usually don't crave. Where most of us want a cup of tea when we have a cold or flu, the Kali Mur will want a toasted cheese sandwich. He wants something that should turn his stomach—that may well end up turning his stomach inside out—yet he still wants it and must have it. He can become quite insistent when it comes to food.

This is an irritable patient who cannot find comfort in anything, including the food he demands. The Kali Mur patient can become very angry very easily, or can fall into spells of self-pity, from which he will exit only for the sake of angry outbreaks.

At his best, he is a rather indifferent patient. One who finds no humor or pleasure in anything, but who will suffer in silence, often with his eyes closed. Who usually wishes to be propped up in bed or to sit by the window in silence. He is disinclined to speak, does not wish to be asked questions. Questions will usually make him angry, especially questions about the wisdom of his demands, especially concerning food.

Physical Symptoms

Let's start with pain. This is a great remedy for those who are in pain, especially if their pain is chronic and mysterious in nature. This is a remedy for rheumatism and for rheumatism that comes on after fever. As a remedy made from a substance that is a building-block of the elastic fibers of the body, Kali Mur is very helpful for patients with joint pains caused by a lack of elasticity in connective tissues or from a tightening of the fascia, the tissue that encloses muscles and organs of the body. Thus the pains associated with this remedy are apt to move from place to place in the body without warning or apparent reason. These patients may feel their pains all the way down into their bones and may cry out in pain. The pain is pulsing and throbbing in nature.

Kali Mur can be very helpful in cases of strains or sprains that do not heal or are slow to heal. For chronic injuries caused by repeated injury to specific parts of the body. All pains associated with Kali Mur will be worse from motion (sometimes that characteristic will be the only way to tell this remedy apart from Kali Sulphuricum, which can be used to treat similar pains but is better from motion). Look for white discharges or a thick white coating on the tongue as a indicator for the need of this remedy.

Kali Mur is useful for rheumatic pains that come on every night that, although better for rest, are worse from the warmth of the bed. Pains that force the patient to get out of bed. The pains tend to force the patient to sit up—he or she is always better from being in a sitting position. Pains that may be described as "lightninglike" because they move about the body, especially down the legs into the feet. This is an excellent remedy for writer's cramp, especially if the hands ache from overuse and the hand and finger joints crack during use. Note that the patient's hands (and feet) may feel cold during periods of pain.

Thus, Kali Mur should be thought of as a good general pain remedy, especially when the onset of pain can be traced back to a specific injury or to an illness from which the patient never fully recovered.

This important aspect of Kali Mur's sphere of activity—its ability to restore to health the patient who has been placed in a form of suspended animation due to an injury or illness—is also illustrated by the fact that Kali Muriaticum is an important remedy for patients who have experienced ill effects after vaccination. Think of this remedy for the person (or pet, for that matter) who has become listless or weak after a vaccination. Just as it will help the patient whose system cannot restore itself after infectious disease, it can help bring back a sense of vitality to the patient whose system has been overtaxed by vaccination. This is an important use for Kali Muriaticum and should be remembered.

In the home, Kali Muriaticum will most often be used in the second stage of a cold, flu, or ear infection.

Let me be clear about what that means. In homeopathic medicine, illnesses like colds are said to have three stages. The first is the onset, in which the symptoms begin, either suddenly or slowly. The patient begins to feel weak, or his throat suddenly begins to hurt, or a fever begins.

In general, the second stage of an illness begins with the onset of discharges. This means when the mucus starts to flow, in most cases. During the second stage, the mucus will be clear, or white, or less commonly, gray. When the mucus becomes yellow or green it is an indicator of the third stage of an illness.

Kali Muriaticum is a remedy for the second stage of illness, when the discharges begin. Look for the discharges to be white or, less commonly, gray in Kali Muriaticum patients (which is to say, in the patients for whom this will be a likely remedy). Look for those discharges to be thick and slimy, even lumpy. All of this indicates the fact that Kali Mur would be a good choice of a remedy to set things right.

Kali Muriaticum is an extremely good remedy for young patients with ear infections or ear pain that extends down into the eustachian tubes, especially children with chronic ear infections. Consider Kali Mur for middle and inner ear infections that congest the ear, make it feel swollen and painful down deep into the head. Look for the glands behind the ear to be swollen. Listen for the patient to complain of a cracking sound in his head every time he blows his nose or swallows. The patient may have trouble hearing due to congestion and will feel that his ears are "stuffed up." Even the external ear may be swollen.

Kali Mur is a remedy to remember for all eye, ear, nose, and throat conditions of younger patients. Think of it for swollen tonsils and sore throats, particularly those accompanied by the traditional white coating of the tongue, tonsils, and throat, that leave the patient hoarse and worse from swallowing. For adenoidal patients. For patients with laryngitis whose throats are coated white, as are their tongues. For patients with coughs, even whooping cough, when the expectorant is white and thick. The cough can be so intense that the patient fears that his eyes will come out of his head. (Homeopath William Boericke noted a "protruded appearance of the eyes" in his patients needing this remedy.) Kali Mur can also be helpful for bronchial asthma and for the second stage of bronchitis, when thick white phlegm forms. The phlegm is sticky and difficult for the patient to cough up. When he succeeds it tends to fly out of his mouth in milky-white, thick lumps. This is a remedy to consider for cases of bronchitis in which the patient's chest feels raw, or when there are flashes of pain and heat in the patient's chest.

The colds cured by Kali Mur carry the same set of symptoms as the ear infections and sore throats. The patient feels that his head is "stuffed up." He hears cracking in his ears when he blows his nose or swallows. He loses his senses of smell, taste, and hearing. He will be improved by resting, but usually by resting in a seated position and not by lying down flat. He may even sleep in a sitting position, as this will help him breathe and help with the drainage of the mucus. Discharges will be white, thick, and slimy.

Kali Mur is helpful in cases of cold sores, or of *aphthae,* the white ulcers that form on the interior sides of the mouth and/or on the tongue.

Modalities

Patients needing Kali Mur will be worse during the night, usually beginning around 5:00 P.M. and growing worse and worse until midnight. Although symptoms will remain aggravated until 4:00 A.M., they are at their worst state at midnight. Consider this remedy for any condition that returns every evening and those that are always worse at midnight.

Kali Mur patients are better from resting, but not from lying down. They are better from staying in a sitting position. Although they are better from resting, they are worse from the heat of the bed and may be forced to get up. Kali Mur patients often find the best relief from their aches and pains by getting out of bed and sitting in a chair. They should be allowed to do so.

They are worse from cold in any form: from cold drafts and moving or open air, from cold applications and cold drinks. They are also worse in damp weather or from dampness in the environment. They will crave warm things, warm food and drinks, which may or may not agree.

They are better from being rubbed, and will respond well to touch in most cases, although some may refuse to be touched by others and will rub their own pains away.

Relationships

As a remedy for the second stage of illness, Kali Muriaticum works well as a follow-up to all the other cell salts, especially Ferrum Phosphoricum, which it often follows in treating upper respiratory infections of all sorts.

In cases of stomach flu or nausea and vomiting from any cause, Kali Mur and Natrum Sulphuricum can be alternated every hour. It can be alternated with Natrum Muriaticum in cases of head colds, especially those that begin with fits of sneezing and tearing eyes.

Cases of chronic rheumatism that follow the general Kali pattern can often benefit either from Kali Muriaticum or Kali Sulphuricum. In these cases, a single symptom will identify which of the two should be used—patients who are improved by motion should be given Kali Sulph, those who are improved by rest will need Kali Mur.

Dosage and Potency

Kali Mur is a short-acting remedy that may be repeated as needed for both acute and chronic conditions. Schuessler most often used the remedy in the 6X, 9X, and 12X potencies. In cases of sore throat, it is suggested that 3X potency be dissolved in warm water and used as a gargle.

This is a remedy that is to be thought of as being for acute and chronic conditions equally. It works well with all other cell salts and can be used in concert with any of them, especially in stubborn cases that are slow to heal. Think of this remedy for any patient with any condition that is hard to move forward to healing, that seems "stuck" in a syndrome of symptoms. In these cases, use the 6X potency two or three times daily until improvement begins, and then cut back to once daily until health is totally restored. In acute cases, do not hesitate to use Kali Muriaticum hourly, or even more often, until improvement begins.

6. KALI PHOSPHORICUM

Overview

Kali Phosphoricum is one of three potassium-based remedies included in Schuessler's cell salt pharmacy. Kali Phos is taken from the chemical compound potassium phosphate, also known as "phosphate of potash." It is a compound of potassium and phosphoric acid. It has a chemical formula of K_2HPO_4. While the compound is soluble in water (insoluble in alcohol), the remedy is made through trituration with milk sugar.

This remedy was fully proven and researched clinically by Schuessler, although homeopath H. C. Allen contributed to our knowledge of the remedy and its uses.

Kali Phos is the premiere homeopathic and biochemical remedy for the condition once known as *neurasthenia*, which is now a somewhat antiquated term for those who suffer from nervous conditions associated with a sense of dread, lassitude, exhaustion, and irritability. It often occurs in conjunction with headache, vague aches and pains, and physical weakness.

Among Hahnemann's remedies, Kali Phos' closest parallel is found in the remedy Pulsatilla, which shares Kali Phos' changeable emotional nature, its warm-bloodedness, its dread of being "closed in," and its tendency toward peevishness.

The Kali Phosphoricum patient will have an issue of warmth. This is a patient who is warm-blooded, worse from being too warm or, especially, from being trapped in a closed or too-warm room, and who is better in open air. And yet, this is a patient who is also lacking in vital heat, who suffers greatly if he or she becomes too cold. Therefore, this is a patient who seeks balance in terms of temperature, both internal and external, who is overly sensitive to changes in temperature in the way that other patients will feel the same sensitivity because of changes in weather from dry to damp or changes in light from day to night. As the Kali Phos can suffer from being too warm (a sensation that will be similar to the claustrophobic patient's dread of being in a too-small place) and from getting chilly, the typical Kali Phos patient will seem to always be opening or closing windows, turning on and off fans, and putting on and taking off sweaters in an attempt to find the right, or "safe" temperature in which he or she can feel at peace and unstressed.

> Indeed, this oversensitivity, applied to any or all aspects of life—physical, mental, or emotional—is keynote to the Kali Phos patient. It is central to the issues that Kali Phos speaks to, along with a sense of emotional exhaustion, physical sensitivity, and an ongoing feeling that everything that does not actively support and nourish the patient stresses him to the point that he is pushed beyond his ability to cope.

Indeed, this oversensitivity, applied to any or all aspects of life—physical, mental, or emotional—is keynote to the Kali Phos patient. It is central to the issues that Kali Phos speaks to, along with a sense of emotional exhaustion, physical sensitivity, and an ongoing feeling that everything that does not actively support and nourish the patient stresses him to the point that he is pushed beyond his ability to cope.

This is, above all else, a remedy that speaks to the nervous system and to "nervous" patients. Potassium phosphate is a constituent of all the tissues in the body, especially to nerve, muscle, and brain tissue, so it should come as no surprise that the remedy taken from this potassium compound should help those with ailments involving the nervous system. In the same way, since this remedy also belongs to the family of phosphorus-based remedies, it should come as no surprise that sensitivity, particularly an emotional oversensitivity and an overly sensitive response to changes in the environment will be a part of this remedy's portrait, just as it is of all other phosphorus-based remedies.

And as this is a Kali group remedy, containing potassium in the compound from which it is made, it shares the tendency toward sluggishness that is keynote to these remedies. In the case of this particular remedy, this sluggishness displays most often in the emotional sphere, with a depression that can be long-lasting or even crippling. But this sense of depression—Kali Phos' particular take on the idea of sluggishness—can carry over to the physical sphere as well. The Kali Phos patient will typically feel this emotional depression or sluggishness by a loss of mental acuity and also by a feeling of physical exhaustion and actual muscle strength. In this way, the Kali Phos patient becomes true to the Kali type, and remains stuck in a fixed position of helplessness until the remedy gives the patient the shove needed to break through the pattern of depression that can grip and grip hard, long-term.

Kali Phosphoricum is often a remedy for elderly patients, who have not only lost their muscle tone but also their willingness to try to regain it, choosing instead to withdraw from the world and from the life that they now perceive as too much of a struggle to be worth the fight.

The color associated with this remedy type is yellow, often a golden yellow. Bodily secretions are often yellow. Even expectoration in cases of cough and cold will be bright yellow. And look for a yellow coating on the patient's tongue.

A certain almost carrion scent is keynote to this patient as well. The patient takes on a smell that is fetid, like the smell of old onions, as the system becomes more and more sluggish and more and more muscle tone is lost. All secretions and discharges will take on this smell. Even the diarrhea that can become chronic in these patients will have the smell of death about it.

This is a patient who is lacking in vital force, who is in a state of perpetual exhaustion, wasting what little energy he or she has in fretting, fussing, and worrying, in seeking to find warmth (emotional and physical). In doing so, the patient becomes ill easily, catches every cold, every flu germ, and is further weakened with each new ailment.

These are children who are underweight, as if they are undernourished. Who seek comfort in the arms of any adult. These are adults who lead what the poet Henry David Thoreau described as "lives of quiet desperation," who take insult from each new jolt of bad news, each new twist and turn of fate and traffic jams, growing weaker with each new offense. These are elders who feel that life has passed them by and has kicked them hard in their rear end as it passed.

Conditions that Suggest Kali Phosphoricum

Allergies, especially seasonal allergies; asthma; bedwetting; concussion; chilblains; depression; diarrhea; gangrene; headaches, especially those associated with menstruation; hysteria; insomnia; melancholia; neuralgia; neurasthenia; nightmares and night terror; sensitive teeth; toothache, accompanied by frontal headache.

Mental and Emotional Symptoms

It should come as no surprise that the mental and emotional symptoms of the Kali Phosphoricum type of patient are dominant over the physical symptoms, although they are less likely to be those symptoms for which the patient seeks help. The Kali Phos patient often yields to his or her mental and emotional state of depression, accepts it, and does not see the possibility for change and therefore will not enter into treatment for it. Instead, they will seek help for usually rather minor physical complaints or, worse, go without treatment because their mental and emotional issues are all too often seen as linked to the age or gender of the patient and not as issues that can and should be resolved. Too often women needing Kali Phos are given hormones and/or tranquilizers, and elders needing the remedy are simply warehoused and ignored. They are left to live their lives in shadows, as lesser and weaker individuals than they could be, instead of being allowed to recover from what can only (homeopathically, at least) be seen as a form of real illness.

As other cell salts act as a tonic on the physical level, Kali Phos acts as a tonic on the emotional level, the mental level, and tonifies the nervous system as well, bringing a vibrancy and vitality to patients who otherwise remain in a state of mental and emotional sluggishness.

The Kali Phosphoricum patient is anxious, nervous, on alert for no good reason. And as the patient stays in a state of constant anxious alert, with alarms going off for no good reason, his or her system—both physical and emotional—pays the price for staying on red alert too long and begins to break down over time. Just as allergies (and it should come as no surprise that the hyperalert Kali Phos is given to allergies and sensitivities of all sorts, especially seasonal allergies) are a product of overresponsiveness on the part of the immune system, which is seeing danger where none exists, the Kali Phos' exhaustion and many of his or her physical complaints are the result of the patient's emotional and mental hypervigilance. Overly sensitive Kali Phos types break down their vitality by burning out their life energy through a sense of fear and foreboding. These are largely future-oriented types, who dread what is to come, or what is happening right now, but out of their control. They may give way to paranoia, and most certainly will give way to fear, even obsessive fear or phobia.

Words are very important to Kali Phos types, as is communication. They will tend to be at either end of the spectrum on this matter, and will either tend to talk or write constantly, overexplaining their viewpoints, or will refuse to talk or communicate in any way. They can be shy people. In spite of their natural shyness, they may expound on and on. They may talk in their sleep.

And while words are important to them, words can be hard for them to hang onto. The Kali Phos types will often have memory loss linked to words. They will not be able to think of the word they need in the middle of their sentence. When writing, they will leave out letters or whole words, may truncate entire sentences or paragraphs. They will use the wrong word, grow frustrated, and then speak or write all the faster or simply refuse to communicate further.

Along with placing an importance on words, they feel that sounds are important, and are very sensitive to them. They can be sensitive to music and be emotionally reached or moved by music, even when all else fails. They can find great solace in music or take great pain from it. They are sensitive to noise and cannot bear unpleasant or too-loud noises. (Note that the noises can be either external or internal. Kali Phos types tend to have noises in their ears—ringing, buzzing, cracking, and the like. These noises can be very troublesome to the Kali Phos patient.) This is, of course, linked to the phosphorus-type sensitivity to the environment, to beauty itself. Every phosphorus-based remedy will feature an aspect of this sensitivity, to color, to sound, to taste and smell, to beauty and ugliness. All are sources of sensitivity to the range of phosphorus-based remedies.

And like the other phosphorus-based remedies, the Kali Phos is better for company. The patient's symptoms will quite literally grow worse when he or she is left alone. They want attention, want human contact and touch. The Kali Phos, however, will be easily stimulated and may become worked up by the presence of company, to the point of exhaustion, a sort of nervous exhaustion that leads to insomnia. Therefore, the caregivers of Kali Phos patients have to learn to dole out company and control the amount of contact the Kali Phos has with those who upset or overstimulate the patient. These are patients, especially when very young and very old, who must be carefully prepared for sleep, with the proper sounds, the proper rituals, to get them to sleep at all.

The nervous, hyperattentive Kali Phos will be given to insomnia, to nightmares, and to night terrors. These are patients whose emotional symptoms are always worse at night. Young patients especially will dread the moment when the caregiver leaves them alone. They will have difficulty in getting asleep and in staying asleep. They wake easily. They will want attention if they wake, will want to be touched, soothed, and even carried. They will want to be reassured that they are safe. They will tend to talk in their sleep. They will have a pronounced tendency to yawn.

Kali Phos types are also known for their tendency to be changeable when it comes to states of emotion. Kali Phos patients are weathervanes (again, easily compared to Pulsatilla types in the homeopathic pharmacy) in that they may be happy one moment and sad or angry the next, without apparent cause. Caregivers are often left to wonder what it is they did to evoke such a strong emotional response, for better or worse, from the Kali Phos patient.

Physical Symptoms

While Natrum Muriaticum is consider the premiere cell salt remedy for those with headaches, Kali Phos is another remedy worthy of consideration, especially for women's headaches that play a regular part in their menstrual cycle. Remember this remedy as well for female patients whose menstrual cycle appears too early or too late, and who become emotionally distraught when their cycle is delayed. It is also to be considered for women whose periods are too heavy and when the flow is accompanied by the foul smell associated with the remedy.

Kali Phos is also said to be the chief remedy for so-called "nervous headaches" that are a part of the overall neurasthenic portrait. It is especially helpful for headaches that have an emotional connection—headaches from anger, stress, overwork, or exhaustion. This is a good remedy for headaches that come on from study and the stress of exams, so students should remember to use it at the end of each semester.

Look for the patient with a headache who needs Kali Phosphoricum to yawn during his or her headache—yawn repeatedly and in a pronounced manner.

Kali Phos is also an important remedy for patient with allergies of all sorts, especially those with seasonal allergies brought on by an oversensitivity to the environment. Look for the keynote yellow discharges as an indicator that Kali Phos is the remedy of choice for a case of seasonal rhinitis. Kali Phos is especially indicated for patients who suddenly develop an allergy and display the emotional symptoms of the remedy: mental and emotional exhaustion, anxiety, depression, and so on.

Remember Kali Phos as a remedy for little children who are asthmatic or who suffer from allergic asthma. Physically, these will tend to be thin children with underdeveloped chests and slim arms (I should note that, while the other Kali remedies tend to be rather heavy, the Kali Phos patient can be quite slim). It is also the first cell salt remedy to consider for cases in which the young patient chronically wets the bed, especially if the urine is bright yellow in color. The same would hold true for cases of incontinence in elderly patients.

Kali Phos is also an important remedy for diarrhea, especially when the stool contains the bright yellow discharge that is keynote to the remedy type. The stool is painless and watery. It may occur while the patient is eating. (This is an important remedy for the symptoms associated with cholera.) The stool can be bloody, and will usually be accompanied by a loud discharge of gas. The stool will have the carrion smell associated with the remedy.

Because of this characteristic scent, remember Kali Phos as a good general cleansing remedy. It can be very helpful for those with chronic bad breath or body odor.

Modalities

The Kali Phosphoricum patient is better from rest, from peace and quiet, from attention and company. From feeling comforted and understood. They crave affection and understanding. They respond to touch, to sounds. The patient is better from eating and sleeping. From gentle motion—especially from walking, which can be a balm to the patient physically and emotionally. They are better from leaning on something or someone. Female patients are improved with the onset of their menses.

The Kali Phos is worse from excitement, from stress, from noise. They are worse from unpleasant touch, from being jarred. They are worse from physical, mental, or emotional exertion. They are worse from cold, worse from being trapped in warm, closed, or confined spaces, worse at night and in the early morning. They are worse when left alone.

Relationships

In headaches and in cases of hemorrhages (Kali Phos helps blood to coagulate), use in conjunction with or alternate with Natrum Muriaticum. Kali Phos is also highly complimentary with Magnesia Phosphorica and can be used in alternation with it for cases of female patients with PMS or irregular periods. Use with Mag Phos in cases involving incontinence and bladder issues as well. May be combined with or alternated with Ferrum Phos as a good general tonic to the whole being, physical and emotional.

Dosage and Potency

Schuessler used Kali Phos in all potencies, from the lowest to the highest, but found the 3X potency to be most effective. He repeated the remedy as needed and found that it repeated well for both acute and chronic cases. It is not a long-lasting remedy and therefore must be repeated often, especially in chronic conditions.

7. KALI SULPHURICUM

Overview

The remedy is taken from the chemical compound potassium sulfate or sulfate of potash, which is abundant in nature and found in such substances as lava. Simply put, the source of Kali Sulphuricum is a chemical salt that is created by a combination of potassium and sulfuric acid. Potassium sulfate's chemical formula is K_2SO_4. Although it may be soluble in water, depending upon its source, it is not soluble in alcohol. Like other cell salts, it is potentized through trituration.

As a sulfate-based remedy, Kali Sulphuricum relates to the flow of oxygen to the cells of the body. It is important, therefore, to cell nutrition and to new cell growth. It has a special affinity for the cells of skin, hair, and nails. It also displays an affinity for mucous membranes throughout the body. This remedy also has impact upon the process of respiration.

Those needing Kali Sulphuricum as a remedy most typically suffer from vertigo; palpitations; a sense of suffocation that makes them crave open or moving air; as well as an overall sense of weight, of heaviness, and of physical exhaustion. In addition, the general portrait of this remedy type includes such emotional and mental symptoms as chronic anxiety—anything from a vague sense of alarm to crippling panic, phobia, and deep dread—and sense of emotional weight as well, typified by a certain characteristic sadness often accompanied by tears and depression.

They tend toward pain as well. Toothache is common and this is a good acute remedy for toothache. Headaches are common. But Kali Sulphuricum is also known for pains in the limbs, especially pains in the neck, shoulders, and back. These pains typically wander about the body, shift suddenly and without warning. They are worse, as is the patient in general, at night and in an overly-warm room.

Kali Sulphuricum is an important remedy for colds, coughs, and flu, for any sort of upper respiratory infection.

The first color associated with this remedy is either yellow or greenish-yellow. Patients needing this remedy will have a slimy yellow coating on their tongues. This same color will dominate in all their secretions and discharges, especially mucous discharges.

The second color associated with this remedy, red, is typical of all Sulphur group remedies. Look for redness in all affected areas of the skin. All rashes are red and itchy. All conditions of the skin and mucous membranes will include heat, itch, and redness.

Just as Ferrum Phosphoricum, relates to the first stage of diseases, especially inflammations and infections, and Kali Muriaticum relates to the second stage when colorless/white discharges begin to occur, Kali Sulphuricum relates to the third and final stage of illness. This is the stage when mucous discharges change from colorless to the yellow/green that is keynote to the remedy. Therefore, Kali Sulphuricum often follows Kali Muriaticum (which itself may follow Ferrum Phos), especially in the treatment of patients with upper respiratory infections of all sorts.

Kali Sulph has the peculiar ability (as does Ferrum Phosphoricum, to a lesser

> Kali Sulph has the peculiar ability (as does Ferrum Phosphoricum, to a lesser degree) to make the patient sweat, and in this way it is an important remedy for detoxification of the body. In the same way, look for Kali Sulph to act as a catalyst for the patient's body to expel any sort of toxin, to increase the flow of mucous discharge from the nose, throat, and ears, in order to bring a swift conclusion to the third stage of illness and speed the patient's recovery.

degree) to make the patient sweat, and in this way it is an important remedy for detoxification of the body. In the same way, look for Kali Sulph to act as a catalyst for the patient's body to expel any sort of toxin, to increase the flow of mucous discharge from the nose, throat, and ears, in order to bring a swift conclusion to the third stage of illness and speed the patient's recovery.

In fact, Kali Sulphuricum is an important remedy to keep in mind for all patients who show a marked lack of reaction, who have a slow and sluggish immune response. Who do not respond or react to well-chosen remedies. A dose or two of Kali Sulph will often help other remedies work when they have not worked in the past.

Kali Sulphuricum relates strongly to two remedies that are part of Hahnemann's homeopathic pharmacy. The first is Pulsatilla, which shares with Kali Sulphuricum the sense of dread and suffocation in a warm room and the wandering nature of both the physical and emotional symptoms. The two remedies are so closely related that some homeopaths refer to Kali Sulph as "The Pulsatilla of the twelve tissue remedies." As Pulsatilla is a plant-based remedy, taken from the Anemone Pratensis, or "wind flower" and Kali Sulphuricum is a mineral-based remedy, the two offer practitioners a rather splendid choice between the quicker-acting Pulsatilla and the deeper, slower action of Kali Sulph. While the purpose of this book is to look at the cell salt remedies, it is important to note such parallels, as they offer students of the biochemical and homeopathic materia medica options for inclusion in their home kits. Pulsatilla and Kali Sulph are remedies of similar action but they are not completely interchangeable, so it would be a very good idea for those considering the use of Pulsatilla to first study it in the appropriate text covering the homeopathic remedies.

Kali Sulphuricum also relates to another potassium-based remedy that is not part of Schuessler's canon, Kali Bichromicum,* which shares with Kali Sulph the distinctive green/yellow color of its discharges and its importance as a remedy used during the third stage of an infection. Kali Sulphuricum is not used as often homeopathically as Kali Bichromicum, but it remains a key biochemical remedy.

The information we have on the clinical uses of Kali Sulphuricum come to us from Schuessler himself. It has not undergone provings by other homeopaths. As a remedy that is taken from a combination of potassium and sulfur, look for Kali Sulphuricum to display aspects of both remedy types. From the Kali group, Kali Sulph takes on its sense

---

* There are a full fifteen major potassium-based or Kali remedies in the homeopathic materia medica. They all share some aspect of the "potash" traits, such as a certain sluggishness, and sense of weight and/or dread. Each remedy remains unique, however, because it is a created from a chemical compound and carries with it the aspects of the other substance from which it was created. Indeed, a case could be made that a great many patients could find a valuable source of treatment just within this cluster of fifteen remedies. The actions of our Kali remedies are so wide and deep that at times they could make the other remedies seem unnecessary.

of weight, of dread, of torpor. From the Sulphur group, it takes its sense of itch, its craving for open, cool air, and its general warm-bloodedness. Like other sulfur-based remedies, Kali Sulph types are always worse from having to stand still for any length of time. They may be happy to be up and moving about or their pain may make them want to rest, but, either way, they will always be worse from having to stand up straight and having to stand still for any length of time. They will slump, they will lean, they will try to walk or sit or lie down. But they will not be happy just standing still.

Conditions that Suggest Kali Sulphuricum

Allergies and sinusitis; asthma; baldness(!); colds, coughs, and flu; colic; constipation; dandruff; diarrhea; digestive upset; eczema; flatulence; irritable bowel syndrome; pain in limbs, neck, and shoulders; poison ivy; psoriasis; rheumatism; ring worm; vertigo; whooping cough.

Mental and Emotional Symptoms

The Kali Sulphuricum patient is known for his or her changeability in terms of mood. He or she can change from seeming quite contented one moment to crying the next, apparently without cause. Kali Sulphs, like Kali Phos types, can leave others wondering what they have done to upset them.

And yet, the Kali Sulph types are less sensitive than the Kali Phos, less likely to ride a full roller coaster of emotions, and more likely to be given to long-term depression. They feel a sense of emotional weight, of being stuck in a state of anxiety, depression, and/or emotional exhaustion. They also do not display the pronounced sensitivity to their environment that Kali Phos types will, but instead will be sensitive only to temperature, to feeling too warm or too confined. They crave open, cool, or moving air and feel better in every way, emotionally and physically, for coming into contact with it. Their pains, again emotional and physical, will be exacerbated by entry into a warm, closed room.

Kali Sulphuricum types, especially young Kali Sulphs, tend to display a particular quirk. They will want specific things: specific toys, specific clothes, even specific foods. They will crave and crave these things and demand them, yet when they get them, they no longer want them. They may even throw the desired thing away from them as soon as they get it.

Kali Sulphs tend to be agitated. They are hurried, always rushing from one place to another, from one task to another. They say they are tired, that they want to lie down and rest, yet they never seem to. As soon as they lay down, they are back up again. Look for the Kali Sulph patient to complain that they feel worse when they are lying down and that their aches and pains or emotional upsets force them to rise up again.

Kali Sulph types tend to be startled easily. They tend to overreact to anything that they perceive as threatening in any way. They are jumpy, easily frightened. Young Kali Sulph types may burst into tears when startled.

Kali Sulphs are given to a specific fear of falling, which may manifest in many ways. For young Kali Sulph types, it may manifest in a fear that they will be dropped when they are held, so they may cry when held or clutch onto the person holding them. Adult Kali Sulphs fear heights, bridges, even airplanes, as all play upon their fear of falling. They will usually experience vertigo while in high places and will feel as if they will fly off into space if they get near the edge of a building or bridge. Some may fear that they will not be able to stop themselves from jumping if they get too close to the edge. Vertigo is a key component of this fear. They feel their whole world fly out of control when they are in high places.

Physical Symptoms

Potassium sulfate is a carrier of oxygen, so it enhances the strength of the cells of the whole body and encourages new cell growth. Therefore, those who have a deficiency of this compound display an unhealthiness that is most noticeable in their skin, hair, and nails. Those needing Kali Sulph as a remedy are given to rashes, especially those that are red, hot, and itchy (it is particularly helpful for those who suffer from poison ivy, especially if the discharge from the rash is watery and yellow), to weak and unhealthy finger and toenails, and to baldness or dandruff (also with the characteristic yellowish color). Think of this remedy for those with pronounced baldness in spots. (In cases of baldness, it is said to take a long time to work, but will encourage growth of new hair if given time.)

The skin may be ulcerated or not. If it is, the ulcers will likely ooze a watery yellow secretion. The skin is typically dry, hot, and itchy. Because this is a remedy that will, by its action, enhance and increase sweat, patients needing it will usually not be sweaty, but dry-skinned instead. They may suffer from such complaints as eczema, nettle-rash, psoriasis, seborrhea, or ring-worm, which typically appears on the scalp or in male patient's beards. Kali Sulph will soothe them all, and bring restored health to the skin, the hair, and the nails.

As an acute remedy, it is the first cell salt to think of for the treatment of poison ivy. There are, of course, other remedies in the homeopathic pharmacy that can be very helpful in treating those who have poison ivy. Perhaps most notable is the remedy made from the poison ivy plant itself, Rhus Toxicodendron.

Of all the cell salts, Kali Sulph is the best bet for those who chronically suffer from constipation, diarrhea, or, most important, from irritable bowel syndrome in which the patient alternates between constipation and diarrhea. The stool in the diarrhea stage will pass with much gas, will be liquid and yellow, and will have a very foul odor. Before the stool is passed, as the constipation stage ends, the patient's stomach will be tympanic, swollen, and tight. The patient will feel shooting or burning colicky pains that will indicate the oncoming bout of diarrhea. The diarrhea will strike without warning and the patient will feel better after the bout. In general, the patient will feel better after diarrhea and while moving from diarrhea into constipation and will feel worse as constipation builds and worst of all just before the built-up toxins are released from the body.

Note that since Kali Sulphuricum patients are often deeply allergic (as are many sulfur-based remedy types), their irritable bowel syndrome (IBS) is often linked to food allergies, especially to allergies to wheat and dairy. While the remedy may be very helpful to alleviating the symptoms of IBS, it often will not clear them away completely without the patient also making some changes in his or her diet. As with most Kali-type patients, the Kali Sulph type is often overweight. They are somewhat sluggish by nature and prone to fall into patterns of eating foods that are completely wrong for their systems. In these cases, indeed, in all cases of IBS, it is important to consider the lifestyle of the patient as a whole, especially their diet and exercise patterns. The patient should not simply be given a pill—homeopathic, biochemical, or otherwise—with the expectation that all will now be made well.

Kali Sulph patients are among our most allergic. This is an excellent remedy for those who suffer from chronic sinusitis (again, look not only at the yellow discharge, but also at the patient's diet, and his or her environments at home and work for indications of those things that might need to be changed), for those with seasonal allergies, and, of course, for those who suffer from coughs and colds when the symptoms match the remedy. Be careful in treating with this remedy to always consider that what you may think is a simple cold is in reality the tip of an iceberg of allergy. Kali Sulphs may often fool you. You will think that this is their third cold of the winter when, in reality, it is a chronic respiratory condition and not a cold at all. For cases of asthma, when the chest rattles with mucous and the discharge coughed up is yellow and thick and slimy, think of Kali Sulphuricum. For all cases of chronic allergies, when the color of the discharge matches and the patient is itchy, hot, sweaty or not, thirsty, and irritable, think of this remedy.

Think of this remedy as well in cases of allergy or sinus in which the patient has, over the years, lost his or her sense of smell and/or taste. Kali Sulph can restore both, as it encourages the clearing out of the sinuses and the free flow of yellowish mucus.

It should come as no surprise that those needing this remedy are often given to snoring and may snore very loudly. With the addition of Kali Sulph to their daily regimen and with prudent changes made to their diet and lifestyle, this remedy (along with those other changes) can dramatically reduce this tendency to snore, to the relief of the whole family.

Finally, like most cell salts, this is a great remedy for those with pain, especially chronic pain that shifts its location in the body from place to place without warning. Think of Kali Sulphuricum specifically for cases of rheumatic pains that get worse in the early hours of the new day; that wake the patient from a sound sleep around two or three in the morning, that force them out of bed and make them walk around the house, as only walking soothes their pain. For patients whose pains are worse when they stand still or lie down flat, who need to walk slowly to achieve a degree of comfort.

Modalities

Kali Sulphuricum patients are thirsty. They will crave cold drinks and be better from drinking them. They are worse from warm drinks and dread them.

They are always better from walking. They are worse from standing still and from lying down in a prone position.

They are worse in a warm room and better from going out into open or cool air. They are warm-blooded patients who will have a tendency to feel too hot and who will have their symptoms aggravated by becoming warm.

Their symptoms will be worse in the evening. They are especially worse in the late night, from midnight until 4:00 A.M., when all their pains and symptoms increase.

Relationships

Kali Sulph is highly compatible with Ferrum Phosphoricum and is often given following it to complete a cure. Note that both remedies, however, are appropriate for cases in which sweating is to be induced and, therefore, it might be necessary to alternate the two remedies or to choose between them.

It is also highly compatible with Silicea and the two may be alternated or follow each other in treatment.

Kali Sulph follows Magnesia Phosphorica well in cases of chronic pain. And it may be used in alternation with Kali Muriaticum in cases of a cold that lingers, a patient who is slow to recover, or a patient who suffers from myriad allergies. Natrum Muriaticum is also used in alternation with Kali Sulph for patients with chronic allergies.

Dosage and Potency

Schuessler used Kali Sulph in all potencies from 3X to 12X. It can be repeated as needed in potencies 6X and lower, but doses should be spaced out longer in higher potencies.

This is a long-acting remedy that is slow to act. One dose may continue to act for up to six weeks. Give this remedy as needed, following the symptoms. It is typically given two or three times a day in 3X or 6X until symptoms improve. When improvement begins, lower the dosage to once or twice a day until symptoms subside. Chronic conditions may require lengthy use of the remedy, as it is slow to work.

8. MAGNESIA PHOSPHORICA

Overview

This remedy, taken from the chemical compound phosphate of magnesia, with the complex chemical formula $HPO_4 \cdot 7H_2O$, is created by mixing phosphate of soda with sulfate of magnesia. The product of the mixture is a six-sided crystal with needlelike projections. The product is edible—in fact, it can be found in breakfast cereals and in beer—and has a sweet taste. It is soluble in water, although the cell salt remedy is created through the process of trituration.

Phosphate of magnesia is abundant in the human body. It is found in bones and teeth and in the spine marrow itself, and in the muscles, the nerves, and the grey matter of the brain. Human sperm is especially rich in phosphate of magnesia.

This is the sole magnesium-based remedy listed among the cells salts. While a trace element, magnesium is vital to the human system and only sodium, calcium, and potassium are more abundant in our bodily makeup. As any deficiency of magnesium leads to irritability of the nervous system, it stands to reason that this remedy will be important for those suffering disorders in the nervous system, and this certainly proves to be the case. The other chief component of the compound from which the remedy is made is phosphorus (another factor in building a healthy nervous system, by the way), so it also stands to reason that those needing the remedy are sensitive and somewhat high-strung. This also proves to be the case.

Magnesia Phosphorica could be considered to be Schuessler's greatest contribution to the homeopathic materia medica, as it has become a commonly used homeopathic remedy as well as a part of the biochemical pharmacy. Schuessler's own proving of the remedy was enhanced by another conducted by homeopath H.C. Allen. His study of the remedy's actions supported Schuessler's clinical findings and added to them.

Constantine Hering also added to our knowledge of this remedy and its uses. He said that Mag Phos was particularly helpful to young patients (which is something of a given, as all phosphorus-based remedies tend to be indicated for younger patients more than for older ones). Both Hering and Allen agreed that, while Mag Phos could be of use to "fleshy" patients, it is most often helpful to those who are thin, or as the homeopaths' put it, "emaciated."

Mag Phos is also often more commonly viewed as a women's remedy, because it is perhaps the first remedy to consider in cases of PMS, especially when the symptoms involve cramping pains that are relieved by the application of heat.

In fact, Mag Phos should be the first remedy considered for any case that involves cramping pains in any part of the body, whether that body is young or old, male or female. This is an excellent pain remedy in general, unless that pain in burning in nature (consider the sulfur-based remedies for burning pains, especially if they also involve itching). Consider Magnesia Phosphorica for pains that are darting in nature, that fly from place to place, that are lighteninglike in both their electrical feel and their speed of relocation, that feel as if they are boring into parts of the body, that are spasmodic. For spasms of any sort, in any part of the body, think of Mag Phos.

The pains associated with this remedy usually either begin on the right side of the body or are dominant there. They are made much worse from cold and are relieved by any sort of heat. Usually they are relieved by pressure as well. Look for the patient to have a spell of weakness or to experience a sudden, profuse sweat just before the onset of pain.

Among the cell salts, there is perhaps no better remedy than Mag Phos for children who are teething.

This alone should give you an indication of the mental and emotional symptoms associated with the remedy.

Conditions that Suggest Magnesia Phosphorica

Colic; convulsions; cramps; headaches and migraines; hiccoughs; neuralgia; pain; PMS; sciatica; toothache and teething pains; whooping cough; writer's cramp.

Mental and Emotional Symptoms

Mag Phos is, by and large, a remedy associated with pain. Those needing it are in the grip of pain, and are, therefore, complaining, lamenting, and wishing the pain on someone else. They can be self-pitying, angry, or changeable in their moods—alternating between anger and self-pity. They tend to be adverse to work and to thinking, because their pain interferes with their mental focus. They may be depressed, may have given up ever getting over their pain, as if it has come to form a physical wall around them that they cannot see over.

These are anxious patients, fretful. They are forgetful. Drowsy. They may give the impression that they will drift off to sleep. And yet their pain keeps them awake, even as it further exhausts them.

They tend to either be very talkative—usually about their own pains—or to sit silent. They are meditative patients. They cope with their pain by becoming extremely stoic.

They tend to have fears that are directly connected to their physical pain. They fear being touched (like those needing the homeopathic

> Mag Phos is, by and large, a remedy associated with pain. Those needing it are in the grip of pain, and are, therefore, complaining, lamenting, and wishing the pain on someone else. They can be self-pitying, angry, or changeable in their moods—alternating between anger and self-pity.

remedy Arnica, which is perhaps the premiere remedy for those with pain), they fear movement, and often fear that they will not be able to move, that they will be paralyzed by their pain.

Physical Symptoms

One word: pain. No other cell salt and, indeed, few homeopathic remedies in general are so associated with pain and so helpful for treating those who are in pain as is Magnesia Phosphorica.

Think of this remedy for those who have pain with any of the following characteristics: crampy, radiating, boring, shooting, or neuralgic. For those who suffer pains that run along a nerve in the body, like sciatica. For those who have severe pains in one small spot on their body, or whose pain shifts from place to place, moving along a nerve, or shifting from one area to another as if a charge of electricity had shot through them. For patients who have convulsions from their pain.

Mag Phos is also helpful for pain that occurs along with a sensation of a lump or ball at the site of the pain. Or if the affected area feels constructed, either externally or internally, as if tightened by a belt, a band or a hoop.

The pains associated with this remedy will tend to be more pronounced on the right side of the body. They may flow to the side of the body that is lain on. They may be so severe that the patient trembles when in pain. Facial tics and twitching of muscles may accompany pain. Any sort of trembling or shaking can be associated with this remedy. For this reason, it is a leading remedy for those who suffer from nystagmus, which is a trembling of the eyes or the convulsive shift of the eyes from side to side.

The pains associated with Mag Phos are worse at night, especially from 9:00 P.M. until 3:00 to 4:00 A.M. They may also be worse at 11:00 A.M. They are worse from the patient becoming cold, from cold in any form, cold air, cold water, cold wind. Patients will be much worse, especially, if their feet get cold and wet.

Two things improve the pain: warmth and pressure. Think of the patient with colicky cramps who presses a hot water bottle tight against her abdomen. This is the picture of Mag Phos. The patient wants to be warm, but especially want to have warm applications at the site of the pain. The patient with a toothache that responds to this remedy will want to hold hot water or other hot liquids in his mouth to soothe the pain. The patient with neuralgic pain will want to sit close to a lit fireplace or stove to soothe his pains.

Motion is another key to identifying the need for Mag Phos. It is not so much that motion actually improves the patient's pain as it is that rest makes it worse. These patients often will not be able to lie down at all while in pain, and sitting in a chair will be the best that they can do in order to rest. But most of the time they are driven to their feet by their pain and pace as long as the spell of pain lasts. Dance is somehow important to Mag Phos types (they love to dance as much as the Natrum Muriaticum loves to laugh), so you will even find them dancing as best they can while in pain. Rhythmic motion will help them cope with their pain.

Think of Mag Phos, along with Natrum Muriaticum, for patients who have headaches. Mag Phos headaches can be severe, and can recur periodically. This is an important remedy for patients who have migraines.

Think of this remedy first for patients who have a sensation of chill just before the onset of a migraine, whose hands or feet get cold before the pain begins. Or for patients who report that, just before the onset of a headache, they see sparks of light in front of their eyes, or who see auras of light around objects.

Think of Mag Phos for patients with headaches that sit above their eyes, headaches that are worse on the right side or that move from side to side, most often from right to left. Often, Mag Phos headaches will begin as a boring pain in one specific spot over the right eye and then will travel very quickly to the whole of the face, with the pain dominating in the forehead. But also think of this remedy for headaches that sit on the top of the head; that feel like a cap is pulled down tight on the head. Or for headaches that radiate pain to any part of the body. These pains, like others common to Mag Phos, have the quality of lightning to them. Also think of this remedy for headaches that begin in the back of the head and travel up over the skull to the forehead.

Migraines of this type are often accompanied by nausea. The patient may vomit from the pain of the headache. Note that hiccoughs may accompany the sense of nausea. The nausea may also be accompanied by cramping and shooting pains in the patient's abdomen.

No matter the particular symptoms of the headache, it will be improved by external applications of heat. Look for the patient to want to take a hot shower when he or she has a headache. Look for the patient to put hot applications on his or her head and then to press them hard against the head while the headache continues.

The headache pain will be improved by pressure, and patients will press against the painful part. They will also be improved by avoiding light, by pulling the blinds, and making the room as dark as possible. They will be improved by walking in the fresh air, and, if the day is not too bright, they will want to go out and take a walk to alleviate the pain.

Mag Phos headaches will tend to come on either between 10:00 A.M. and 11:00 A.M. or 4:00 P.M. and 5:00 P.M. These headaches can be severe and long-lasting. They can last hours or more than a day. Mag Phos patients given to migraines may lose days every month to the pain, days when they cannot work, cannot leave their darkened rooms.

The other use for this remedy that sets it apart is for female patients who suffer from PMS. Consider Magnesia Phosphorica for cases in which patients experience cramping pains throughout the abdomen just before the beginning of the menstrual flow. The pain can radiate from the abdomen to any other part of the body. The pain, as always for this remedy type, is relieved by external applications of heat and by pressure applied to the area of pain. Look for the patient to bend forward when in pain. The remedy is especially indicted if flatulence accompanies the pain.

For cases in which Mag Phos alone does not bring relief, alternate with Calcarea Phosphorica. Give both remedies in the 6X potency, Mag Phos before every meal and Calc Phos an hour after eating. This combination of remedies works for patients with any colicky pains associated with PMS, as long as the pains show the usual traits associated with the remedy—radiating pains that are improved by applications of heat and pressure; that can have any additional characteristic except for burning, which counter-indicates this remedy.

This is an excellent remedy for those who suffer from rheumatism or arthritis, as long as the pain associated with the condition matches the pains described for Mag Phos. While this remedy is most often associated with the right side of the body, in cases of arthritis or rheumatism either side of the body may be affected, or the pain may radiate from anywhere on the body, as long as that pain is improved by heat and by pressure (hard rubbing or putting the weight of the body on the painful area).

Think of this remedy for cases of arthritis or of pain in general that can be associated with what would loosely be called "writer's cramp." This is the remedy of first choice for any patient who has pain in his or her hands—however severe—that can be associated with spending long hours holding or using a tool, whether it is a keyboard, a chisel, or a violin. Magnesia Phosphorica can be dissolved in warm water in these cases,* and a washcloth soaked in the liquid can be applied to the painful areas of the body, especially the hands, to help speed relief. The remedy may be applied topically and taken orally at the same time.

When the hand pain and finger joint pain is accompanied by stiffness and numbness, think of Mag Phos first. It may be alternated with Calcarea Phosphorica if Mag Phos alone does not bring relief. Or the patient may take Calc Phos by mouth while applying dissolved pellets of Mag Phos directly to the hands. The best combination to bring relief can be found through exploration.

Mag Phos works well with the other phosphorus-based cell salt remedies in relieving pain. In cases involving chest pain, especially pains in the chest that radiate around to the back or down the sides into the hips and legs, alternate Mag Phos with Kali Phosphoricum to achieve relief and to calm the heart. Note that there can be many

---

* Note that some patients report that they receive a special benefit if they take the remedy Mag Phos orally after it has been dissolved in warm water or even in warm tea.

causes for chest pain, and the majority of them are not serious, but, when chest pains occur, it is important to see a doctor immediately to rule out any heart or circulatory issues that may be the source of the pain. Among the cell salts, Mag Phos stands out as the best remedy for those who suffer from angina pectoris.

I have already mentioned that Mag Phos can be helpful for those who suffer from toothache. This remedy can help tide you over until you can get to the dentist when you have a sudden toothache that is soothed by holding warm or hot liquids in the mouth. In chronic cases, this is the first remedy to consider for what may be more generally considered "mouth pain." For sensitive teeth that are aggravated when anything cold is eaten or drunk, or from inhaling cold air into the mouth. Consider this remedy for cases in which the sensitivity travels from tooth to tooth, or from one area of the mouth to another, or if the pain radiates from one painful tooth to the whole of the mouth or jaw.

This is our premiere cell salt remedy for those in pain. For those with cramping pains in their calves, most especially if that pain is accompanied by a sensation of twitching or shaking. When in pain, patients may feel a throbbing or twitching throughout their whole body. This is a great general remedy for those who suffer from chronic pain in the lower part of their body, from the abdomen downward. For those with sciatica, most especially when it also involves a feeling of sensitivity or tenderness in the feet.

Modalities

It hardly seems necessary to repeat that the Mag Phos patient is improved by heat, by pressure, and by bending over double when in pain. The patient is always better from a hot bath or shower and from rubbing the affected areas of the body. The patient may ask for a massage and will want to be rubbed hard.

Mag Phos patients are worse from cold in any form, from drafts. They are worse when they are uncovered and will want to keep affected areas of the body wrapped tight. They will tend to want to keep their feet covered, as a sensation of tenderness or sensitivity in the feet often accompanies their pain. The same sensation may extend to their hands as well.

Mag Phos patients are worse at night and pains increase at night. Their pain also grows worse as they become exhausted from dealing with it.

This is also a remedy of periodicity. This means that it may seem as if the patient's pain symptoms run on a schedule. Just as a female patient may experience PMS monthly, other Mag Phos patients may have a headache every week or every month, may have arthritis pains that are worse on alternating days. Any periodic pains should suggest Mag Phos as a remedy.

Relationships

As noted, Magnesia Phosphorica works well in conjunction with the other phospho-rus-based remedies, especially with Calcarea Phosphorica and Kali Phosphoricum for cases of patients with chronic pain.

Consider using Mag Phos alternating with Calcarea Phosphoricum for any cases involving toothache or the pain associated with teething in infants. This combination is helpful for any tooth or bone pain in which fever is not present. If fever is part of the picture, consider alternating Mag Phos with Ferrum Phosphoricum.

Mag Phos works very well with Natrum Sulphuricum for cases of colic and abdom-inal cramp that also involve flatulence and vomiting. This combination also works well for those with arthritic or rheumatic pains in the joints of the hand that involve trem-bling as well as pain.

Alternate Magnesia Phosphorica with Kali Muriaticum to bring relief to patients for whom hiccoughs are a chronic complaint, or when Mag Phos alone does not put an end to a case of hiccoughs.

Finally, Magnesia Phosphorica and Natrum Phosphoricum work well in tandem in cases of heartburn that are not cleared away by either remedy alone.

Dosage and Potency

Schuessler suggests that Mag Phos works best in the 6X potency, although all potencies are used.

This is a remedy that can be repeated as needed. It may have to be given repeat-edly, perhaps every half hour, in cases of severe pain. As with all other cell salts, decrease the dosage as the symptoms improve. This is a quick-acting remedy, but its effects are not long lasting. Therefore, repeat the dosage as needed.

9. NATRUM MURIATICUM

Overview

By the time you finish studying Natrum Muriaticum you will wonder why any other remedies are necessary. This single remedy, taken from sodium chloride, the salt that is sitting on your dining table right now, is one of the most important of all remedies, homeopathic or biochemical. Its chemical formula is $NaCl$. As a chemical compound, it is so abundant in nature that it may be easier to list the places where it is not found than the places where it is.

Sodium chloride is easily dissolved in water and can be potentized either by the process of dilution or by trituration. However, there are those who insist that, as a cell salt remedy, the Natrum Muriaticum remedy created by the process of trituration—as the other cell salts are—is more potent than the remedy that is created by simple dilution.

The function of sodium chloride in the body is to regulate the amount of fluid in cells. It is part of the vital function of fluid balance because is has the ability to draw and retain fluid, to attract water, which is vital to the process of cell division.

While the majority of the cell salt remedies were first produced as biochemical remedies by Schuessler and then went on to become part of the homeopathic pharmacy, Natrum Muriaticum was first created as part of the homeopathic materia medica. Hahnemann himself created the remedy and proved its clinical uses. It was one of the most important and most used homeopathic remedies before Schuessler borrowed it for his biochemical treatments, and it remains so today.

Indeed, just as the substance from which it is made is among the most abundant in nature, both inside and outside of our own bodies, the need for the remedy Natrum Mur is ubiquitous among patients. Among the homeopathic remedies, it is said that Natrum Mur will elicit a curative response in more patients than any other remedy. Along with Sulphur and Arnica, it has earned its place among polycrests (remedies of the first order of importance) in the materia medica.

In short, this is a highly versatile remedy.

Think of Natrum Mur for any patient who suffers from edema, from bloating or from swelling in any part of the body. For the patient with high blood pressure, especially those patients with hypertension caused by an overabundance of salt in their diet. For patients who crave salt in their diet, crave the taste.

Natrum Mur relates to patients who have poor nutrition, whose bodies lack the ability to take nourishment from their diet or whose diet itself is bad, filled with refined foods and salt and sugar, and not enough nutritional value to sustain good health. Therefore, look for Natrum Mur patients to have digestive disorders of all sorts. Their muscles are underdeveloped or atrophied. Their bodies may be emaciated or swollen. They are weak, although they have a good appetite and eat heartily. They are among our most thirsty patients. They will tend to want nothing more than to lie down, especially after they have eaten.* They may have spells after eating in which they feel faint. This sense of dizziness may be linked to emotions, especially to strong emotions, to being in crowded rooms, or from emotional and/or physical stress.

---

* This need to lie down is keynote to the remedy and runs through the patient's physical and emotional symptoms alike. The Natrum Mur will want to lie down and rest after coming into contact with the heat of the sun; after having had sex; after eating; after coming into contact with company; after emotional upset; after being made to feel sentimental by music, photographs or talking about memories of old times; and also during spells of pain, especially chronic back or joint pain or headache. The Natrum Mur will see lying on his or her bed not just as a nice idea but as a panacea. They will be improved in every way if they are allowed to lie down. For their sake and for everyone else's it is a good idea if you let them.

This is a remedy type in which the emotional symptoms and physical symptoms are intertwined, and in which the emotional symptoms are every bit as important as the physical. These are patients who present themselves as being indifferent. Indifferent to things that are, in truth, important to them. Indifferent to love. Indifferent to their own family. They are patients who cover a sense of hurt or betrayal with a mask of indifference. And yet, internally, they cling to their sense of hurt, of vulnerability, and, quite often, of anger at having been hurt or betrayed. They are patients with a strong sense of right and wrong, of loyalty and betrayal, who trust slowly and take great pains to make sure that their trust is never betrayed.

Think of the effect that salt has in the human body and you will understand the remedy itself. Salt absorbs, retains. Salt causes the body to retain water, which, in turn, raises blood pressure and causes bloating and swelling in the system. In the same way, patients needing Natrum Mur retain. They retain emotional hurts and slights, glowering over them internally while presenting a mask of indifference. Physically, they retain their aches and pains, while again presenting a mask that suggests that all is well. They are patients who are slow to seek help for their ailments, both because they are slow to trust and treatment involves some degree of self-revelation and of trust, and because in their stoic state of indifference they are slow to admit that their illness will not simply resolve itself if they continue on as if all is indeed well.

> The typical Natrum Muriaticum is stubborn, just as his or her physical symptoms can be very stubborn. This is a remedy for those who suffer from chronic complaints, from headaches that can come to rule the patient's life, from allergies—with the very peculiar keynote that the allergies that respond best to Natrum Mur are to those things that the patient loves most: Natrum Muriaticum patients will tend to develop allergies to beloved pets, favored foods or vacation spots, especially if they are by the sea.

The typical Natrum Muriaticum is stubborn, just as his or her physical symptoms can be very stubborn. This is a remedy for those who suffer from chronic complaints, from headaches that can come to rule the patient's life, from allergies—with the very peculiar keynote that the allergies that respond best to Natrum Mur are to those things that the patient loves most: Natrum Muriaticum patients will tend to develop allergies to beloved pets, favored foods or vacation spots, especially if they are by the sea. This is also a remedy for chronic pain, pain that follows the sun, as we shall see. Pain in the bones, the joints, the glands; pain that can be pressing, pinching or paralyzing in nature; pain that can seem internal or external, that can leave patients feeling merely bruised, as if they have been beaten, or all but paralyzed in their agony.

This is the remedy of choice for old injuries, old ailments that never quite heal, but return periodically to plague the patient. This is a remedy that seems filled with contradictions—it is the remedy of the absent-minded individual who never forgets a slight, but fails to retain much else. It is the remedy for the proper lady who laughs loud at a dirty joke. Who laughs in public but goes into her room to cry. Who presents a mask of emotional invulnerability but fears embarrassment above all else.

Natrum Muriaticum excels as a remedy for those with chronic complaints, but it is an excellent acute remedy as well. There is no better remedy for digestive distress, especially after overeating, and most especially when accompanied by hiccoughs. There is no better remedy for the first stage of colds, especially when the first symptoms of a cold coming on are fits of sneezing. On the emotional level, there is no better cell salt to give when delivering some very bad news. It is also the best remedy for those who have had their hearts broken.

Conditions that Suggest Natrum Muriaticum

Anemia; back, bone, and joint pain; claustrophobia; colds, coughs, and flu; constipation; depression; diabetes; diarrhea; eyestrain; fainting spells; fever; goiter (imbalance of the thyroid of any sort); gout; grief; headaches; heart disorders, especially tachycardia and palpitations; heartburn and general indigestion; herpes, fever blisters, and canker sores; hiccough; involuntary urination; irritable bowel disorder; menopause and menstrual disorders; nearsightedness; skin conditions: corns, eczema, hives, nettle rash, ringworm, scars, warts; sleepwalking; sunstroke; varicose veins; yawning.

Mental and Emotional Symptoms

Foremost of all the emotional states that make up the complex Natrum Muriaticum psyche is grief. There is no more powerful remedy in either the biochemical or homeopathic pharmacies for those who grieve. Natrum Muriaticum is especially indicated in cases of long-term grief, or grief that has become confused with betrayal in the mind of the patient. It is often called the widow's remedy, and is most especially indicated for widows who feel as if they have been deserted by their dead mates.*

This is the first remedy to consider in any case that involves the loss of love, whether that loss comes about through death, desertion, or through the sundering of a relationship. It is especially helpful for cases in which physical illness, most often

---

* Note that the homeopathic remedy Igantia Amara is also often used in cases of grief. However, it is indicated for the emotional upset and roller coaster of emotions associated with the first stages of grief, soon after the death or desertion has occurred. Natrum Mur is more often indicated for cases of long-held grief, when life has been paralyzed and the patient has failed to move forward since the moment of loss. Therefore, in the homeopathic pharmacy, Natrum Mur is considered to be the chronic or constitutional version of the acute remedy Ignatia.

allergies, headache, or more generalized bone or joint pains come on after a loss of love.

Love is a tricky thing for Natrum Murs. They crave it and avoid it in equal measure. This is the remedy for the young person, the teenager, who loves with his or her whole heart, is hurt as a result, and consequently suffers a loss of innocence and trust. For those who love unwisely, especially when it becomes a chronic issue. For those who cling to their love long after the relationship has ended, who can become obsessive in their love, or who can become obsessed with a certain type of individual that they seek out, knowing how the relationship will end before it begins. For those who love unwisely, those who get involved with married people, not just once, but again and again.

It is also the remedy for those who, having been hurt, never love again. For those who transfer their feelings from individuals to causes and cultures, for those who transfer their feelings to animals, especially house pets, to whom they become too attached. For those who grieve over the loss of an animal companion as deeply as the loss of a human companion.

In their grief, Natrum Mur patients present to the world as placid a face as they can muster. They grieve in silence, in private. They cry in private and become very embarrassed if they are caught in the act of grieving, especially if they are caught crying.* They feel at their most emotionally vulnerable when they are crying. (Note that the issue of crying is key to this remedy for grief. One should also consider this remedy for cases in which the patient *never* cries, no matter how deeply he or she feels the loss of love. For the patient whose tears are held deep inside, never to be released, not even when the patient is alone. It is the most important remedy—homeopathic or biochemical—for cases of grief in which the grief itself has been deeply suppressed and never dealt with at all.)

It is an important symptom of their emotional being that Natrum Muriaticum patients do not want to be consoled. They can grow quite angry when they are told that another person knows how they feel—Natrum Murs, in their grief, are quite certain that they do not. They can react with either anger or a surprising indifference when they are comforted and told they are cared for, and that their wellbeing is important to another person. Most often, this sudden emotional retreat has to do with the fact that Natrum Murs fear they will cry if they hear such things, and therefore stop anyone from saying them. Whatever the reason, Natrum Murs do not want to be comforted or fussed over in any way.

---

* Tears are, in general, an important thing to Natrum Muriaticum patients. They want to control their tears, hold them back when in public, only to cry a great deal in private. In the same way, they cry when they laugh, tears stream down their face. Note that this issue with tears connects to the more general issue that the Natrum Mur tends to have with the loss and retention of fluids. They may also urinate involuntarily, especially when they laugh. The colds and allergies associated with the remedy also involve the flow both of tears and of copious amounts of mucus.

On the other hand, they want with all their hearts to be made to laugh. Laughter is the only loss of emotional control that is actually welcomed by typical Natrum Murs. They often exhibit a most unexpected pedestrian or bawdy sense of humor. And, as has been noted, they tend to lose physical control over their body fluids when they laugh. Their eyes may tear, their noses may run, and they may slightly lose control of their bladders as well. For the Natrum Mur, whose central issues involve retention, laughter is a blessed release. No matter how depressed, withdrawn, or indifferent he or she may seem, the Natrum Mur will welcome laughter with a childlike glee.

Natrum Mur types are easy to anger, easy to fright. They will have dreams that upset them, dreams from which they awaken afraid. They dream of robbers, of things being taken from them.

On the emotional plane, this is a remedy for phobias as well, especially for claustrophobia. Natrum Mur patients will feel as if they will faint if they are trapped in too small a place. They will panic, their hearts will race, they will sweat from fear just as their eyes tear from laughter—again, abrupt emotion has the physical result of the release of retained fluids.

Natrum Mur types present a mask of indifference to the world and will often insist that they wish to be left alone. They may physically withdraw from the world, often simply taking to their beds as they do in times of physical pain. And yet, deep within, Natrum Murs seek love, crave love, and desire nothing more than an emotional connection with the world. This complexity makes Natrum Mur types unknowable in some ways, as they will not reveal their needs or wants and yet may expect those around them to know them well enough to give them what they need. This can create friction in the household—the Natrum Mur is further hurt by what he or she interprets as a lack of caring by others who simply don't understand or see the need at hand. As a result, the Natrum Mur becomes increasingly angry or withdrawn, without anyone else (and perhaps even the Natrum Mur himself or herself) knowing why.

At times it can take a keen understanding of human nature to see the need for Natrum Mur as a remedy. Often it is given to patients based upon what they will not say or admit rather than by what they will. Natrum Mur types usually insist that they are quite well, that they do not understand why their friend or loved one has insisted they seek treatment; that they are only doing so for the sake of others and to keep peace in the household.

Only in simple acute cases do Natrum Mur patients admit their misery and ask for help. Even in these cases, their tendency is to want to simply withdraw, go to bed, and be left alone to suffer. Those who fuss over these patients do so at their own peril. When they are acutely ill just send them to bed, give them plenty of liquids and a very funny movie to watch, and they will be fine.

Physical Symptoms

Where to begin? Starting with the top of the head and working down, think of this remedy (along with Magnesia Phosphorica, which may be alternated with Natrum Mur if the symptoms suggest that it should) as the leading cell salt remedy for those with headaches. For those given to migraines. This is a great remedy for those who suffer from periodic headaches, such as headaches in female patients that accompany their monthly menstrual cycle. For those who suffer from pounding headaches, headaches that are congestive in nature and usually located in the forehead or in the temples. For headaches that accompany constipation, especially if both are chronic conditions.

For acute headaches, think of Natrum Mur for headaches that come on after the patient has been in the sun too long, or for headaches from eyestrain, reading too much, or close work like sewing. Tears will accompany the headache in these cases.

These patients will, as always, want to lie down while they have their headaches. They will be improved from sleeping and are often worse in the morning, only to grow even worse as the sun rises in the sky. Headaches that are worse in the day, better at night. Headaches accompanied by photophobia.

Alternate Natrum Mur and Calcarea Phosphorica for cases of headache in which the pain is so bad that the patient vomits water or clear, thick fluid. Alternate the two remedies if headaches are accompanied by twitching.

Think of Natrum Mur for headaches that begin with or are accompanied by a sensation of gauze in front of the eyes, when the vision dims, or when there is a discharge from the eyes, either tears or a clear, thick mucous discharge, that accompanies the headache pain. (Think of this remedy for congestive headaches caused by or accompanying the symptoms of nasal allergy. For these cases, the remedy Kali Sulphuricum may be alternated with Natrum Mur.)

This is an excellent remedy for dry eye, for eyes that are chronically irritated, dry, and red, with itching and burning pains, especially if these symptoms accompany chronic allergies. This is also the first cell salt to think of in cases of conjunctivitis. For pain in the eyes that is accompanied by itching, burning, and redness.

It is one of our best general remedies for those who suffer from allergies.* For old,

---

* There is a special trait to the Natrum Mur allergy: Natrum Murs can develop an allergy suddenly and without warning. These patients inevitably become highly allergic to something—a beloved pet cat, or a food, such as bread—that they dearly love, forcing them to have to separate from it. This not only reinforces the Natrum Mur issue with love and betrayal, it also further separates them from those around them. They retreat further into themselves and their rooms as the symptoms of their allergies increase both their physical discomfort and their sense that happiness and affection of any sort can only have a bad outcome.

chronic cases in which the patient has lost the sense of smell and taste. For colds that begin with wild bouts of sneezing followed by a flow of thick, clear fluid, like raw egg white. For patients who speak with a nasal tone because their noses and sinuses are completely blocked. For allergic symptoms that involve the ears, with a feeling of congestion in the ears, a roaring in the ears. A cracking sound in the ears when the patient chews. The patient will yawn, perhaps constantly and chronically, to try to open his or her ears. The patient's sense of hearing, as well as smell, taste, and sight, might be partially shut down by the symptoms of allergy.

Natrum Mur patients, especially those suffering from chronic complaints, will often have faces that reveal their need for this remedy. They have dry mucous membranes. Often their skin is greasy in parts and very dry in others. Look for their lips to be very dry, often cracked; their foreheads to be greasy and shiny. Their throats and mouths are dry, so they are thirsty, constantly thirsty for cold things, especially for cold water. Natrum Mur types are given to fever blisters and cold sores on their lips and in their mouths. This is the leading cell salt remedy for herpes occurring in any part of the body. In general, there is a look of unhealthiness about their skin, especially on their faces.

Think of Natrum Mur for cases of heartburn from overeating when the patient wants to lie down and rest, and in cases of chronic digestive disorders that involve constipation, heartburn, and headache, especially when the patient's diet consists of wheat (Natrum Murs love bread, especially bread and butter), salt (they may actually salt their bread and butter), sugar, alcohol (especially wine), and processed foods. Natrum Murs are often not big meat eaters, preferring carbohydrates, pasta, and especially bread and potatoes to red meat.

In digestive distress, the Natrum Murs will combine heartburn with palpitations or racing of the pulse, which will be improved if they lie down. They will belch and/or hiccough, will experience a flow of stomach acid in their throats. Commonly, the Natrum Mur with chronic digestive disorders will sweat on his or her face while eating. The Natrum Mur will typically feel better when his or her stomach is empty, but will be unable to resist his or her hunger and will not only eat, but overeat.

Natrum Murs come in all shapes and sizes, all ages and genders, but often they may surprise you that they are not heavier, given the amount of food they eat and the high-caloric foods they prefer.

Always, with this hunger, is a great thirst. Natrum Mur patients want cold drinks, not hot. They want things that will quench their thirst. They like sweet drinks, iced tea, sodas, even a cold beer, but will always tend to prefer cold water to anything else.

This is an important remedy for female patients who have lost all interest in sex. Who have an aversion to sex and to the opposite sex. For women who suffer from a painful dryness of the vagina, which can make intercourse painful. For young girls who have a delayed onset of their menses. (This is another remedy for those who are late in achieving life's milestones: late in speaking, late in walking, and, in this case, late in the onset of the monthly cycle.) It is also an important remedy in cases of female infertility.

Note that Natrum Mur also has its uses in the sexual sphere for male patients. It is a remedy for men who have seminal emissions after sex has taken place or during the night. It can also be an important remedy for male patients with impotence or delayed orgasm.

Finally, Natrum Muriaticum is an important remedy for those who suffer pain, especially chronic pain. For arthritis and gouty arthritis. For pain in any part of the body, but especially in the arms, legs, and knees. Dry skin in the affected parts can be an indicator of the need for Natrum Mur, as can the chronic appearance of hangnails. Pain will be accompanied by numbness and tingling. Parts of the body easily "go to sleep" if the patient puts his or her weight against them. The affected parts, especially the legs and feet, will feel chronically cold as well. The muscles in the legs, especially the hamstrings, feel tight, too short, and weak, as if they could not hold up the body. The patient's ankles may feel weak, may "turn" easily. This is the first remedy to think of for cases of old injuries to joints, especially the knees and ankles, that have never healed properly and that continue to be reinjured and grow weaker with each new trauma. This is also the first remedy to think of in cases involving pain in and between the toes—especially in cases of gout in the big toe.

The affected joints, especially the knees, will crack when the patient moves them. Think of this remedy for cases of arthritis in the finger joints when the joints crack loudly and the pain is accompanied by hot and sweaty palms.

This is an excellent remedy for lumbago, for chronic lower back pain, especially in men of middle age or older who carry their weight in their stomachs and, as a result of weakened abdominal muscles, weaken and injure their backs. Their pain, of course, improves when they lie down, especially if they lie down on a very firm mattress or even on the floor. Think of this remedy for any case of back pain in which the patient can stoop quite easily and fluidly, but then cannot straighten his back to stand up again. Look for the patient to hold his back with his hands, to put pressure on his back in order to move about.

Modalities

Natrum Mur patients are better, in general, from any fluid flow from their bodies: from sweating, from crying, from nasal discharge. They are better from bathing, from being in cool air, and from fasting (even though they will not want to). They are better if they

skip a meal. (Indeed, Natrum Murs are usually better in general from not doin,
they want to do and instead doing what is better for them: from avoiding the love .d-
tionships they are drawn to, the foods they crave, and the emotional habits they
choose.) They are better from clothing that fits rather snugly and supports them. They
are better from sleeping and should be allowed to lie down and rest in peace and quiet.
They are usually better from applying pressure or by rubbing any affected parts of their
bodies. They are always better from laughing.

They are worse from too much time in the sun, although they may crave it, especially because it will help them sweat. They are worse from being by the seashore,
although they usually desire to be there. They are worse in the daytime, especially from
9:00 A.M. to 11:00 A.M., although they are improved in the early morning, before
breakfast and the beginning of the day. They are worse from any sort of emotional disruption, from feeling deep or passionate emotions, and from any sort of consolation or
sympathy. They are worse from too much noise. They are worse at the time of the full
moon.

Relationships

Natrum Muriaticum can be used in alternation or combination with either Kali Sulphuricum or Kali Muriaticum for cases of allergies and colds that involve the ears, the
eustachian tubes, and the hearing. Alternate or use in combination with Calcarea
Phosphorica for headaches in those who are high strung or emotionally passionate. Use
in combination with or alternating with Magnesia Phosphorica for chronic headaches
or migraines. Also use with Mag Phos in cases of chronic headache in female patients
when the headaches are tied to the monthly cycle, usually just before the onset of the
flow. Think of Natrum Phos and Ferrum Phosphoricum in alternation at the onset of
upper respiratory complaints.

For cases of long-term grief, alternate Natrum Muriaticum with Calcarea Phosphorica. Do not give either remedy too often in these cases, but allow each dose to act
before either repeating it or alternating to the other remedy.

Dosage and Potency

Despite its humble origins in terms of chemical compounds, Natrum Muriaticum is a
deep-acting and long-lasting remedy. One dose may act for up to forty days. Schuessler
most often suggested that Natrum Mur be given in 6X potency, although it is commonly given in 3X and 12X potencies as well. Note that, as a homeopathic remedy, it is
used in all potencies from lowest to highest. It may be repeated as needed in acute conditions. However, in chronic cases, it should not be given too often and may work best
in alternation with other cell salt remedies.

10. NATRUM PHOSPHORICUM

Overview

Sodium phosphate, also called "phosphate of soda," has a chemical formula of $Na_2HPO_4 \cdot 12H_2O$ in its sodium phosphate, dibasic dodecahydrate form. The substance is abundant in the human body and is found in the corpuscles of the blood, and muscles and nerve tissue, as well as in the brain and in intercellular tissues. In nature, it is found in sea water, in saline springs, and salt lakes. It is present in bone ash. It is insoluble in alcohol but is soluble in warm water. However, the cell salt is made through the process of trituration.

The remedy Natrum Phosphoricum was proven by homeopath E. A. Farrington, and clinically tested by Schuessler who noted that, as a phosphorus-based remedy, it is of particular value to young patients—with infants, Schuessler used this remedy in a 1X potency—and in those whose ailments are the result of a buildup of acid (particularly lactic acid) in their system. It is also valuable for conditions caused by an overabundance of acid in the system, like gout, where the acid in question is uric acid.

Therefore, Natrum Phosphoricum is, among the cell salts, the best remedy to use in cases of gout, although Natrum Muriaticum is perhaps more helpful in cases of long-term gout. The two remedies may be used in alternation in stubborn cases.

Much of the action of this remedy will suggest that it is phosphorus based. Not only does it have an affinity for youth, but it also has some of the modalities that often suggest Phosphorus. The Natrum Phosphoricum patient is sensitive, like the Phosphorus. He or she will tend to be afraid of the dark, will be fearful, and will have his or her symptoms aggravated when a thunderstorm approaches.*

But Natrum Phosphoricum is taken from a chemical compound that also includes sodium, so many of the traits associated with sodium-based remedies will be apparent as well. The inorganic salt that is the basis of the remedy is used by the human body to regulate the amount of water in the blood and to balance the amount of other fluids in the body, including bile and pancreatic juices. It also keeps these fluids at the proper consistency and functions to maintain the proper acid and alkaline balance. Therefore, a state of acidity—one that can be very unhealthy for the total system—is a chief indicator for the need of this remedy.

---

* The homeopathic remedy Phosphorus, while not a cell salt, is related to several of our cell salt remedies in that the substance phosphorus is part of the chemical compound from which the cell salt is created. Thus, you will find that attributes of the homeopathic type will cross over into the symptom picture of the cell salts that contain phosphorus. Most patients needing these related remedies, for instance, will tend to be young, sensitive, worse from cold, and better from warmth, comfort, and attention.

The acid state can unleash a number of symptoms, from indigestion linked to sour belching and vomiting to diarrhea, cramping pains, and joint pains and body aches. The color that indicates the need for the remedy is yellow. The patient's discharges are yellow and sour. The discharges, most typically urine, will also burn, as they are acidic. The patient's skin can take on a yellowish tinge as well, as can the whites of the eyes.

Natrum Phosphoricum does not have the widest range of uses of any of the cell salts. Its uses are rather narrow in terms of range, as they tend to fall into one of two camps: either the patient suffers from chronic digestive disorders that are based upon an abundance of acid in his or her system, or the patient is suffering from pain that can be lumped within the diagnoses of arthritis or, more commonly, gouty arthritis. Either way, overacidity plays an important part in the cause of the symptoms, making Natrum Phosphoricum a vital remedy among the cell salts.

> Natrum Phosphoricum does not have the widest range of uses of any of the cell salts. Its uses are rather narrow in terms of range, as they tend to fall into one of two camps: either the patient suffers from chronic digestive disorders that are based upon an abundance of acid in his or her system, or the patient is suffering from pain that can be lumped within the diagnoses of arthritis or, more commonly, gouty arthritis. Either way, overacidity plays an important part in the cause of the symptoms, making Natrum Phosphoricum a vital remedy among the cell salts.

Acidosis is the general medical term for an overabundance of acid in the human system. It most often is broken down into to two major categories, although other forms of acidosis are possible. The first is "respiratory acidosis," in which the lungs fail to remove all the carbon dioxide from the body. This disrupts the acid-alkaline balance in the body (a human body must maintain a pH reading between 7.35 and 7.45 to be considered healthy). Respiratory acidosis can be chronic, which takes a long time to develop, or it can be acute. In chronic cases, it can be caused by such diverse diseases as asthma, scoliosis, or even by chronic overweight. In these cases, the body compensates for the increased acidity by having the kidneys work overtime to produce chemicals that restore the acid-alkaline balance and a stable condition usually results. Acute conditions are much more dangerous, because carbon dioxide is quite suddenly not being removed from the body in sufficient amounts and the kidneys are not given sufficient time to restore balance. Symptoms of either acute or chronic respiratory acidosis include lethargy, mental confusion, shortness of breath, and an almost overwhelming sleepiness.

The other most common form of acidosis is called "metabolic acidosis," and refers to an overacidic state of the blood. It can, like respiratory acidosis, be a rather simple, stable condition or it can be quite serious, even life threatening. It can be caused by such underlying conditions as diabetes or kidney failure, or as a side effect of taking some allopathic drugs, even some simple, over-the-counter medications like aspirin. Like that patient with respiratory acidosis, the patient with metabolic acidosis also tends to be lethargic, sleepy, and confused. But look for him to have a unique characteristic breathing pattern that is rapid and shallow.

While these two broad categories of acidosis are those most commonly accepted by allopathic practitioners, naturopaths, nutritionists, and homeopaths alike agree that more and more patients are displaying the signs of chronic acidosis. Their diets and environments are increasingly filled with toxins, and their bodies are having more and more difficulty in removing these toxins from their systems. As a result patients' bodies are ever more acidic and therefore ever more vulnerable to diseases of all sorts.

Overacidity can be linked to myriad conditions because an overabundance of acid forces the body to react in one of two ways, neither of which can be considered healthy or can be maintained long-term while still keeping the body's systems in order. Once acid levels reach the point that the excess can no longer be excreted from the body (most often in urine or sweat), the body will attempt to balance itself. One way it does this is by entering into a state of "autotoxification," in which it begins to store the acid in body tissue. An example of this is gout. Gout is caused when the body stores excess uric acid crystals in body fat, until that storage tissue is filled. At that point the acid crystals are stored in the joints, resulting in the swelling and pain associated with the disease.

Another way the body tries to cope with overacidity is through the process of "buffering." In this case it "borrows" important minerals—mostly sodium, calcium, magnesium, and potassium—from elsewhere in the body to neutralize the acids in the system. The first process results in a toxic system that is filled with poisons that have been stored as safely as possible for minimal damage to the vital organs. The second results in the depletion of the whole of the body, and its ability to fight disease and its overall functions are weakened. Either way, the presence of excess acid in the human system can lead to chronic weakness, illness, and an early death. The body's need to rid itself of toxins and in doing so, maintain a healthy acid-alkaline balance is paramount to well-being.

Therefore, while the actions of the remedy Natrum Phosphoricum may not be as dramatic or wide-ranging as those of other cell salts, they are vital to the health of the body. When it is called for, Natrum Phos stands alone as the remedy that can create that vital balance between acid and alkaline.

Conditions that Suggest Natrum Phosphoricum

Acidosis; arthritis; constipation (chronic); goiter; gout; heartburn; indigestion; postnasal drip (chronic); rheumatism; stomach upset; worms and other parasites.

Mental and Emotional Symptoms

Like all sodium-based remedies, Natrum Phosphoricum carries with it a degree of indifference that can either mask or tamp down the usual emotional sensitivity that you will find in a phosphorus-based remedy. Therefore Natrum Phosphoricum types will tend to display their sensitivity on a physical level, and will be very sensitive to changes in the weather, especially to an oncoming storm, and to changes in temperature, with their tendency toward a lack of vital heat.

An exception to this can be music. Just as laughter can open the floodgates of emotion for Natrum Muriaticum types, music can break through the wall of indifference that surrounds many Natrum Phos types. They can become quite restless when listening to music, quite agitated. Music can also unlock deep emotions, particularly deep sorrow. Natrum Phos patients may cry when they hear music that moves them.

The Natrum Phosphoricum, like other Natrums, is fearful, however, and most often this fear is placed in the future, in the inescapable feeling that something bad is about to happen. Therefore, while it is not a remedy for the patient who is as depressed as the Natrum Muriaticum patient can be, it is a remedy for the patient who experiences free-form anxiety. This is a patient who may experience a low-level form of anxiety at all times, although the sense of anxiety can become more pronounced at night. Night terrors are common to the type, as are nightmares and fear of the dark. These patients will also hear footsteps at night, see ghosts, monsters, and the like. They will insist that the shape of furniture they see in a darkened room is the shape of hiding people or monsters. They fear intruders.

The Natrum Phos can also show the same emotional and mental symptoms as the patient suffering from acidosis: a certain sluggishness of thought, a sense of confusion, a certain dullness in both mind and spirit.

While Natrum Muriaticum types will want to lie down, Natrum Phos types will want to sit. They are disinclined to walk, to exercise, and will like nothing more than to sit quietly.

Physical Symptoms

In its use as a remedy for physical symptoms, Natrum Phosphoricum is first and foremost a remedy for those with indigestion. It can replace any over-the-counter antacid, especially for those who have to chew antacids every day of their lives. It is a powerful remedy—both in acute and chronic cases—for those whose digestion is overly acidic. For those who have indigestion that includes heartburn, belching with a sour or acid taste, and nausea that may be accompanied by a sick headache. For those who regularly have heartburn that begins two to three hours after eating, or that is made worse by eating fatty foods. Especially from eating meals containing butter, milk, sour foods, vinegar, fatty foods, and cold drinks (which may at first soothe the condition, only to aggravate it later, even causing the patient to vomit, once they are warmed in the stomach). They are among the most sensitive patients when it comes to sugar. They are aggravated by sugar and should avoid it. Therefore, foods like ice cream, which are cold, fatty, dairy, and sugar-based, are the foods that will most greatly aggravate the Natrum Phos patient's condition and should be totally avoided.

Consider this remedy for cases in which indigestion is accompanied by a sense of heat in the abdomen, chest, and throat; that may also be accompanied by a flushing of the face, which is red and hot. (Note that even if the whole of the face is red, the area around the nose and, especially, the mouth, will stay very pale, even white.)

Consider Natrum Phos first for cases of indigestion that also involve chronic constipation that only very occasionally alternates with a single, sudden bout of diarrhea. The diarrhea, caused by an excess of acid, will result in a stool that is jelly-like, mucus-filled, and painful to pass. It will be sour smelling and green or greenish-yellow in color.

For cases of chronic indigestion, especially those that have been complicated by the continued use of antacids, consider alternating Natrum Phos with Natrum Sulphuricum, a remedy whose action often completes the cure begun by Natrum Phos. For cases that follow the pattern of symptoms indicated here, begin treatment with Natrum Phos alone, adding Natrum Sulph in alternation if improvement has not begun after several days of treatment.

As yellow is the color commonly associated with the need for the remedy, the patient's tongue will typically have a thick yellow coating. Commonly the Natrum Phos patient with chronic indigestion will have chronic postnasal drip as well, with thick yellow mucus draining down the back of his or her throat. The throat is dry, the patient is very thirsty. Note that, as an acute remedy, Natrum Phos is an excellent choice for patients with sore throats that are dry, that are worse from swallowing solids and better from swallowing liquids, and that feel as if there were a lump or a plug in the throat.

This is the premiere cell salt remedy for patients with worms or with any other intestinal parasites. Keynote to the use of the remedy is that the patient will pick his or her nose. And I mean really pick at it, bore into it with a finger. The nose and sinuses are chronically blocked in such cases, but the drainage flows down the back of the throat and not from the nostrils. The patient may also suffer from another symptom of parasites, itching and burning of the anus, especially when the patient is in bed at night—this symptom may contribute to the Natrum Phos' tendency toward aggravation at night and restless sleep.

Natrum Phos is perhaps most often used in combination with Ferrum Phosphoricum. These two phosphorus-based remedies enhance each other's ability to treat a multiplicity of disease states, most notably those associated with inflammation and pain. Therefore, Ferrum Phos is most associated with Natrum Phos in the treatment of arthritis and gouty arthritis, but may be considered in any case in which a sensation of heat and burning accompanies the other symptoms.

Natrum Phos is perhaps our best cell salt remedy for those who suffer from gout, and as gout is not an epidemic in our culture (due, in no small part, to our overreliance on diuretics in the allopathic treatment of those with hypertension), it is an important use for the remedy.

When the human system is functioning as it should, uric acid in the body is kept soluble in the blood by the presence of sufficient amounts of sodium phosphate and by the body temperature itself. Should there be a deficiency of sodium phosphate in the blood, uric acid builds up, and the body, recognizing it, transforms the acid into an insoluble salt and stores it in crystalline form in body tissues as part of the process of autotoxification. Adding sodium phosphate in the potentized form of the cell salt Natrum Phosphoricum allows these crystals to be dissolved once more and removed from the body in urine and sweat. Thus, Natrum Phos is our most powerful remedy for the treatment of chronic gout.

It is also a remedy for any sort of arthritic and/or rheumatic pain that follows its general symptoms: pain worse before a storm, pain worse from motion or physical exertion, pain improved if the patient sits quietly.

Natrum Phos has a special affinity for the ribs, especially for the ribs on the left side of the body. The patient, like the acidiosis patient, will have trouble breathing and will take shallow and rapid breaths because deep breathing hurts the ribs and fascia. This is generally a left-sided remedy, with pain either originating on the left side and moving to the right, or pain that is worse on the left side than on the right. The pain will also be increased if, while in bed, the patient turns and lies on his or her left side.

This is a patient who lacks vital heat, who is always chilly and always worse from becoming chilly. Who is worse in open or moving air, who wishes to be in the warm room that other types avoid. The patient's pain is improved by warmth, improved by staying perfectly still, by not even breathing too deeply, by speaking softly or staying silent.

This is an excellent remedy to think of for cases in which pain dominates in the toes (especially the large toe) and the fingers. When the pain extends to the hands and wrists and the feet and ankles. These pains can extend up the arms and/or legs, with a sensation that is more like weakness than actual pain. The arms and legs feel tired, weak, as if they are unable to support the body or perform their functions.

The Natrum Phos patient wants to sit down. The sitting position is a key to understanding this remedy type and to recognizing the need for it. Consider this remedy for those who fall asleep sitting up in the early part of the evening. (Especially if the symptoms of chronic indigestion and belching are then followed by a great desire to fall asleep in front of the television while sitting in a comfortable chair.) Consider this remedy for those who, once they have awakened in their chair, go off to bed, only to find that they have a much more restless sleep lying down than they do while sitting up.

Modalities

Natrum Phos patients are sensitive patients. They are very sensitive to music, which can either greatly improve or aggravate their symptoms, depending upon the individual patient's reaction to specific music.

They are also very sensitive to temperature and to changes in the weather. They are made worse by cold, by drafts, by open or moving air, and made better by warmth, especially by being in warm places, with one very major exception: the Nat Phos patient will be aggravated by lying down and by the warmth of his or her bed.

They are worse when a storm is coming and will feel their pain increase as it approaches, only to improve once more once the storm has passed.

Patients are, in general, better during the day than at night, although their aggravation will come on more from darkness than from night. As long as they are warm and the room is well-lit, they will usually not feel the aggravation that comes on with darkened rooms and long shadows.

Natrum Phos patients also have an interesting dual modality when it comes to eating. They are worse from fasting and will feel the need to eat even if they know that they will suffer from it. Initially they will feel much better after eating, but they will feel a general aggravation two to three hours later if they have eaten things they either cannot digest or that contribute to the general state of overacidity that is the root of their ailments.

Relationships

While all the cell salt remedies work well with each other, the phosphorus-based remedies work especially well in concert with each other. Natrum Phos and Ferrum Phos are two remedies that are especially well paired, especially when any sort of inflammation accompanies indigestion. Think of these two remedies in combination or alternation when a patient with indigestion also displays a red face or red, burning ears. The two remedies can be very helpful when indigestion is accompanied by acid reflux, especially on a continuing basis.

In cases of gout that Natrum Phos alone does not cure, alternate with Natrum Sulphuricum, as Nat Sulph often completes cures that Natrum Phos begins.

Dosage and Potency

This is a rather slow-acting remedy that usually requires some repetition before improvement of symptoms begins. Schuessler most often prescribed it in 6X potency, although the 3X, the 4X, and the 12X are also commonly used. Repeat as needed, two to three times a day in chronic cases, more often for acute indigestion, until improvement begins, then lower dosage to once a day as needed. With indigestion and pain, improvement usually will be noticed within two days. Improvement may take much longer for cases of chronic gout.

11. NATRUM SULPHURICUM

Overview

Natrum Sulphuricum, taken from the chemical compound sodium sulfate, is one of our oldest homeopathic remedies, perhaps one of the oldest medicines on earth. It has a chemical formula of $Na_2So_4 \cdot 10H_2O$. Natrum Sulph was an alchemical remedy before it was homeopathic. It was first studied by the alchemist Johann Rudolf Glauber in 1658. He named it *Sal Mirabile*, although it ultimately came to be known as *Sal Glauberi* or simply as Glauber's salt. He used his remedy as a purgative or a laxative or a diuretic.

Sodium sulfate naturally occurs in seawater, like the other sodium-based cell salts. It is also found in mineral spas, in this case most notably those in Saratoga Springs, New York. As with Natrum Muriaticum, sodium sulfate is easily soluble in water, but the remedy is created through the process of trituration.

Natrum Sulphuricum is considered to be the perfect remedy for the *hydrogenoid* constitution, which is to say that this is the remedy of first choice for those whose illnesses are caused by living in damp places, in basements, in wet environments. Those whose health is compromised by living near water, by the sea. Those whose illnesses are made worse from being in damp places, or even from eating foods near water or from eating fish—this last may seem ridiculous, but such is the extreme sensitivity to dampness of the hydrogenoid patient. They are worse from any change in the weather, can feel the change from dry to wet coming on by the increase in their symptoms, and always feel their best in dry, warm weather. The weather that aggravates can be damp or wet in any form—many Natrum Sulph patients, particularly those who suffer from asthma, will become much worse in foggy weather.

Indeed, the whole idea of fluids and the balance between wet and dry is key to understanding the remedy. It is important as well to the chemical compound from which the remedy is made. Both sodium sulfate and sodium chloride (the chemical compound of the remedy Natrum Muriaticum) are sodium-based substances, but their functions are quite opposite. Both substances absorb water due to the presence of sodium, but they do so for opposite reasons. Sodium chloride absorbs water to retain it for use within the body. Sodium sulfate absorbs it to eliminate it from the body. Sodium chloride is necessary to the creation of new cells, while sodium sulfate is important to aid in the disintegration and elimination of old, dead cells.

Sodium sulfate, therefore, functions throughout the body, especially in the liver (which reinforces the fact that Natrum Sulph is an important remedy for cleansing the body of toxins, as it stimulates the liver), pancreas, intestines, and the bladder. Without the presence of sodium sulfate, the bladder would not be stimulated and voluntary urination would not occur. This suggests that Natrum Sulphuricum will prove an important remedy for those with diabetes (which, of course, should only be treated by medical professionals), for those who have to rise up out of bed throughout the night to urinate, as well as for those who, failing to rise, are incontinent in the night.

It should come as no surprise that keynote to the Natrum Sulphuricum type is a watery discharge, which may be clear, white or, more typically, greenish-yellow. Another chief physical characteristic is found on the tongue, which usually is coated with a thick greenish coating, but may also have a brownish or grayish tinge.

The most important single symptom common to the type, however, is its extreme sensitivity to damp, to becoming wet in any way. It is, therefore, the remedy to think of for patients with rheumatic pains of any sort in any part of the body that are extremely sensitive to dampness and to changes in the weather from dry to damp. Also think of Natrum Sulphuricum for patients who suffer asthma, when attacks are brought on by damp. And this is an excellent remedy for those with sciatica, when the associated pain follows the same sensitivity to dampness and, especially, when the pain is truly maddening; when the patient cannot find a position, sitting, lying, or standing, that offers any degree of comfort or relief.

This idea of being uncomfortable in general will play out in many of the emotional, mental, and physical conditions helped by the use of this remedy. It is an important remedy for those who find that, night after night, they have an uncomfortable night's sleep. They have trouble falling or staying asleep and wake through the night (perhaps to urinate). Think of this remedy as well for those who awaken very early for no apparent reason, and for those who awaken from sleep unrefreshed.

Natrum Sulph types also tend to be uncomfortable in their bodies. As this is a cell salt associated with lax muscle fibers

> Natrum Sulphuricum is a remedy for the melancholy patient, for the patient who feels an inner restlessness, who feels out of step in his or her own life. This is a remedy for the patient who is depressed and responds to external stimuli with an almost manic response. This is the remedy for those who suffer from seasonal affective disorder (SAD), and who are strongly affected by a lack of sunshine in the winter months. The Natrum Sulph is always sad, slow, and sluggish on gray days.

and, often, with being overweight, patients needing Natrum Sulph often are dissatisfied with their physical bodies and unhappy with the way they look and feel. They have the tendency toward irritability, toward feeling that something is missing. They tend to awaken each day with a sense of quiet dread for what the day will bring. Physically, this discomfort typically shows itself in the fact that Natrum Sulphs are given to having either cold hands, cold feet, or both. They feel a certain vulnerability that is brought on by this sensation of cold, especially if their feet are both cold and wet. In this case, the Natrum Sulph type will feel a sense of weakness and pain through his or her whole body and will sense a deep wave of fear and dread.

This remedy is helpful for certain skin conditions as well, including patients with warts, with skin tags. It is also, perhaps, the most important remedy for stubborn old cases of gout that are not cured by the use of Natrum Phosphoricum alone. In these cases Natrum Sulph can be used after Natrum Phos or in alternation with it to flush the stored uric acid out of the body once and for all.

Finally, Natrum Sulphuricum is the single most important cell salt remedy for another physical complaint: think of this remedy first for all cases that involve an injury to the head, all cases of concussion. It has been clinically shown to be very helpful in cases involving brain damage, especially when the injury results in changes in personality.

Conditions that Suggest Natrum Sulphuricum

Asthma (caused by damp); bedwetting; costochondritis; diabetes; diarrhea (chronic); flu; gout (chronic); head injury; headaches and migraines; nephritis; overweight; rheumatism; SAD (seasonal affective disorder); sciatica; warts.

Mental and Emotional Symptoms

Natrum Sulphuricum is a remedy for the melancholy patient, for the patient who feels an inner restlessness, who feels out of step in his or her own life. This is a remedy for the patient who is depressed and responds to external stimuli with an almost manic response. This is the remedy for those who suffer from seasonal affective disorder (SAD), and who are strongly affected by a lack of sunshine in the winter months. Natrum Sulphs are always sad, slow, and sluggish on gray days. They react as negatively emotionally to damp days as they do physically. They are particularly down on foggy days.

They respond to sunlight with a lifting of the spirits. That which ameliorates their physical symptoms—namely sunny, dry, and warm weather—improves their emotional and mental symptoms as well.

They also respond strongly to music, like the Natrum Phosphoricum patient. But while the Natrum Phos responds either positively or negatively to music depending upon the volume, the emotional content, and the memories the music evokes, the Natrum Sulph always reacts negatively to music. Even lively music makes the Natrum Sulph sad. They find no solace, no joy in music.

The Natrum Sulph patient can become deeply depressed, especially the Natrum Sulph who is given to chronic insomnia or to sleep that fails to refresh. This is a remedy for the patient who contemplates suicide, who feels that he must use all of his self-control to keep from shooting himself. This sense of a constant need for emotional restraint is keynote to this remedy and a strong indicator for its use. Again, the same conditions that incite his physical pain will also cause his emotional or mental distress: gray days, damp weather, fog, and, especially, insomnia.

This internal distress may go unnoticed by those who know the Natrum Sulph. Like all Natrums, the Natrum Sulph often masks his or her feelings, and instead seems the most industrious of people. The Natrum Sulph, often motivated by his or her inner feelings of meaninglessness and melancholy, will want to keep busy, will all but beg for tasks he or she can perform, and will work hard the whole day through. This is part of the mechanism of restraint that allows Natrum Sulph types to cope with their inner struggles. They can be perceived as restless people, even a bit fussy. They may also seem to be a bit unfriendly, because they are not given to easy conversation, and may not wish to be spoken to, especially in the morning.

Note that, although they can be quite industrious, Natrum Sulphs find their work tiresome. They may consider it next to impossible to focus on any task that requires a mental effort.

It is also common to the type that they may be seen by others as mild, even shy. They are quiet people who, suddenly and for no obvious reason, are capable of explosive temper tantrums. As is common to all sodium-based types, they may show indifference to those they love. They may be estranged from their family members, no matter how much they might love them.

Think of this remedy when a patient's personality changes after a concussion or brain injury, or following any sort of physical trauma to the head. Emotional changes of any sort can indicate a need for this remedy: sudden changes in likes and dislikes in food, relationships, and, especially, music. In the same way, it can be very helpful to those who suffer any sort of memory loss after physical injury.

Physical Symptoms

Let me clarify one important thing right up front: while typical Natrum Sulphuricum patients will react negatively to damp, they do not have a negative response to cold. They are as happy on a cold, dry, sunny winter day as they are in summer. It is the degree of humidity that matters, not the temperature. In fact, given that this is a sulfur-based remedy, it should logically follow that the Natrum Sulphs are warm-blooded types. While this is not the case—in general, the Natrum Sulph patients are rather chilly types (most especially with cold hands and feet)—they do tend to get too warm easily and prefer being in open, fresh air, even if being in open air means that their hands and feet will get cold. They also crave cold things to eat and drink, particularly cold water, just like the Natrum Mur and the Natrum Phos patients.

This is a left-sided remedy, in which the chief complaints will tend to be worse on the left side of the body. It has a special affinity, as does Natrum Phos, for the left side of the chest and can be very helpful to patients who experience costochondritis, a painful inflammation of the fascia connecting to the ribcage on the left side of the chest.

Because Natrum Sulphuricum acts to stimulate the liver, the pancreas, the intestines, and the bladder, it helps the body eliminate toxins from the system. It helps regulate urine flow and restore voluntary control of urination to those who are incontinent. It is the remedy to consider both for those who have trouble urinating and those who suffer from polyuria, an overabundance of urine. Because Natrum Sulphuricum plays such an important part in the elimination of toxins through urine, it is a vital remedy for those who have stubborn or chronic cases of gout. In these cases, it should be used in alternation with Natrum Phosphoricum, or better still, after Natrum Phos has been given a chance to work on its own. This is because Natrum Phos will dissolve the crystals of uric acid that the body has stored and Natrum Sulph will then remove them from the body in urine. This process cleanses the overabundance of uric acid from the system and ends the pain and suffering of gout. So taking Natrum Sulph alone will not always cure gout, as it will not dissolve the crystals, and taking Natrum Phos alone may not be enough to bring about a cure, since it does not have Natrum Sulph's ability to sweep toxins from the system via urination. They are best used with Natrum Phos beginning the case and Natrum Sulph ending it. Note that, when first taking Natrum Sulph, a change in pattern of urination is a solid indication that the remedy is working.

Just as Natrum Sulphuricum plays an important part in removing any buildup of uric acid from the system, it can also help cure illnesses caused by a buildup of lactic acid. In these cases, it again works well in combination with or alternation with Natrum Phos.

And, just as it can help clear away acids from the system (always following Natrum Phos, which is our best antiacid cell salt) Natrum Sulphuricum is extraordinarily good at ridding the system of an overabundance of bad cholesterol. Think of Natrum Sulph particularly for those patients who have high levels of triglycerides in their system. Many patients who need Natrum Sulph are overweight and in rather poor physical shape in terms of exercise, so this remedy can act as a tonic to their system, not only removing the emotional sense of weight that is common to the type, but also their physical heft as well. In fact, Natrum Sulph and Natrum Phos again work well in combination for those who are obese, to help reestablish healthy patterns of rest, sleep, activity, and diet. Taken daily in alternation, they can be helpful for those who need to reestablish a healthier lifestyle.

Natrum Sulph is also the first remedy to think of for all cases of asthma that are made worse by damp or foggy weather. Think of it also for cases of bronchitis and even pneumonia when the left lung is chiefly affected. All three conditions will share the same general symptoms: worse from damp or foggy weather; a hoarse voice; a constant cough that may bring up ropy expectoration containing a greenish pus; a general sensation of soreness in the chest, particularly on the left side of the chest, that is better from pressure, better from the patient lying on that side or by holding his or her chest when he speaks or coughs; and a cough that is always worse in the early hours of the morning, specifically from 4:00 A.M. to 5:00 A.M. Look for the patient in question to try to breathe slowly and deeply as a means of breathing without coughing and a means by which he or she can bring enough oxygen into his or her lungs.

Respiratory symptoms often alternate with digestive disorders. This is a remedy in which diarrhea is common, even chronic. Diarrhea occurs after each fit of coughing, is induced by coughing. Stools are sudden, greenish, watery, and painless. They are passed with a good deal of gas. The patient, it should be noted, will feel much better after passing stool. In chronic cases of diarrhea, the patient will rush from his or her bed to the bathroom, or will have a bout of diarrhea just after stirring in the morning. (Note that the tendency toward having a bowel movement first thing in the morning just after waking is common in the sulfur-based remedies.) Gastric symptoms will be accompanied by a tongue that is coated with a thick and dark greenish-brown or greenish-gray covering. The gastric symptoms may also be accompanied by a toothache or by an increased sense of sensitivity in all the teeth, or a sensation that the teeth have grown, are too large or too long.

In acute circumstances always consider Natrum Sulphuricum for cases of influenza that follow the pattern of combined respiratory distress and diarrhea, especially if the flu has come on in damp weather or after the patient has been in a damp environment or gotten drenched.

Finally, since it is a remedy for those who are exquisitely sensitive to wet weather and damp environments, it stands to reason that Natrum Sulph would be helpful for those who suffer from rheumatism. And this is certainly true. It may be used for any who suffer from rheumatic pains that follow the general modalities of the remedy.

But Natrum Sulphuricum is especially suited to those patients who suffer from sciatica, especially those who are all but crippled by it, who can find no position, standing, sitting, or lying down, that will bring relief. It is especially indicated for sciatica in the left side of the body. It can also be very helpful for those who suffer from hip pain that is typified by a constant difficulty in getting up from a sitting position. Either the hip pain or the sciatica will cause the patient to have to frequently change position, which relieves the pain, but only for a moment. The patient will rub the affected area, will put pressure on it, and may even lie on it to bring relief.

Modalities

Natrum Sulph patients are better from cold air, from open air. From cold drinks and food. In dry weather. They are better from sunshine and on sunny days specifically, and from light, generally speaking. In times of pain, they are better from frequently changing positions.

Natrum Sulphs are always worse in the morning, from 4:00 A.M., when they may awaken from sleep for no reason (only to lie awake until they finally give up and get up), until breakfast time. They are always better for having breakfast and should never skip it. They are irritable in the morning and do not want to be spoken to until they have eaten breakfast.

They are worse from damp in any form: damp weather, damp basements, and damp locales like the seashore. They are worse from coming into contact with the night air. Worse from lying on their left side. Worse on gray days or in darkened rooms. They are always worse from music, which upsets and depresses them.

Note that Natrum Sulphuricum has an annual time of aggravation. Look for the Natrum Sulph to experience an increase in his or her chronic ailments or a distressing acute condition each spring, as the dampness associated with the transition from winter to spring is difficult for the type. The time of year when the snow melts and is replaced by rain is especially trying, emotionally, mentally, and physically.

Relationships

As noted, Natrum Sulphuricum works especially well in conjunction with Natrum Phosphoricum, especially in cases involving chronic gout or obesity or high cholesterol.

Consider giving this remedy in conjunction with Kali Phosphoricum for patients who suffer from restless sleep and nightmares.

Give this remedy in alternation with or as a follow-up to Ferrum Phosphoricum for cases of flu that involve fever, respiratory distress that is worse on the left side of the chest, and diarrhea.

Dosage and Potency

Natrum Sulphuricum is most often given in the 3X, 6X, or 12X potencies, with 6X being most common. Schuessler gave the remedy in very low 1X or 2X potencies in repeated doses. It is a remedy that repeats well and may be given as needed. In chronic cases, it can be given two to three times daily and is well suited to taking an hour after meals. As improvement begins, the number of doses should be decreased until cure results.

12. SILICEA

Overview

Silicea, taken from the substance silica, or flint, is unique among the cell salt remedies. First, it is the only cell salt that is taken from a single source and not from a chemical compound. Also, silica, along with sodium chloride, is among the most common substances on earth. Where sodium chloride is abundant in the waters of the ocean, silica is a constituent of the sand along the seashore. Much of the earth's mantle underneath the oceans contain silica, as do sea sponges and plants growing both in the sea and on dry land.

Silica is a building block, giving strength and stability to all things that contain it. Plants, animals and the earth itself depend upon silica for strength and support. Silica is absorbed by plants to give strength to their stems. Silica is not soluble in water or alcohol. The remedy Silicea is created through the process of trituration.

Silica is abundant in the human body. It can be found in traces in blood, bile, and urine and is contained in connective tissues throughout the body, in the spine and brain itself, in nerve tissues and membranes, in the skin, the hair, and the nails. In other words, it serves the same purpose in the human body that it does in all of nature—it gives support and strength. It is a vital component in the development of tissue in the growing fetus and is a necessary ingredient in the healing process and in the ongoing creation of new cells.

Silicea, the remedy taken from the substance silica, is also unique. Like Natrum Muriaticum it is a remedy that was developed by Samuel Hahnemann, who was the first to see the medicinal potential in this common substance, and not by Schuessler, who borrowed the remedy from the preexisting homeopathic pharmacy and added it to his own.

As a homeopathic remedy, Silicea stands with Natrum Muriaticum, Sulphur, Phosphorus, and Calcarea Carbonica as a true *polycrest*, a remedy of the first order of importance, whose action carries through to every system and organ of the body. Further, like the other true polycrests—the handful of remedies among the many thousand in the homeopathic pharmacy—Silicea is a remedy that speaks to a part of the human condition that is so wide and so deep that the vast major-

> Silicea has the power to have an impact upon virtually all aspects of the human system, especially upon bones, joints, skin, mucous membranes, and glands. The picture of the patient needing this remedy is a portrait of malnutrition, as Silicea reigns supreme in terms of assimilation and those needing it are those whose systems have lost their innate ability to nourish themselves.

ity of humans would have some healing response from taking it. Although it may not be the remedy of best choice in many cases, it will still be beneficial for many, many diverse patients suffering from a multiplicity of conditions by virtue of its universality.

To understand the uses of the remedy, one only has to look at the function of the substance silica and then contemplate what might result if it was lacking.

Silicea has the power to have an impact upon virtually all aspects of the human system, especially upon bones, joints, skin, mucous membranes, and glands. Patients needing this remedy are portraits of malnutrition because Silicea reigns supreme in terms of nutritional assimilation, and the systems of those needing it have lost their innate ability to nourish themselves. (This will especially be true for children who need this remedy. In these cases you may see such indicators as rickets, a swollen abdomen, and thin legs and arms. This is the chief remedy to think of when a child shows signs of failure to thrive.) Often the signs of a need for Silicea will be seen in the patient's hair and nails, both of which will seem unhealthy. The hair is sweaty—head sweat is a keynote symptom for this remedy type—and lank. The patient may also be losing his or her hair, as this is the remedy for premature baldness or baldness due to malnutrition. The nails will be weak. Look for the patient to have white, clouded areas on his or her nails, and for fingernails and toenails to break, chip, or peel easily. The patient's fingertips will be dry and cracked, even infected. This is the chief remedy to consider in cases of whitlows or felons, which are infections at the sides of the fingernails. (Calcarea Fluorica is the other remedy for this particular condition and these two remedies can be used in combination or alternation when whitlows are present. Silicea follows Calc Fluor very well and often clears away the symptoms that Calc Fluor fails to cure.)

There are many different indicators of a need for Silicea. Silicea types are chilly—so chilly that often there is nothing that can be done to make them warm. They are chilly in spite of closing the house up tight, in spite of wrapping up, in spite of exercising. Nothing stirs their vital heat, nothing makes them feel truly warm. They hold themselves rather rigid, in a defensive posture, due to the fact that, cold as they are, lacking in vital heat and general vitality as they are, they cannot relax.

Thus the Silicea type is often both restless and exhausted.

This is a remedy that is slow and deep-acting. In this it mirrors the disease states that the remedy impacts. Silicea is more often used in chronic cases than in acute cases. Patients who respond to Silicea more often than not have an illness that was slow in forming and long in developing. Once it takes hold it severely limits their ability to live their lives. These are the children of famine and of war. These are people who live in want, in poverty. In our country, more often than not, they are those who may look as if they are well fed, but who are not. Their diets consist of cheap fast foods, which give them the same distended stomachs as the children of famine but with the swollen, even obese bodies common to those who eat an overabundance of salt, sugar, and fat. They those who are slow to develop—children with bones that do not form, with fontanelles that stay open beyond the expected stage of development—late with all milestones in life as if they lack the strength to keep up. They are those with wasting diseases of all sorts, chronic afflictions of the immune response. Every injury is slow to heal, if it heals at all, and every injury threatens to become infected. These are patients whose systems bear the brunt of vaccinations that have caused them deep harm. Their bodies and minds are locked in combat with life itself, their ability to adapt has been replaced with an ongoing sense of dread and doubt. They may lack backbone, be cowardly, or, more commonly, passive-aggressive, because they cannot bear to take a stance. They shrink from confrontation, and yet hold a small, hard core of pure will and remain stubborn even in moments of apparent cowardice. These are easily underestimated, both in terms of their mental, emotional, and physical strength and in terms of their survival skills.

In other words, the need for Silicea is displayed most clearly in a certain *lack* on the part of the patient. They lack strength on the mental, the emotional, and physical planes of existence. Where other remedies—particularly the calcium-based remedies—may show a similar slowness in terms of development and weakness in terms of bone growth, no other remedy shows such an all-pervasive sense of deficiency as does Silicea. And since Schuessler's theory of biochemical medicine is largely based on this notion of deficiency, perhaps no other remedy so clearly demonstrates the power of the cell salts as Silicea. Like Natrum Muriaticum, Silicea is so commonly needed and useful in conditions both general and highly specific that one could easily come to the conclusion that no other remedy is really needed—that Silicea alone is the universal remedy needed to put all things right.

And most certainly there are worse things you could do than give most people a dose or two of Silicea. Silicea is a very good remedy choice for those of us who impede ourselves through lack of strength, lack of self-confidence, or lack of sheer intelligence, for those of us who trap ourselves in a forest of details, focusing on the minute details of our lives and not on the wholeness of life, who live not in the moment but in dread of what is to come in the next moment, who eat the wrong things, fail to care for our bodies as if they were meant to last a lifetime, drink alcohol we can't handle, get involved in relationships we can't cope with, and work our way up to positions in our careers in which we feel that we will be discovered for the counterfeits and failures that we truly are at any moment—in other words, for all of us.

Conditions that Suggest Silicea

Acne; AIDS; anemia; bedwetting; body odor; boils; bone disease; bunions; carbuncles; cataracts; chronic fatigue; conjunctivitis; constipation; especially chronic; cough; diabetes; fainting; foreign objects in body: splinters, shrapnel; fractures, especially those slow to heal; glands swollen; headaches; homesickness; infections that are slow to heal; joint pain, especially in the hips and/or the knees; injuries, especially cuts; keloids and scar tissue; malnutrition; neuralgia; obesity due to poor diet and malnutrition; passive-aggressive behavior; rheumatism, especially chronic; rickets; sinusitis, especially chronic; strains and sprains; sweat on head and feet that is smelly; tooth decay; vaccinations; whitlows; worms and parasites; writer's cramp.

Mental and Emotional Symptoms

While it is certainly true that the typical Silicea patient will be stronger on the mental and emotional level than on the physical level, he or she also displays weakness in terms of the mind and spirit. The typical Silicea presents himself as a shy person, a person who is willing—perhaps overly willing—to please. Who is overly sensitive to all stimuli, especially to noise; who startles easily and, when startled, responds by becoming in turns anxious and irritable. Who might be described as more peevish than truly irritable.

These patients have trouble concentrating, trouble completing tasks, because they tend to get lost in a maze of details, and see only the details and not the finish line. They want to think clearly, but are unable to do so. In this way, they may be said to be lacking in vision. They cannot see the task through to completion, but can only work from crisis to crisis, detail to detail.

And yet, time and again, when dealing with Silicea types, I have seen their core, no matter how small, of pure flint. Those who require Silicea understand the importance of silica, the importance of structure and strength, and they cling to what bit of it they can. This gives them a wonderful and unexpected thread of stubbornness in their nature. They present themselves as completely yielding but harbor a secret need to stay true to themselves, and, in doing so, often take on passive-aggressive behavior patterns. They tell any person who they sense is stronger or dominant over them that they will do as they have been told and then continue on, working as before, under their own secret guidance. Silicea is the remedy for those who cannot abide confrontation, who cannot stand on their own two feet and take a stand, but who, nevertheless, stubbornly cling to their own beliefs, quietly rebelling against all in authority.

Silicea types can be difficult patients. They do not take the remedies they report that they have taken and do not get the results they claim to have experienced from the remedies that they actually have taken. They are not exactly liars, although they do tend to tell lies. Instead, they believe that their survival depends upon presenting themselves to the world as perfect lackeys, but they know on some deep level the fate of all lackeys and hope to avoid it. This is the remedy needed by those who have lived through revolutions and wars and famines and fires, who have experienced real trauma and real hunger and wasting and loss, so it is not surprising that even those who have not been placed in such traumatic situations will still mirror the behaviors of those who have. This is a remedy that deals with the fundamental issue of survival and it reveals the patterns of behavior that are required by those who struggle to survive in doing so.

Children needing this remedy—and it is quite commonly needed by younger patients—often cry when spoken to. These are babies who wake at every sound, startle easily, and cry as a response to being startled. (Note that all Silicea types tend to have keen hearing and are overly responsive to sounds of all sorts: human voices, music, and so on. Of all five senses, hearing is the most developed in most Silicea types.)

Silicea patients are filled with anxiety and riddled with fears. They fear strangers, and will often feel as if they are being watched. They have, along with this fear of being watched, a huge fear of public speaking, or of being the focus of attention. They have a fear of falling. They have a fear of thunderstorms, and, especially, of lightning. They fear sharp things, especially knives. They have a fear of being cut that can border of fascination. They may have a secret desire to cut themselves, to slowly slit open their skin. They tend to be afraid of leaving home, of travel. They do not like to travel and do not travel well or happily, and wish to be at home.

Silicea patients are highly suggestible, even if they do retain their stubborn core. They are easily convinced and easily motivated by guilt. They tend to feel guilty, even for things that they have not done. Silicea types often equate contemplating an action with actually attempting it. Thus they feel guilt over sexual imaginings and yearning, guilt because they have contemplated murder.

Their sensitivity and anxiety can lead to a long-lasting sense of depression as well. They can be rather sad people, given to sadness linked to their sense of guilt, most especially after any sexual act, even masturbation. Their sense of sadness is magnified when they are left alone. While Silicea types never wish to be the focus of group attention, they do not wish to be alone either. These are people who are depressed if they are forced to live alone or work alone. They want the company of those they love and can be quite clingy as a result.

Physical Symptoms

Think of Silicea first in all cases of chronic disease that are caused by malnutrition or that involve a delayed or depleted healing response. It is a good remedy to use with all other cell salts in cases of this sort, even if other cell salts seem better indicated. It can be used in combination or alternation with all the other salts and works well with them. As it is the product of a single substance and not a compound, adding Silicea to the case should be seen as adding the adjunct supplement of silica anywhere it is needed. This is a simple remedy, slow to act, but powerful and completely gentle. In this, it again reveals itself to be perhaps the biochemical remedy most central to Schuessler's concept of combining the idea of homeopathy with that of nutritional supplements.

The Silicea type can often be identified by his or her sweat and scent alone. Perspiration is always a key to the type. Some will sweat only on the top half of their body, and will show an excess of sweat on their head and under their arms. Others will sweat only on their heads or on their feet, or in one place or the other. It is common in patients needing this remedy that they will have a head that sweats while they sleep, and in spite of this, will need to keep their heads covered, as this sweat is not a sign of being overheated. Think of this remedy for sweaty patients who are cold, never warm. Think of this remedy for patients whose feet sweat to excess and whose sweaty feet are very smelly. Think of this remedy for all patients whose sweat is extremely smelly.

This is the first remedy to think of for those who have body odor, especially if that odor continues even after they have bathed. (The sulfur-based remedies will also carry this characteristic symptom. Sulfur types will have a distinctive sulfur, or "rotten egg" smell to them, while Silicea types will have a more offensive smell—think of the smell in old tennis shoes.)

The symptom of sweat and smell can be played out in two ways. Most commonly, this is the remedy suggested by those who sweat to excess. But it is also the remedy to think of for all cases in which illness has come on from the suppression of sweat, and for patients who do not sweat at all. In a culture that values dry underarms, we have created a number of patients who are chronically ill due to their reliance on antiperspirants that suppress the body's need to release toxins through sweat. Silicea is the remedy for those who have illnesses caused by suppressed sweat, especially by suppressed foot sweat.

Silicea is also the remedy to think of for any wound or cut that becomes infected, or for wounds that do not heal. Think of this remedy for cases of keloids, scar tissue that forms that is raised and red. Silicea will help the body to reabsorb the issue and allow the scars to heal.

Think of Silicea for all abscesses and boils, especially those that are filled with white pus. Silicea always will act to bring pus forth, to cause its formation to rid the body of toxins. In this action, Silicea is opposite that of Calcarea Sulphurica, a remedy that inhibits the suppurative process. For this reason, these two remedies should not be used concurrently in any case involving infections. Silicea's action is to encourage the formation of pus—especially white pus—and to eliminate it from the body, while Calc Sulph's action is to prevent its formation. They do not blend well. For cases in which abscesses need to ripen and expel their load, the remedy of choice is Silicea. For cases in which wounds fester, where the pus is yellow, or when infection has continued a long time, or the formation of pus has ceased but the wound is not healed, the remedy is Calc Sulph.

Just as the remedy Natrum Sulphuricum will push liquids out of the body, Silicea will work to expel all foreign material from the body. Therefore, it is the remedy of choice for cases of such things as splinters. Homeopathic literature is filled with stories of old shrapnel that has, after half a lifetime, been expelled from the body of an old soldier through the use of this remedy.

Silicea is the remedy of first order for swollen glands anywhere in the body, especially glands that are chronically swollen. It is helpful in cases of chronic rheumatism and neuralgia in which the patient is constantly cold, and is improved when his or her head is covered, and when the patient is made as warm as possible, when affected parts are covered, even wrapped up tight. This is a remedy for patients with soreness of affected parts, with a tendency toward infection, with headaches that are improved by covering the head and by putting pressure against the painful part, headaches that are worse on the right side of the head. For patients with unhealthy skin, skin that is covered in lumps and scars, and acne with whiteheads on the face and shoulders and back. For patients with weak backs, and especially weak arms and legs. They may have underdeveloped muscles in the arms and/or legs. Look for patients to walk as if they were just learning how. Look for their arms and/or legs to tremble.

As this is also a remedy known to be important for those who suffer from malnutrition, think of it in all cases in which a given patient's diet is lacking in nutrition, regardless of whether it is the result of the quality or quantity of food eaten. It is an important remedy for chronic constipation, especially if the patient has a frequent urge to pass stool but is unable to do so or is only partially able to do so, and as a result, feels the constant urge.

It can also be helpful to those who are chronically constipated but who, from time to time, have a sudden bout of diarrhea, especially when the stool has an intense cadaverous odor to it.

Modalities

Silicea patients are always better in summer, worse in winter. They are improved during hot, humid weather. They are better from warmth, from direct applications of heat, and from being wrapped up tight with blankets, clothing, or bandages. Their heads, especially, will feel better from being covered, which will not only improve conditions such as headache but will make them feel better as a whole.

They are made worse by change, especially by a change in the weather. But many Silicea patients will feel deeply challenged by change of any sort, any upset to their schedule. They hate to travel and feel deep yearnings to be home. They are also worse from any form of excitement, from any passionate displays of emotion on the part of others. They are worse from loud noise or bright lights. Worse from being startled. Worse from being touched, especially from being shaken or jarred. Worse from being left alone. They do not tolerate alcohol in any form and should avoid it.

They are worse in cold air, better in a closed room. Worse from suppressed sweat and better from sweating. (They are also better from urinating.) They are particularly worse if their foot sweat is suppressed or if their feet get cold or wet. They become sick easily if their feet get cold and/or wet. They are worse at night and, especially, in the early morning. Worse during the time of the full moon, which drains them. They are always worse from cold things and from becoming cold.

Relationships

Be careful in using this remedy concurrently with Calcarea Sulphurica in cases involving suppuration for the reasons noted above.

This aside, Silicea blends well with all other cell salts for cases in which a patient displays a sluggish immune response or any sign of malnutrition, especially as seen in the skin of the face, the hair, or the fingernails or toenails.

Dosage and Potency

Schuessler used Silicea most commonly in the 6X and 12X potencies. Remember that this is a slow-acting and deep-acting remedy, so do not continue to repeat the dosage, thinking that it is not acting, without giving it sufficient time to act. Do not repeat too often in chronic cases. Give the remedy no more than twice a day; repeat for a longer number of days or weeks rather than too often during any given day. This is predominately a remedy for those with chronic complaints and therefore should not be repeated with the frequency that one might use with a remedy more commonly associated with acute conditions.

PART THREE

Common Applications for Cell Salt Remedies

"The inorganic substances in the blood and tissues are sufficient to heal all diseases which are curable at all. If the remedies are used according to the symptoms, the desired end will be gained by means of application of natural laws."

—W.H. SCHUESSLER

CHAPTER SIX

Using Cell Salts
at Home

Ⓗow you use the cell salts in your home will be largely determined by where you place them in the balance between homeopathic remedies and nutritional supplements. Those who think of them as supplements will tend to take them in clusters, as supplements are taken, either before or after meals. Those who think of them as being more similar to homeopathic remedies will tend to take them in accordance with the Three Laws of Cure, the rules by which all homeopathic remedies are given.

The Law of Similars

The first of these laws is the Law of Similars, which I have written about earlier in these pages. That law is stated as "Like cures like." This is, of course, the heart of homeopathic philosophy, but it is the heart of homeopathic practice as well. If we were to apply our use of cell salts to it, we would have to seek, first and foremost, to choose the remedy or remedies from among the twelve that are most similar in their actions to the symptoms of illness at hand. And that works on all three levels of being, with mental, emotional, and physical symptoms all being weighed. If one remedy could be found that would, in the totality of its actions, be most similar to the totality of the symptoms at hand, that remedy would be considered curative to the case. Giving it alone would be enough to bring the patient's system back into balance.

That is the Law of Similars in action, the central idea being that the energy of the remedy balances the vital force of the patient, allowing for the restoration of health.

This law, of course, does not take the concept of deficiency into consideration. Those who do consider deficiency will tend to use the remedies more like nutritional supplements, as it is quite possible for a given patient to be deficient in more than one thing at a time. Just as a given patient may take both vitamin C and vitamin B_{12}, it is also, so this reasoning goes, quite possible for that same patient to take both Natrum Muriaticum and Silicea at the same time. Indeed, it would be preferable if the patient were thought to be deficient in both tissue salts.

But this brings up another of our Laws of Cure. The second law, Simplex, tells us that we should use only one remedy at a time. Which brings up the concept of *poly-pharmacy*.

Polypharmacy

Now, if there was anything about allopathic medicine that irritated Samuel Hahne-mann the most, it was likely the whole idea of polypharmacy. Those who read his mag-num opus *The Organon of Medicine* for the first time are usually surprised to realize that the first half of the book is not about homeopathy. That the entire first half of the bible of homeopathy isn't about homeopathy specifically, but is, instead, about the whole idea of medicine, and how medicine can be practiced in order to meet the goal of offer-ing the patient a cure that is at once "rapid, gentle and permanent."

For Hahnemann, one of the most important aspects in attaining this goal was and is the strict avoidance of polypharmacy. By always giving only one medicine at a time.

Why? Because all medicines do more than one thing. All have myriad actions in the human system. Anything that can be considered medici-nal is medicinal because it is a catalyst to change in the human system, because it shakes the patient out of the rut of his illness. In doing this, any medicine will be the cause of a number of changes. The drug that lowers blood pressure by calming the heart also has the action of lowering the pressure in the eye, and a hundred other things. Both allopathic and homeopathic medi-cine recognize this fact, but each system deals

> Hahnemann would argue that, no matter whether you are practicing allopathy or homeopathy, you need to map the whole sphere of action of any medicine or remedy and be quite aware of the full potential of that medicine before you give it.

with the fact that all medicines act in numerous ways in a different manner. In homeo-pathic medicine, the various changes that a given remedy can induce are studied and recorded in the most detailed manner possible in the materia medica. In allopathic medicine, these same changes are studied, but the primary focus is to identify the desired action of the medicine. All other changes caused by that medicine are named "side effects," and are basically considered to be, more or less, what a retailer would call the "cost of doing business." In other words, patients are instructed to put up with the side effects in order to enjoy the primary action of the remedy, the reason the medicine was prescribed in the first place.

The trouble with this approach is that side effects can be tricky things. They differ from person to person. One person may be able to take a given medicine without much difficulty, while another may find the side effects to be intolerable. There is no way of predicting what will happen.

Hahnemann would argue that, no matter whether you are practicing allopathy or homeopathy, you need to map the whole sphere of action of any medicine or remedy and be quite aware of the full potential of that medicine before you give it. Further, he would say that both allopathic and homeopathic medicines should be given on the basis of the whole of their activity and not just for the sake of a single action. (Paying attention to only one of multiple actions forces us all to agree to the nonsense idea that side effects are acceptable—or makes us deal with them as the Wizard of Oz instructs when he advised, "Pay no attention to the man behind the curtain."). Sometimes in allopathic medicine, we find that the side effect of a given medicine becomes, over time, the reason why it is given. An example of this is Minoxidil, which was originally given as a vasodilator, a remedy for hypertension. When it was found to have the side effect of growing hair, its purpose shifted to being a medicine for baldness. How much better if it had been used for patients struggling with high blood pressure and baldness in the first place.

Now this may be a rather benign example, but, in general, think how much better it would be if we could target our drugs less directly and instead use them more generally. In that case we could make use not only of the primary effect but also of all the side effects. We could match the medicine not just to the single symptom, but to the patient as a whole. It would make allopathy a much safer and more effective form of medicine.

This leads us back to polypharmacy, the use of more than one medicine at a time. The problem with polypharmacy goes back to the fact that every medicine does more than one thing, has more than one action. If you give one medicine you must be aware of all the things that it could potentially do, and you have to watch to see exactly what it does do, in each particular patient. The changes may be slight or they may be dynamic.

One medicine alone can potentially change the life of the patient who takes it, for better or worse. So, if one medicine has four, five, six actions, makes half a dozen changes, what happens if you give more than one medicine at a time? How can you know which medicine is creating which particular change? And since each can create multiple changes on its own, how can you ever know how two medicines will interact? What might the two of them do together that neither of them would do alone?

This is the curse of polypharmacy; it leads us into situations in which we no longer know what medicine is doing what and what symptoms (as they shift) are natural and to be expected, and what symptoms are being caused by the medicines. Allopathy has a solution for this as well—but, unfortunately, it is the same old solution that got us into this mess. Just as the allopaths created the new term "side effects" for all those things the medicines did that they did not particularly want them to do, they created a new term *iatrogenic* for all the disease states that are created inadvertently by medical treatments (as opposed to mechanical injury, infectious diseases, or genetic predispositions). Just as the allopaths try to create an environment in which side effects are seen as not only tolerable but actually acceptable, they also seek to make us feel that it is entirely appropriate for us to develop new diseases that are caused by the treatments we are given.

I don't find it acceptable. And for this reason, I stand with Hahnemann in upholding the Law of Simplex (that which tells us to only use one remedy at any given time), whether I am using homeopathic remedies, Bach flower remedies, or cell salts.

After all, putting true crises aside for a moment, I have to ask the question, what is the real advantage of using more than one remedy at a time? Especially in the case of chronic illness, is there any advantage to rushing into multiple treatments? It seems to me that starting with a single remedy offers both the patient and the practitioner a way to note and understand the full range of a given medicine's actions before deciding whether to add another remedy. It seems to me that most of us agree that less medicine is the best medicine, that we should only take medicines we actually need, and that we should know the full range of actions of each medicine we take and why we are taking them. If this is the case, why wouldn't we always want to start out with one dose of one remedy and then wait a bit to see what changes it creates? Anything else seems rash at best. At worst it seems to be courting disaster (and by "worst" I guess I mean "allopathic polypharmacy," which in my opinion is about as bad as it gets in terms of medicine).

> It seems to me that starting with a single remedy offers both the patient and the practitioner a way to note and understand the full range of a given medicine's actions before deciding whether to add another remedy. It seems to me that most of us agree that less medicine is the best medicine, that we should only take medicines we actually need, and that we should know their full range of actions of each medicine we take and why we are taking them.

Alternation or Combination?

I have consistently used the phrase "in alternation or combination" in these pages. By choosing this phrase, I have left it in the hands of the reader—the practitioner, if that reader takes it upon himself or herself to actually administer any form of medication—to make the decision as to how these remedies can best be used.

Admittedly, I have, in some very specific cases, suggested that certain remedies be used in combination. In the same way, in similar circumstances, I would recommend the use of more than one homeopathic remedy, alternating rapidly between them, or would recommend the use of more than one Bach remedy. These are cases of emergencies, when time is of the essence and the choice of a single remedy is very difficult. In the vast majority of cases, however, I find it not only preferable, but actually more effective to use all things homeopathic one at a time.

In the case of cell salts, that means that if I think that more than one cell salt remedy is called for in a given case, I start with one of them—the remedy that seems most directed to what is happening right now, right in this moment, or that reflects the dominant symptom or symptoms. I give that remedy for the first two or three days in chronic cases, for the first few hours in acute cases. Then, after I can get a picture of just what impact that cell salt has on the patient and how it does or does not improve his or her symptoms, I add the second remedy in alternation, keeping the doses a few hours apart, so I can observe the impact of each dose and watch how the patient's symptoms shift and improve over time.

To put it simply, as a rule of thumb when dealing with the cell salts, I think that a single cell salt is best, when possible. If I feel the need to use two, I think they are better used in alternation than in combination. And I think that I would be very hesitant to use more than three remedies in alternation at any given time. I would save the use of any combination of two or three remedies for emergency situations, when time is of the essence.

Admittedly, this flies in the face of the stated philosophy and practice of biochemics, which tells us that it is quite all right to use multiple remedies at the same time. Since the cell salts occur naturally in the human body, you are, in giving them, only returning to the body substances that it needs, that it craves, and in using multiple remedies, you are only giving the body the means by which it can build healthy new tissue and remove dead cells more effectively.

There is even a product on the market that combines all twelve of the cell salts—all in 6X potency—with the idea that, together, they act sort of like a multiple vitamin. The bottle states that the mixture is for: "Relief in cases of general weakness, weariness, stress, vague/undefined symptoms, or for use as a general tonic." Suffice it to say that since the substances combined in that mixture are in the form of cell salts, and therefore are homeopathic remedies no matter how low their potency, I have issues with the whole idea of this approach, which basically is utilizing polypharmacy. But I leave the decision concerning its use up to the reader.

The Third Law of Cure

Hahnemann's third law of cure has two parts. It is called the Law of Minimum, and it states first that you should always treat a given patient by using the lowest possible potency of medicine that will be effective. Now, it is true that this statement has more to do with homeopathic medicine than with cell salts, since there is a much greater difference between a 30C and a 200C potency than there is between a 3X and a 6X potency. So, this aspect of the Law of Minimum does not significantly apply to the cell salts, as all are given in very low potency. But the second aspect of the law is most appropriate. It states that we are to limit the number of doses to the least number that will get the job done. No more.

This also tends to fly in the face of the concept of giving the cell salts in an open-ended manner, and forces us to choose whether we are to use them as if they are nutritional supplements or as if they are homeopathic remedies. Although you can consider them to be both, to be the perfect balance between the two, you cannot in truth find that same balance in giving them. Some practitioners, likely those who would use the "multiple vitamin" mixture of all twelve remedies, indicate that the cell salts are as harmless as vitamins and may be given as such, taken daily for the rest of your life if you like. Others, myself among them, would ask once more, what is to be gained in giving

> We now think of medicine, which we once thought could cure us, as something that can sustain us. We believe that if we do not constantly take medicines—more and more and stronger and stronger medicines—we will surely die. This is not the kind of thinking that leads to health, but only to more and more treatments that leave us sicker than before. Hopefully, those who turn to the cell salts will not add to this misdirected thinking by overusing these simple little medicines as well. The thought process through which a treatment is given and a medicine is used is a powerful thing. Be sure of what you are doing before you give any medicine, no matter how harmless it may seem.

any medicine of any sort when it is not needed? Can anything good come out of taking it, no matter how benign it may be, if you do not need to take it? Once health is restored, once the patient is brought back into balance, it seems common sense that treatment should cease. The body should be trusted to retain the balance it has achieved. If this proves false and treatment is needed in the future, it can begin again, but only at that point. We have to get away from the idea that medical intercession is always a desirable thing; that if one medicine is good, two are better; and that if a 3X potency is good, 6X is twice as good. All of these are falsehoods, in my opinion. They all lead down the path on which we begin to think that side effects are inevitable, that diseases caused by medical treatments are acceptable, and that, in the end, the best we can hope for is to manage our illness and control our pain, instead of holding on to the idea that we can one day actually be well.

We now think of medicine, which we once thought could cure us, as something that can sustain us. We believe that if we do not constantly take medicines—more and more and stronger and stronger medicines—we will surely die. This is not the kind of thinking that leads to health, but only to more and more treatments that leave us sicker than before.

Hopefully, those who turn to the cell salts will not add to this misdirected thinking by overusing these simple little medicines as well. The thought process through which a treatment is given and a medicine is used is a powerful thing. Be sure of what you are doing before you give any medicine, no matter how harmless it may seem.

Using Cell Salts at Home

So the first step in deciding how you will use the cell salts at home is for you to decide whether you will approach them as nutritional supplements, as W.H. Schuessler would have directed, or as homeopathic remedies, as Samuel Hahnemann would have insisted. No matter which method you decide to use, things proceed from there in pretty much the same way.

Cell salts are available in nearly every health food store in the country, certainly any health food store that carries homeopathic remedies.* Just like any other homeopathic remedy, they are considered over-the-counter medications and are available to anyone who wants them without a prescription.

Now, when the time comes to use the cell salts, the first step is one of case taking. In taking the case, you must first determine the situation at hand. What has taken place? Is this an acute or a chronic situation? This is more complicated in my description about it than it will usually be when you are actually doing it. You will see that your child has skinned a knee, has awakened with a sore throat, or is teething. These are all acute situations and all are situations in which the cell salts can be put to good use.

The chronic situations in the home for which it is appropriate to use the cell salts include chronic digestive disorders—constipation, bloating, or acid reflux—or skin conditions, or cases of simple allergies like seasonal allergies (these may seem acute, in that they occur for only a few days in the spring, but are, in reality, chronic conditions—as all allergies always are).

Usually acute ailments will last less than two weeks and will resolve themselves. In these cases, you are usually working to help speed healing and to bring comfort to the patient throughout the healing process. But these are the illnesses that take us by surprise, indeed, that take our immune systems by surprise. They are sudden and short-term and are easier to cure than a chronic illness, in that the goal of treatment is simply to return the patient to the level of health enjoyed before the ailment started. If you are treating a patient with a cold or flu, you are seeking only to help them recover from those symptoms and, at the end of treatment, be at the same level of health they were before the onset of symptoms.

---

* Turn to the Appendix for a list of Internet sources of cell salt remedies. They can be ordered individually or in kits for home use.

In chronic conditions, things are more complex.* In many chronic conditions, the factors that created the situation at hand are not so easily identified. Many involve stress, lifestyle choices, age, weight, diet, exercise (or lack thereof)—multiple factors that result in chronic dyspepsia, chronic asthma, chronic conditions of the skin, chronic aches and pains associated with the muscles and/or joints, and on and on. These are harder to get a handle on, both in terms of cause and in terms of treatment. And they are harder symptoms to remove. You may find that improving them is remarkably easy, but removing them is very, very hard. In these cases you have to know when you have reached your level of skill and when to call the doctor. In fact, whether you are using the cell salts, the homeopathic remedies, the Bach remedies or other floral essences, nutritional supplements, or herbal remedies, you must always keep in mind that none of these things can be used as effectively in the hands of a well-meaning parent or loved one who takes on the role of the practitioner as they can be by a trained medical professional. It is therefore important that, in the first place, your doctor knows of your use of any form of medication beyond those that he or she has given you (there is no place for secrets when it comes to medicine) and, in the second place, that you know when to treat things on your own and when to call the doctor. The cell salts are a wonderful and safe form of self-treatment. They are not, especially in the hands of the unskilled student, a panacea.

> If the patient has several symptoms, try to find out which is the worst, which dominates from his or her point of view. Try to find out in what order they appeared, or if any of the symptoms are linked, if they alternate or connect together in any way. Notice the patient's manner, how he or she answers the questions, how they speak and how they behave. Learn to observe.

Case Taking

In beginning the case taking, you will have to observe and judge the situation. Learn right up front to observe as best you can all that is going on—not only the physical nature of the patient's symptoms, but also his or her emotional and mental reaction to those symptoms. Break down the case into the component symptoms. What, if it can

---

* Part of what makes treating patients with chronic conditions more problematic is that the goal of treatment is more difficult. In acute cases, you are only seeking to return the patient to the level of health he or she had before the onset of recent symptoms. In chronic cases, you are seeking to improve the general health of the patient. Not only to rid the patient of symptoms that have been in place for some time now, but also to so strengthen the patient's system that the symptoms will not return and he or she will, in essence, be healthier than before. This can be quite complicated and may require a great deal of patience on the part of the practitioner and the patient alike.

be known, is the cause of the symptoms, and what individual symptoms is the patient experiencing.

Make a list of the symptoms. In most cases, it will be best to actually write a physical list. In simple acute cases, usually those involving a simple mechanical injury, this won't be necessary, and the case taking and remedy selection will happen more quickly than I can write about it. But in other acute cases it is best to make the list, even for those of simple colds or earaches. List the symptoms down the page. Seek the same information about each individual symptom by asking the patient:

Sensation: How does it hurt? What is the nature of the pain?

Location: Where does it hurt? Get as specific as possible.

Duration: When did it start hurting? How long has it been hurting? What were you doing when it started hurting?

If the patient has several symptoms, try to find out which is the worst, which dominates from his or her point of view. Try to find out in what order they appeared, or if any of the symptoms are linked, if they alternate or connect together in any way. Notice the patient's manner, how he or she answers the questions, how they speak and how they behave. Learn to observe.

Take time to observe the patient's physical being. Check the affected area for discoloration, for swelling, for any change.

Check the tongue in all cases of indigestion of any form, as well as in all cases of colds, flu, and other similar illnesses. The tongue is one of our best indicators when it comes to the selection of a remedy. Always check the patient's tongue in all chronic conditions. When you are in doubt as to what to do next, check the tongue. Learn the colors of the coating and what remedies they suggest. Learn what swelling of the tongue indicates. What a clean tongue indicates.

In the same way, learn the discharges and what they indicate. With only twelve remedies and with each linked to a particular color or colors of discharge, this is a fairly simple task to accomplish. Soon, you will know what a red, hot, flushed face indicates, what swelling without inflammation indicates, what a yellow tongue indicates. These are guiding symptoms that will lead you to a remedy.

Modalities

Next, try to find out the modalities of the case. Modalities are those things that make the symptoms better or worse. These are very important and will guide you in the selection of a remedy or remedies.

Work first from the point of view of each of the symptoms that you have already listed. What makes each one feel better or worse? Common catalysts to improvement or aggravation are hot or cold applications, motion or rest, specific positions of the body, times of day or night, weather conditions or changes, and changes in the environment (hot, cold, wet, dry, and so on). Gathering the modalities of the case will help you gather the sort of information that will lead you to the right treatment.

Make sure you also gather the modalities that concern the patient as a whole after you have gathered the information about each individual symptom. While an injured knee may feel better from applications of ice, the patient, as a whole being, may want to be in a warm room or wrapped up tight. Or the patient who has to keep a hot application clutched tightly to his or her back may also want fresh open air in order to feel better as a being. So be sure to compare the modalities of the case, as they apply to the symptoms and to the patient as a whole.

From this gathered information—about the onset of the case (and its cause, if it can be determined), the details of the symptoms and the modalities of their discomfort, as well as the general information regarding the behavior of the patient and what makes him or her feel better as a whole being—you should have enough information to make the selection of an indicated remedy or remedies. Again, remember to use the tongue as an indicator if you are unclear as to which remedies are suggested.

At this point you will have to make the final decision as to how you will use the remedies, as supplements or as homeopathic remedies. This decision will determine how you proceed. In most cases, the remedy or remedies used may be given by mouth and may be dissolved in warm or cool water (in many cases as the patient prefers), and used topically as well. A clean towel can be dipped in the dissolved remedies and applied directly to the site of the injury or symptom. Even digestive symptoms or allergies or headaches will respond better if the treatment is topical as well as by mouth. In some cases, you may choose to give one remedy topically while using another internally. This can work well in cases of mechanical injury in which the affected area is limited, but the impact upon the patient's being is profound. One remedy, such as Ferrum Phosphoricum, can be used topically at the site of the injury, while another, like Kali Phosphoricum, can be given for the emotional trauma that accompanies the physical trauma. Or more than one remedy can be dissolved in water and given internally and topically at the same time. These are the decisions that you will make in the future based upon the experiences you have gathered in the past. I can only suggest that, in most cases, it is better to err on the side of giving too few remedies and doses than to err by giving them too liberally (certainly in most cases that you are attempting to treat in the home, as opposed to calling 911). While the cell salts are gentle and low in potency, aggravations are not unknown.

Aggravations and Provings

An aggravation is a temporary increase in discomfort, in the aches and pains of the case, before they are improved. They usually indicate that the treatment given was a bit too hurried or too high in potency or dose. They are not dangerous; in fact, they can be a very good sign, because the case that is aggravated after the remedies have been given is very likely to be greatly improved shortly thereafter. Some practitioners actually look for the aggravation as a sign of cure. (I personally would like to see those same practitioners go through aggravations when they are ill and watch others rub their hands together in glee while they watch them writhe in pain. I tend to think that, after such an experience, they would not seek to create aggravations any longer. Instead, they would seek a simple, gentle, and rapid cure.)

This is, to me, another argument for beginning the case with a single dose of a single remedy to see what happens. The likelihood of an aggravation is far less this way, and the actual impact that the cell salt has on the case can be traced. Other remedies can be added, if needed, in the hours or days following the original treatment.

Whether giving a single remedy or a combination, the question that next arises is one of repetition. When do you give the next dose? The answer to that depends upon the impact of the first dose. If the patient's symptoms shift and hopefully lessen as a response to the first dose, then you need not give a second dose until symptoms begin to recur. That may be in a matter of a half hour, an hour, or half a day. Always follow the symptoms when determining the number of doses that a patient needs.

In the same way, always follow the symptoms when choosing a remedy, or when deciding to change remedies or add remedies. Watch how they shift, lessen, and otherwise change. These changes can either be an indication that the remedy you have given is doing good work, in which case the choice is whether or not to give another dose, or they can be an indication that the remedy is not helping or not helping enough, in which case you must consider changing the remedy or giving a second remedy in alternation or combination with it. Again, these decisions may be made in a matter of minutes, hours, or days, as the situation dictates. As the discomfort of the patient dictates. And, again, never hesitate to ask for help, to seek the advice of a medical professional when appropriate.

Since many people use the cell salts nutritionally and, therefore, give the same remedy repeatedly for a long period of time, we need to be aware of the notion of provings and how they apply to the use of these remedies.

Provings can happen either accidentally or on purpose. All homeopathic remedies—and the cell salts are homeopathic remedies—go through a proving process as part of the "research and development" phase of their potentization. Before they are given as remedies, all homeopathics are tested. This means they are given to healthy people (homeopathic medicines are the only medicines that are tested on healthy humans, as opposed to sick patients or laboratory animals) to see what changes they can bring about. These tests are double-blind studies in which some people are given a placebo and others are given the remedy. All who take part then keep a strict diary of all the changes they experience. This information is gathered and, in some cases, repeated again and again until the full effects of the remedy can be traced. Then it becomes a part of the homeopathic pharmacy.

Accidental provings happen when a remedy is given too often. You see, the real power of homeopathy is in the repetition of dosing. When you give a remedy once, you show its capability in the case at hand, but when you give it again and again, you show its real power. Even remedies that are not similar enough in their action to cause change in the case will, if you repeat them enough, start to work artificially, start to graft the symptoms of the remedy onto the case. That is another reason why I always begin with a single dose of a single remedy: to see how the patient will feel as a result, not only of that remedy but of that single dose. From there I move forward carefully, always watching the symptoms and how they are changing, watching the patient to see whether or not he or she is improving as a whole being (looking better, behaving better, becoming stronger) as a result of the doses. In fact, I tend to look at every dose as a single dose, not as a part of a series of doses. I tend to never repeat what does not have to be repeated.

Those who do not use the cell salts in this manner run the risk of proving the remedies—of having them create new symptoms that are the action of the remedy and not of the disease. (This is the homeopathic version of the iatrogenic diseases of allopathy, with the difference being that the symptoms disappear when you stop giving the cell salts that are causing the symptoms, which is not always the case with iatrogenic diseases.) While provings can be uncomfortable, they are not dangerous. The worst thing about them is that they are confusing. You can, as the practitioner, become very confused as to why the symptoms are changing as they are. As a rule of thumb, if new symptoms appear after giving repeated doses of a remedy or remedies, always check the information you have on the remedies you are using. See if those new symptoms are listed as being among those treated by the remedies. If they are, you are likely seeing a proving and should hold back on your doses.

In all cases in which provings are suspected, don't give the next dose for a while. Hold back and watch. If the symptoms fade and the patient improves without that next dose, then wait some more and see if the patient needs another dose or if the healing process is complete. If the original symptoms return, give the next dose and again wait to see if improvement begins. As a rule of thumb, always seek improvement, and lay back on the remedy once you have gotten it. Don't give it again unless or until the symptoms begin to return. And please note that I specifically used the word "improvement" and not "cure." What you seek is an improvement of symptoms, not their total elimination. Improvement means that the remedy is working and deserves time to complete its action. That is the goal of the dose, not a total cure. It may take several doses, multiple remedies, or just enough time without doses for a cure to take place naturally. Follow the symptoms, seek the improvement, and trust the body to heal itself. This is the best advice I can give in the use of these or any other remedies.

And remember that more cases are ruined by the use of too much medicine than by any other method. This is true in allopathic medicine just as it is in homeopathic. Keep this in mind whether you are using cell salts or more highly diluted remedies. Trust your patient's ability to heal more than your own ego's need to be the source of that healing. Give only the doses that are needed and only when needed and provings won't happen and aggravations will be few and far apart.

Potency

The issue of potency is one of the reasons to use the cell salts in the first place, because it is of much less importance when dealing with the cell salts than it is with the homeopathic pharmacy as a whole. When you have that whole pharmacy at your disposal you must deal with thousands of remedies, each in a multiplicity of potencies from very low to very high. Therefore, you must choose carefully from among them to make the healing process rapid, gentle, and permanent.

With the cells salts, we have only a dozen remedies, and all of them are kept to potencies of 12X or under. Still, even with this simplified approach to homeopathic treatment, we have to consider potency.

In all cases, the 6X potency is considered to be the general starting point for treatment. The home base. Most cell salts are most commonly available in 6X and it is usually a good, safe, and effective potency to give. But keep this in mind: for cases in which emotional or mental symptoms are important, use a higher potency, use 12X. For cases in which skin conditions are important, such as poison ivy, go lower and use the 3X potency. This is because if you go with a higher potency with skin conditions, the body will cause the rash to spread, in the process of expelling the symptoms. This will make the patient a good deal more miserable than he already is before he is made well. So suit the potency to the symptoms. Emotions are best soothed by higher dilutions. Conditions based very much in the body, like skin conditions, some digestive complaints, and specific allergens (like allergies to cats) work best in low dilutions, even down to a 1X.

But when in doubt, stick to the multiples of 3: 3x, 6X, 9X, 12X. For cases in which you want to start out very gently, start the case with a single dose of 3X and build upward, on the multiples. Then, after waiting, if the improvement this brings is not sufficient or does not last sufficiently long, going up to 6X and again watching, and so on. This is a good, safe method of treatment, especially for chronic cases.

This brings us to another rule of thumb, which has to do with the treatment of acute conditions versus that of chronic cases.

While it flies in the face of logic, acute cases tend to take more doses of more remedies to clear them away than chronic cases. It is in acute cases that I tend to alternate (you may want to combine) a larger number of different remedies than I will with chronic cases. In chronic cases, doses are given further apart, but since acute cases often involve more severe discomfort they require doses that are given more rapidly or require the use of more rapid alternation of remedies. Patience is required in chronic cases. What was slow in coming will also be slow in going. In chronic cases in particular, too many doses of too many remedies given too close together can result in confusion that will require time and skill to resolve. Better instead to avoid the confusion through patience.

Completing the Case

Knowing when to stop giving a remedy can be difficult, especially if you are giving the cell salts nutritionally. The question is one of goals.

Compare cell salt treatments with diets. When we start a diet we always start out with a specific goal in mind. There is a weight we weigh and a weight we want to weigh. We adjust our eating and our exercising so we can lose enough weight to hit the goal. Once we attain the goal, we make changes in our program of diet and exercise so we can maintain it.

The same goes for cell salt treatments. In just the same way, with all cell salt treatments, especially those that are for chronic complaints, there will be that moment when the specific goal has been met and health has been restored. At that moment, the plan must change from one of attaining the goal to one of maintaining it.

That may mean that the remedy must also change. Often the remedy Calcarea Phosphorica is used at this point, as it is our general remedy involved in the maintenance of health or in recovery. Or Calcarea Fluorica may be called for, as it often is. Or the same remedy that was curative may be needed, but in lower potency or in doses that are much farther apart. Or no remedy may be needed. (My preference, by the way, whenever possible is that no remedy be used unless it is absolutely needed. I see little reason for us to become slaves to a new type of pill, and instead prefer not to use pills of any sort when they are not needed.)

In all cases the moment that the goals have been reached is the moment when the case should be taken again, hopefully for the last time. Work down that list of original symptoms again. If all have been cleared away and the patient is free of pain or limitation and capable of living life unfettered, then let him do so. If the illness itself has passed but it has left the patient depleted, then consider a new remedy, such as those listed above. If the patient is greatly improved but the illness lingers, consider the same remedy in a new potency or in continued doses, or consider adding a new remedy in alternation.

But if that hoped for thing has happened, and the patient has been made well, then shake hands and part company. The patient is well and you have done your job. Remember, more cases are ruined by too much medicine than by too little.

Lessons Learned

I believe that, even in the home, or even in terms of self-treatment, there is a place for case management. There is a requirement to learn both from successes and from failures, a need to learn and to continue learning from both what has worked well and what has not. Each offers important information. Always make sure to take the moment that it takes to reflect over the case after its completion. Ask yourself what you did and what you might have done better. Only by taking this moment can you be sure that you will do better next time.

Used carefully and appropriately, I believe that the cell salts offer a simple and yet surprisingly powerful tool for healing, whether you ultimately choose to use them like nutritional supplements or as homeopathic remedies. They are both, after all, and will respond to both viewpoints. It is more important that you use them within the context of your capability, that you do not work beyond your level of understanding than that you adhere strictly to Hahnemann's concept of what is and is not homeopathic.

One last thought, however—and it is important. It has to do with when you actually sit down and learn about the cell salts. Most of us make the mistake of waiting until our child is awakened in the early hours of the morning with an earache to try and figure out which remedy has a bright red face that is dry and hot, because our child happens to have a face that looks that way. If you wait until then to try and learn about the cell salts, you would likely do better to go to the emergency room and try and learn about them some other time. Those who try to learn homeopathy in a crisis are those who are likely to fail to use the remedies correctly. This is the most important thing that I can tell you. Sit down and learn about the cell salts, the symptoms they have, the way they look and act and smell, when they are not needed, when all is well. That way, when a crisis comes, you will have the knowledge at your fingertips and can go and

> Those who try to learn homeopathy in a crisis are those who are likely to fail to use the remedies correctly. This is the most important thing that I can tell you. Sit down and learn about the cell salts, the symptoms they have, the way they look and act and smell, when they are not needed, when all is well. That way, when a crisis comes, you will have the knowledge at your fingertips and can go and get your kit and treat the patient with some degree of knowledge and calm. This is what will yield the best results, I promise you.

get your kit and treat the patient with some degree of knowledge and calm. This is what will yield the best results, I promise you. This will make the time you spent with this book and others like it well worth the investment: when you feel fevers fade, see pained expressions smooth into calm repose, and notice eyes become bright once more. All because *you knew* what to do.

Chapter Seven

A Reference Guide
to the Cell Salts

As there are only twelve cell salts, it is easy enough to have each of them on hand at all times in a home kit. Each remedy can vary in potency from 1X to 12X, which ups the ante for a full-range kit from a dozen to a gross of remedies, but generally speaking, a 6X potency will be good for home use (any alternate potencies for use in specific cases or for specific remedies will be noted).

In the pages that follow you will find a simple list of common conditions and the remedies that are most often linked with those conditions. Keep in mind, however, that even though the cell salts are used nutritionally, they are low-potency homeopathic remedies and should be respected as such. The use of too many different remedies or of remedies that are repeated too often can lead to a case that, instead of clearing up nicely, becomes more and more confusing. Before giving any remedy or remedies listed here, make sure to read more about them in Chapter Six of this book or in a more detailed materia medica. Before giving a remedy, it is important to check to see if that remedy is a good match for the patient *in toto;* that it matches not only a single symptom, but also the patient's state of being as a whole. By doing this, you can be sure that you will make the best choice possible from among the cell salts in any instance of home use.

FIRST AID

There are two important things you have to remember when it comes to first aid treatments.

Number one is to remember that, just because you have opted to use cell salt remedies to treat those who are in need of first aid, it does not mean that you do not need to do any of the logical and sensible things that should accompany any first aid treatment. In other words, remember to assess the patient who is in need of first aid and respond to that patient's needs. Wounds need to be cleaned, patients calmed, bodies need to be moved or not moved, as the situation dictates. Do not come to think of the cell salts as a cure-all, something that can be used in place of common sense. Used correctly and appropriately, they can be of great help in common household ailments and emergencies. Used outside the context of common sense, the cell salts will seem to fail as remedies, not because they have not "worked," but because they have not been given the opportunity to work as they are meant to.

> Remember to assess the patient who is in need of first aid and respond to that patient's needs. Wounds need to be cleaned, patients calmed, bodies need to be moved or not moved, as the situation dictates. Do not come to think of the cell salts as a cure-all, something that can be used in place of common sense. Used correctly and appropriately, they can be of great help in common household ailments and emergencies.

Which brings us to point number two: when using the cells salts, or, indeed, any form of over-the-counter medicine, make sure to never work beyond your skill level. If you have a patient with a simple cut or bruise, or who suffers from a cold in the nose, it is all well and good to keep them rested and comforted, and to treat them with cell salts until their health is in good order once more. If, however, you have a patient who is gravely ill or has been the victim of severe physical trauma or high fever, do not hesitate to go to the emergency room or call 911. In cases such as these, the cell salts can provide stop-gap remedy until help arrives.

This having been said, consider the following remedies in first aid situations.

General Remedies for Physical Trauma

Physical trauma can range from minor to more serious injuries. This section covers simple falls, blows, and bruises, from playground injuries to banging your knee on the kitchen counter to car accidents. Any form of mechanical injury to any part of the body may direct you to choose among these remedies, as they are our general "first aid remedies."

Ferrum Phosphoricum

To ease the actual effects of a blow, reach for Ferrum Phosphoricum, which is the first remedy to think of in all cases of mechanical injury, especially if the skin at the site of the injury is red and swollen. Also think of Kali Muriaticum, which is an excellent general remedy for physical injury, as well as an excellent follow-up to Ferrum Phos. Give Ferrum Phos first, with doses up to every fifteen minutes until improvement begins, in 6X, 9X or 12X potency, whatever you have on hand, the higher the better. Ferrum Phos responds to the first stage of the injury, when the site of the injury feels hot, swollen, and very painful. Kali Mur is more often associated with the second stage of injury, when the affected parts feel achy and stiff. Because of this, I do not suggest that the two remedies be used concurrently or in alternation at the time of the injury. Ferrum Phos should be given first, and Kali Mur added (either alone or in alternation at that point, as symptoms suggest) as the symptoms shift from the initial trauma to a more prolonged state of pain. If the patient feels the pain only upon motion and rests comfortably when not in motion, then you must alternate the two remedies to give relief.

Kali Phosphoricum

This remedy has a special place among the remedies for those who are injured or wounded. As a wound or injury of any sort can provoke a great deal of emotional upset all around, it is my suggestion that Kali Phos be considered as the remedy for all—the patient and the caregiver alike—who become emotionally upset by the circumstances of the injury. This is especially true when the patient is a child and the caregiver is that child's parent. A dose of Kali Phos can help the caregiver cope emotionally with what is an extremely traumatic situation: watching a loved one suffering, frightened, and in physical pain. Just as Kali Phos is the remedy to think of for the emotional effects of physical pain, it is the remedy of choice for keeping the caregiver in a state in which they can function logically and effectively and keep enough emotional distance to be helpful in this very stressful situation.

Natrum Muriaticum

For long-standing injuries or for injuries that leave a specific part of the body weakened, with a tendency to reinjure, Natrum Muriaticum is always indicated. Note that Natrum Mur is especially helpful in cases involving injury to joints, particularly the knee, ankle, and hip joints, and to the back. Natrum Muriaticum is very helpful for those with chronically weakened backs. Think of Natrum Mur (in combination with Silicea, as needed; see below) as the best remedy for the third stage of injury. Use Ferrum Phos for the first stage, the stage of initial impact, Kali Mur for the second stage, the stage of pain, and Natrum Mur for those injuries that are not totally healed by these first two remedies, those injuries that leave the patient in a state of chronic weakness or pain. In these cases, both Natrum Mur and Silicea are needed, and can almost be thought of as one remedy.

Natrum Sulphuricum

For physical trauma that results in deep changes in the patient's behavior (especially in injury to the head), the remedy is always Natrum Sulphuricum. This is always the remedy for any sort of wound that leaves the patient changed, that impacts him or her emotionally and spiritually as well as physically. Natrum Sulph may be used in combination with Natrum Mur if the state seems chronic, or with Kali Phos (see below) if the patient is highly agitated.

Kali Phosphoricum

For the emotional trauma that accompanies an injury, think of Kali Phosphoricum. This is the remedy for those who become upset, frightened, or anxious due to their injury. Who are frantic and need to be comforted. It can be used in combination with any of the other remedies listed here to help center and calm the patient as he or she heals.

Calcarea Phosphorica

This is perhaps our most important remedy when it comes to bones: to the formation of healthy bones and to the healing of injuries to bones and all hard tissues in the body. Calcium phosphate is a component of both bone and teeth, and is therefore vital to their formation. Once it has been potentized it is also an important remedy for injuries to bones. It is also a component of soft tissues and a component of blood. As Calcarea Phosphorica promotes the growth of new, healthy cells, blood cells included, it is an important general remedy for the restoration of health and the prevention of disease. Calc Phos acts as a general tonic to the system and can be given along with any other cell salt to enhance its power. It works to stimulate healing and to prevent disease.

Calcarea Sulphurica

Use the remedy Calcarea Sulphurica to help the system cleanse itself and to clear any infection that is building. If the wound has been neglected, if it has not been properly cleaned and the patient has not been attended to as he or she should have been, always think of Calc Sulph, and use it in conjunction with Ferrum Phos and Kali Mur. Especially if the wound is becoming inflamed, if it is red and swollen and hot, alternate or combine Calc Sulph with Ferrum Phosphoricum to help stem the inflammation. Calc Sulph may also be used either before or after Silicea in cases of wounds that are becoming infected or that have failed to heal properly once pus has been expelled.

Silicea

Always think of Silicea in any form of injury that is slow to heal, or for any patient whose ability to heal from any illness seems compromised. Remember that Silicea is a slow-acting, deep-acting remedy and that you may have to repeat it in regular doses for some time before the healing process is complete.

Kali Muriaticum

This is the remedy to remember in all cases that have to do with swelling. For the swelling of tissues that results from all blows, cuts, and bruises. For all hemorrhages, especially those that bleed dark blood, and for wounds that clot but do not heal. For all hard swellings of the skin that occur along with injuries of any sort.

Specific Remedies for Physical Trauma

For injuries to the bones: Calcarea Phosphorica and Silicea, used separately or in combination, are the two most common general remedies. (See Fractures, below.)

For injuries to soft tissue—skin, tendons, and ligaments: Think of Silicea as a follow-up to two initial remedies, Ferrum Phosphoricum and Kali Muriaticum, used in alternation or combination.

For injuries that are slow to heal: Silicea may be used in combination or alternation with any other indicated remedy or remedies.

For any injuries that are threatening to become infected: Use Calcarea Sulphurica if the infection is threatening but has not yet begun, as it may prevent the formation of pus. If pus has formed, give Silicea as the remedy to ripen the wound and expel the pus. Calcarea Sulphurica is also helpful in healing old wounds that have not healed properly. It will prevent reinfection. For injuries in elderly patients: consider Natrum Muriaticum and/or Silicea. The two remedies may be combined or used in alternation with patients who are slow to heal from injuries, or who seem resigned to the discomfort of their injury.

For injuries in which the pain returns after the injury has apparently healed: Natrum Muriaticum or Silicea. You will see this important combination suggested again and again for cases of injuries of all sorts. These remedies work best in alternation, in my opinion. Give each twice a day, four to five tablets at a time. Give the Silicea an hour before breakfast and dinner and Natrum Mur an hour after those meals.

Fractures

Fractures—broken bones—can be complete or incomplete, simple or compound. The nature of the fracture itself will help you determine the cell salt remedy or remedies that should be used. Keep in mind that in all cases of fracture, a trip to the emergency room is called for.

Incomplete fractures, also called "greenstick fractures" are those in which the bone is only partially broken, and are, therefore, the least serious. A complete fracture is one in which the bone is completely broken.

Simple fractures are those that involve only the bone, cases in which the soft tissue is still intact. Compound fractures, in which not only the bone is injured, but also the soft tissue, tendons, ligaments, and, most often, the skin, are the most serious. In cases of compound fracture, there can be a danger due to blood loss. There is also an increased danger of infection if the skin is broken. In all cases of fracture, the greater danger to the health of the patient may not be the broken bone itself, but the splintered fragments of bone caused by the break that can cut blood vessels and nerves.

All cases of compound fracture involve not just consideration of the bone, but also treatment of the wound involving one or more of the remedies listed in the section on wounds (see below).

While the cell salts are certainly not a replacement for more traditional treatments in cases of fracture, they can help speed the healing process and make sure that the bone, when healed, is as strong as it was before the break. They can also help make sure that bone fragments are safely reabsorbed into the system.

General remedies for fractures include Silicea, Calcarea Phosphorica, Calcarea Fluorica and Natrum Muriaticum.

Silicea

In all cases of fracture, whatever other remedy or remedies you may use, make sure to use Silicea. From the time of the break until the bone is completely healed, Silicea will be called for to make sure that the bone heals completely and that the bone is strong.

Calcarea Phosphorica

This is the general remedy for any injury to bones and should be given in all cases of fracture, whether simple or compound. Like Silicea, with which it pairs very well, Calc Phos will add strength to the bone and speed healing, while supporting the overall strength and vitality of the injured patient.

Calcarea Fluorica

Calcarea Fluorica is also considered a good general remedy for fractures, and may be selected in place of Calcarea Phosphorica if the patient's overall symptoms suggest its use. Calc Fluor is especially helpful in cases of greenstick fractures, when the bone is bruised or partially broken. (Calc Phos is, however, the more general remedy for use in cases of fractures.)

Natrum Muriaticum

For fractures that are deeply painful, think of Natrum Muriaticum in addition to or in alternation with any of the three general remedies. Add the Natrum Mur if the patient does not want to move in his or her pain, if he or she wants to lie down and be left alone. Natrum Mur is a good third-stage remedy to think of in all fractures if the bone or joint seems permanently weakened by the injury.

Specific Remedies for Fractures

When broken bones do not heal as quickly as they should: Alternate or combine Silicea and Calcarea Phosphorica. Whenever the speed of healing is an issue, or when healing is incomplete and the patient depleted, think of adding Silicea into the mix. Just as the addition of silica to a plant's stem gives that stem strength to support the whole plant, the addition of Silicea to an injured patient's system will strengthen the patient's whole system and make healing both faster and more complete.

For past injuries to bones that have left the bone weakened and prone to reinjury: Combine or alternate Natrum Mur and Silicea. Natrum Mur, as has been noted, is always the remedy to think of in old injuries, in injuries that tend to recur again and again. The combination of these two remedies, therefore, makes a powerful tool for any injury that has left the patient with a chronic complaint, weakness, or pain. This is an especially good combination for elderly patients.

Head Trauma/Concussions

Any injury to the head can be cause for alarm, although most result in nothing more than a lump. Special caution should be taken if the patient shows any signs of concussion, including headache, general trembling, palpitations, vertigo and/or fainting, chills, cold sweats, and nausea. If the patient loses consciousness, however briefly, he or she should receive emergency medical treatment immediately.

General Remedies for Those Who Suffer a Trauma to the Head

Use Ferrum Phosphoricum, followed by or in combination with Kali Muriaticum, for traumas to the head. I know that much has been written about the fact that Natrum Sulphuricum is the specific remedy for all cases of head trauma, but Natrum Sulph is especially helpful for cases in which the patient seems somehow *changed* as a person following the injury. Most cases of head trauma, indeed, of concussion, do not result in this, so the best place to start is always with the same combination that is our general tool for injuries: Ferrum Phos for the first stage of the injury, especially when swelling results; and Kali Mur as the follow-up remedy, when the lump has raised on the head. Both remedies can be dissolved in water and applied externally as well, as part of the cold compress applied to the site of the injury.

Specific Remedies for Those Who Suffer a Trauma to the Head

If the injury to the head seems to impact the patient as a *being*: Natrum Sulphuricum is always the indicated remedy. This is the remedy for the third stage of the injury, if the blow to the head seems to be creating chronic changes to the patient. Think of this remedy if the other cell salts fail to bring about a state of complete health or if the patient has any emotional or mental issues caused by the blow to the head. Use especially if the situation seems to be becoming chronic.

For the patient who is manic or anxious following an injury to the head: Kali Phosphoricum should be added to the remedies used. Kali Phos can be given by mouth while Ferrum Phos and/or Kali Mur is used topically in the wet compress. Kali Phos can even be dissolved in warm tea and given to the patient in slow sips as needed to help restore a sense of calm.

If the patient experiences changes in vision after injury to the head: Magnesia Phosphorica should be used in addition to other indicated remedies.

Wounds

Simply put, wounds are any break in the skin that exposes the body to infection. The cause of the wound and the nature of the wound itself can help simplify the selection of an appropriate remedy.

Incised wounds are made by sharp objects that slice into the skin, leaving a clean cut. Lacerated wounds involve a ripping or tearing of skin, leaving a ragged-edged cut. These two forms of wound suggest the same group of remedies.

They also require the same first-aid precautions in addition to the cell salts. When dealing with any wound, the first step in treatment is to try and stop the bleeding. In cases of simple incised or lacerated wounds, this can usually be done by applying simple, gentle pressure on the wound and/or by raising the affected area upward. External applications of cold water or ice can help to stop the bleeding as well.

The next step is always to clean the wound, to clear away any debris that may be in the wound. Running water works well to clean a wound.

The third step is to bandage the wound to prevent infection and/or reinjury.

As always, it is important to judge the severity of the situation to decide when a visit to the emergency room is needed, as some wounds will need stitches in order to heal correctly.

All wounds need attention as they heal. Make certain to keep the wound clean and to check for signs of infection as it heals.

General Remedies for Cuts and Wounds

Kali Muriaticum, Ferrum Phosphoricum, Magnesia Phosphorica, Calcarea Sulphurica, and Silicea are the remedies to look to in cases of cuts and wounds.

Of these, the two most used general remedies will be Kali Muriaticum, for the swelling of the wound and Silicea, to promote healing. Together these remedies will promote the growth of healthy new cells and promote the expulsion of all that is unhealthy in the body.

When in doubt, you can always start the treatment with Ferrum Phos and Kali Mur, as you would with any other injury. But if the cut is clean and simple, if it does not involve inflammation, heat, swelling, and redness, Ferrum Phos can be skipped (unless the wound is bleeding a good deal, when Ferrum Phos again becomes a suggested remedy), and Kali Mur can be the remedy of first choice. In all cases, Silicea is a good choice as an adjunct remedy to either or both Ferrum Phos and Kali Mur, as it will help the skin heal and will help prevent the formation of a scar.

Specific Remedies for Cuts and Wounds

For any cut that bleeds very freely, for cuts that seem to bleed more than they should for the size and depth of the injury: Natrum Muriaticum. To help stop bleeding from any cut, add Ferrum Phosphoricum to the choice of remedies.

For cuts that seem to hurt more than they should, given the size or depth of the injury: Natrum Muriaticum, Magnesia Phosphorica.

If the patient responds to the pain by lying down to rest: Natrum Muriaticum.

If the patient paces the floor in pain or sits up in a chair: Magnesia Phosphorica.

For injuries from animal or human bites (lacerated wounds): Magnesia Phosphorica is the remedy of first choice. It may be added to Kali Muriaticum in combination or alternation in all cases of lacerated wounds.

For cuts that are becoming infected: Calcarea Sulphurica. This remedy is very important in the beginning stages of infection. Used immediately, it will cleanse the affected area and clear away an infection. This is an important remedy to consider in all wounds in which the skin has been broken.

For any cut that is slow to heal: Silicea. Silicea is the last-stage remedy to be used in almost all cases of cuts or wounds. Its use will help the skin heal completely and will help prevent scarring.

Puncture Wounds/Splinters

Puncture wounds, the final category of wounds, are caused by narrow, sharp objects, such as needles or nails. For our purposes, insect bites will also be categorized as puncture wounds.

As with any other wound, it is important that the puncture be kept clean, and that any bleeding be stopped. The two issues of import when dealing with punctures are that they are notoriously slow to heal and that they can present a danger of infection. They need to be kept clean (even insect bites), and to be watched as they heal.

General Remedies for Puncture Wounds

Silicea is the major general remedy for puncture wounds. Silicea will promote speedy healing of the wound. As with all case of wounds, Ferrum Phosphoricum may be considered for the time just after the actual injury when the wound is fresh, especially if the skin is red and swollen. Kali Muriaticum, as always, is a good follow-up remedy to Ferrum Phos in cases of wounds. But just as in cases of cuts, Ferrum Phos may often be omitted. In cases of insect bites, the combination of Ferrum Phos and Silicea is often sufficient and Kali Mur is not called for.

If the puncture seems to be becoming infected, add Calcarea Sulphurica to the mix. But, if you do, remove Silicea. Silicea and Calc Sulph can be used in *alternation*, but not in *combination*, as they have an opposite impact on the body—Silicea promotes the gathering of pus to expel it from the body, while Calcarea Sulphurica inhibits the formation of pus. Which you use at any given time depends upon the situation. For wounds that are moving toward infection but are not yet infected, Calcarea Sulphurica is an excellent remedy that can help to avoid infection. For wounds that are already infected, in which pus is formed, Silicea will help the body expel the pus and heal the wound. For wounds that do not fully heal in spite of treatment, follow the Silicea with Calcarea Sulphurica again to complete the healing process.

Specific Remedies for Puncture Wounds

For splinters, for any wound that embeds foreign matter in the skin: Silicea. As Silicea is known to be the remedy of first choice to help the body expel any embedded foreign object, it can be very helpful for splinters that are caught down deep under the skin.

For insect bites: Magnesia Phosphorica is an excellent remedy, especially if the insect bites are small, red, and look rather like a rash. The remedy can be dissolved in cool water and applied externally on a cool, damp cloth. It can be taken internally as well, or Natrum Muriaticum can be taken internally while Mag Phos is applied directly to the skin.

For insect bites that are painful: Natrum Muriaticum.

For insect bites that are itchy or make the skin very tender: Kali Phosphoricum.

Bruises

Bruises, which result from physical trauma to the soft tissue of the body that does not break the skin, are also called contused wounds. Because they are wounds, they need the same basic remedies that are used for other wounds. Ferrum Phosphoricum, followed by Kali Muriaticum, should be the remedies of first choice if swelling of tissues has taken place, as it commonly does with a bruise. Other remedies to keep in mind include Natrum Sulphuricum, Kali Phosphoricum, and Calcarea Phosphorica, which should be used in the treatment of all bruises.

Ferrum Phosphoricum

For bruises that are accompanied by swelling, heat, and inflammation, think of Ferrum Phosphoricum first. Note that Ferrum Phos can be dissolved in water for topical application to wounds. Use a good half-dozen pellets of 6X, 9X or 12X potency—again, the higher the better in this case—for topical applications. Ferrum Phos is the remedy to be used just after the physical injury has occurred.

Kali Muriaticum

For bruises that are black and blue, Kali Muriaticum is the remedy of choice. If the swelling is hard to the touch. Kali Mur, like Ferrum Phos, can be dissolved in cool water and applied topically to the bruise. Kali Mur is the remedy of choice for this second stage of the contusion, after any initial inflammation has passed.

Calcarea Phosphorica

Cal Phos should be included in any treatment of any bruise. It may be combined or alternated with Ferrum Phosphoricum and/or Kali Muriaticum in the treatment. It may be used at any stage in the treatment, although it is most often used as a final remedy after Ferrum Phosphoricum has already been used to clear away inflammation. Alternated or combined with Kali Muriaticum, it speeds the reabsorption of blood from the bruise and promotes the growth of healthy tissue.

Natrum Sulphuricum

For cases in which the patient is severely bruised, when he has been beaten or in a severe accident, consider the remedy Natrum Sulphuricum. Just as this is the remedy of choice for cases of concussion, it is also very helpful for the patient who has been overwhelmed by his injuries, and who is not "acting like himself."

Kali Phosphoricum

Use the remedy Kali Phosphoricum for cases in which the patient feels emotionally bruised, whether or not he or she is physically bruised. Kali Phos can be used in conjunction with any of the other remedies listed for the patient who feels raw, anxious, or overwhelmed; who considers himself or herself to be emotionally bruised. For instance, Kali Phos can be given internally, while Ferrum Phos or Kali Mur (or both in combination) is applied externally in a wet compress.

Shock

The physical state of shock occurs—often in conjunction with a physical injury of some sort—when blood flow to important parts of the body is interrupted, either from blood loss or from a sudden drop in blood pressure. In either case, the symptoms most often associated with shock include a sense of anxiety or surprising calm; rapid, shallow, breathing or panting; a pulse that is rapid and shallow; and a sudden cold sweat on the body, accompanied by nausea and vertigo. The patient in shock may faint. He or she may be disconnected with the events that caused the shock. The patient may also be exceedingly thirsty.

Note that shock may have a physical or an emotional cause. And that the best remedy to use is most often determined by the emotional symptoms displayed by the patient.

Note also that shock may be dangerous. Physical shock may indicate the need for emergency medical treatment.

Our most important remedies for shock are Kali Phosphoricum, Magnesia Phosphorica, and Natrum Phosphoricum. Other indicated remedies include Natrum Muriaticum and Natrum Sulphuricum.

Kali Phosphoricum

This is the general remedy for those in shock when there are no defining symptoms. Kali Phos is always the remedy of first choice when the patient is in a state of agitated shock, when he or she is overly emotional or emotionally raw. It is especially called for if the patient feels cold due to shock.

Magnesia Phosphorica

For cases in which the patient in shock is "twitchy," the best remedy is Magnesia Phosphorica. This is the remedy to think of for the patient who needs to "steady" his or her nerves, whose body jerks and jumps, in whole or in part, due to the shock of events. This is the remedy as well for the patient whose hands, or other specific parts of the body, tremble due to shock. (Note that Kali Phos can also be helpful for trembling and should be used in combination with Mag Phos in cases of shock that involve involuntary trembling of the whole body.) Think of this remedy when shock is accompanied by sleeplessness.

Natrum Phosphoricum

For the patient who is in a state of "nervous exhaustion," consider the remedy Natrum Phosphoricum. This is a good follow-up remedy (usually for Kali Phosphoricum) for the aftereffects of shock, for the depletion and exhaustion that follows physical and emotional shock. In fact, this remedy may be needed by the caregiver and patient alike to help deal with the long-term impact of events.

Natrum Muriaticum and Natrum Sulphuricum

Both of these sodium-based remedies come into play in cases of shock. For the patient in shock who seems withdrawn, in denial of the situation, who only wants to be left alone, give Natrum Muriaticum as an acute remedy. Natrum Sulphuricum is a good follow-up remedy to Natrum Mur in cases of shock in which the patient remains indifferent to his or her situation and out of touch with himself or herself emotionally. Note that Natrum Mur is especially helpful in cases of shock that also involve grief, such as the death of a loved one. In these cases, Natrum Mur can help with long-held feelings of grief, sorrow, and betrayal.

Emotional Trauma

Emotional trauma is a more general category than shock (see previous page). These are the remedies most commonly used in cases of emotional upset, whether they are caused by bad news, by a nightmare, or by the circumstances of daily life, such as being the victim of a crime, a near miss on the highway, or any other situation that leaves the patient physically unharmed but emotionally vulnerable and raw.

Note that, when it comes to emotional upset, the general rule in dosing is the higher the potency the better. With the cell salts, that means using all the remedies listed below in 12X potency. The potency can be much higher when using the homeopathic equivalents.

General Remedies for Emotional Trauma

Kali Phosphoricum and Natrum Muriaticum are the major remedies for emotional trauma. This should come as no surprise, as each of these remedies has symptom portraits that emphasize or combine the physical with the emotional. Together they represent a yin/yang of emotional response, with Kali Phos typically being the remedy for the patient who shows his or her emotional distress, who is highly charged emotionally, while Natrum Mur commonly being the remedy for the patient who, while upset, masks it as best as he or she can. This may not always be the case. Natrum Murs can be highly charged emotionally, if they are pushed past their emotional limits. They can, for instance, cry publicly, even though such a loss of control may well send them running from the room. They are more likely to openly display such powerful emotions as anger and rage while masking their feelings of fear, anxiety, and grief.

Note that Natrum Mur, often followed by Natrum Sulphuricum, is an important remedy to keep in mind for those who act inappropriately in a given situation. For those who find themselves laughing at funerals, when they are deeply upset. When the action runs counter to the emotion.

Specific Remedies for Emotional Trauma

For cases of emotional trauma in which the patient is highly agitated: Kali Phosphoricum is the major remedy. The Kali Phos will likely be a blur of emotion and of physical movement. This is a weathervane of a remedy, with emotions shifting as often and effortlessly as the wind. Those around the Kali Phos may often wonder what it is that they said or did that so offended or hurt the patient. These are patients who cry easily, laugh at odd times, and display a raw emotional vulnerability.

Note that while we typically think of the Natrum Muriaticum types as being more stoic than the Kali Phos, they can become highly agitated as well. They often will react with rage when they feel betrayed or abandoned, or when they feel pushed to the wall emotionally. In these cases, they may seem more like Kali Phos types than Natrum Mur types, as their inner sense of vulnerability comes to the surface.

For cases in which a patient is highly agitated, consider combining the two remedies and use Kali Phos and Natrum Mur concurrently.

Consider adding Magnesia Phosphorica to the mix when a highly charged emotionalism keeps the patient from sleeping and, instead, drives them to twitch or move about or fuss with their hands, wringing them.

For cases of emotional trauma in which the patient seems indifferent, unconcerned: Natrum Muriaticum. This is the standard behavior pattern for the Natrum Mur patient. Indifference is the mask that they typically will wear when emotionally upset. Later, they will tend to blame those who failed to read their minds and understand their needs in times of vulnerability.

For cases of emotional trauma in which the patient suffers from fear: Silicea. The Silicea type is, by nature, timid and shy and given to fear, either vague, general fears associated with anxiety, or very specific fears, such as public speaking, that can cause the patient to have crippling panic attacks. Silicea is to fear as Ferrum Phosphoricum is to fevers—it is our best generalized remedy when we do not and cannot understand the nature or cause of the fear, but only can recognize that it exists. Whether the fear state is acute or chronic, give Silicea. Silicea can be used in combination or alternation with any of the other remedies for those who fear, and is especially helpful in dealing with long-term, deep-seated fears.

For the patient in whom emotional trauma manifests over time in a set of specific fears: Kali Sulphuricum. The Kali Sulph type will tend to link the emotional upset with a specific detail, a specific place, person, sight, or smell. He or she will develop a fear of bridges, heights, enclosed places, specific colors, animals, or foods because these act as a trigger that will cause the circumstances of the original upset to recur. Silicea can be used in combination with Kali Sulph for these patients, as can Natrum Phosphoricum, especially for younger patients. Both Natrum Phos and Kali Sulph will tend to have specific fears, of thunderstorms, of the dark. Both will want to have company and comfort.

For the patient who suffers from fears that are absolutely groundless, who fears unlikely things: Calcarea Fluorica, Kali Phosphoricum.

For the patient who is irrational in his or her fears, who has fears that involve a wild imagination, consider Kali Phosphoricum, Natrum Phosphoricum, and Calcarea Phosphorica.

For cases in which emotional trauma is accompanied by terror: Kali Phosphoricum, Natrum Muriaticum and Silicea. The Kali Phos connection is typical of the type. The patient is anxious and fearful and cries easily, wanting comfort. The Natrum Mur connection may be harder to spot, because the Natrum Mur type will often seem indifferent to upsets. However, this is a remedy that feels deep fears, and can respond to terror by shutting down, physically and emotionally.

The Silicea type responds to a sense of terror with physical weakness. Terror drains the Silicea patient of his or her vital force, weakening them into a state of physical exhaustion or illness. Silicea is a remedy for those who experience terror by shutting down, by letting go.

Note that Natrum Phosphoricum is another remedy to keep in mind for states of terror, especially when it is linked with very specific fears, such as of ghosts or the dark. It is often needed by young patients who have deep fears, night terrors, and fears of being left alone. Natrum Phos and Kali Phos combine quite well in these cases and can be used in alternation or combination. When alternating, start with Kali Phos and add the Natrum Phos after a few days if symptoms have not cleared.

If the sense of terror comes on very suddenly: Natrum Sulphuricum. This remedy will be especially helpful if the emotional trauma is accompanied by physical trauma, or if the state of terror comes on as a result of physical trauma.

For the patient who is hysterical: Kali Phosphoricum is once again the general remedy. If the patient is having an acute attack of hysteria, Kali Phos will always calm things down. If the patient is given to repeated attacks of hysteria after an emotional trauma, give Natrum Muriaticum or alternate between the two remedies. For the physical impact of an attack of hysteria, or for the patient who is exhausted after hysterics, give Natrum Muriaticum. Alternate it with Natrum Sulphuricum if the patient does not seem himself after the hysterics have ended.

Note that if the single attack of hysterics goes on and on and the patient cannot be comforted or calmed, a single dose of Silicea, given after Kali Phos, often sets things right. The dose of Silicea, of course, may be repeated if need be.

For cases of emotional upset that result in physical exhaustion: Silicea. Do not underestimate the use of Silicea in cases of emotional upset. It can be an extremely good remedy for those who react to emotional trauma by becoming irritated, or who have difficulty in thinking due to their upset (Magnesia Phosphorica will share this symptom). Especially think of Silicea if the patient's emotional state seems to be draining his or her physical strength, if the patient seems to want to waste away as a result of emotional upset or loss.

Also, for cases in which emotional upset becomes chronic, especially those associated with a loss of love, combine or alternate Silicea with Natrum Mur. As always, this combination is helpful to all patients, but it is especially useful for those who are older. Younger patients who have suffered a loss of love often will require Natrum Phosphoricum or Kali Phos instead of Natrum Mur, although Silicea will still be strongly indicated.

For cases of emotional trauma in which the patient becomes obsessed with the cause of their upset: Kali Phosphoricum. Think of this remedy for both acute and chronic cases in which the patient broods; when he cannot think of anything except for his emotional trauma. If the upset keeps him from sleeping or makes his behavior manic, consider combining or alternating with Magnesia Phosphorica. If the condition becomes truly chronic and the patient broods over the situation that caused him emotional harm, combine or alternate Kali Phos with Natrum Mur. Natrum Mur follows Kali Phos in these cases, and completes its actions well.

For the patient who, after an emotional trauma, becomes forgetful: Calcarea Phosphorica. Calc Phos is another important remedy for those who grieve. Often the coping mechanism displayed by the Calc Phos will be to simply forget—not only the specific cause of the emotional upset, but other aspects of his or her life as well. It is keynote to understand the difference between the Cal Phos and the Natrum Mur patient regarding grief, as both types mask their hurt. The Natrum Mur masks his hurt from others, but the patient himself is all too aware of it. The Calc Phos patient, on the other hand, does the opposite. He makes himself completely unaware—to the greatest degree he can achieve—that anything is amiss.

For the patient who sees things, who has hallucinations while in a state of panic: Combine Kali Phosphoricum with Natrum Phosphoricum. All the phosphorus-based remedies tend to be more emotionally sensitive than the other remedies. This is particularly true of Kali Phos and Natrum Phos. Both types will see ghosts, will start easily at every noise, and will wind themselves up to the point that they will insist there are monsters under the bed and robbers downstairs. While either remedy may be used alone in these situations, the combination of the two is most effective.

For the patient who is anxious, who feels that "something bad" is about to happen: Ferrum Phosphoricum is the remedy of first choice. Just as it is the remedy to think of first in cases of physical injury, it can be very helpful in the first stages of emotional injury as well. In the same way, it is an excellent remedy for the patient in a panic attack or a state of vague, free-form anxiety in which he or she is concerned about the near future.

Note that, on a more chronic level, Natrum Phosphoricum patients are very concerned about the future and what will become of them. This remedy can be very soothing to children who fear they will be abandoned or worry that their parents will die. In the same way, it can help those who worry about the future based upon present or past upsets. It follows Ferrum Phos well in these cases and can be used with it in alternation or combination, as needed.

Specific Remedies for Patients with Characteristic Behaviors

For the patient who:

Talks too much (babbles) when upset: Ferrum Phosphoricum.

Always talks too much: Natrum Muriaticum.

Refuses to speak at all when upset: Kali Phosphoricum.

Talks nonsense: Kali Phosphoricum.

Talks in his or her sleep: Magnesia Phosphorica.

Sighs constantly when upset: Natrum Muriaticum.

Sighs habitually: Natrum Phosphoricum.

Whines when upset: Natrum Phosphoricum.

Screams when upset: Kali Phosphoricum.

Yawns when upset: Kali Phosphoricum.

Gets sleepy when upset: Magnesia Phosphorica. Note that Mag Phos is the remedy for those who respond to emotional trauma by becoming sleepy, but not by actually sleeping. The Natrum Muriaticum patient is much more likely to actually go to sleep when upset, or to feel as if he or she is becoming physically weak as a result of an emotional trauma. The Mag Phos reaction to high emotion will be one of two possible behaviors: either the patient will want to stay very still and will react with the state of sleepiness, or he or she will become agitated and will have to move about and pace the room. The Natrum Mur will always react by wanting to lie down and rest, if not sleep.

Chatters his or her teeth when anxious: Kali Phosphoricum is the indicated remedy.

Trembles when upset: Magnesia Phosphorica, especially if the patient's hands tremble.

Carries things from place to place, room to room, and does not know why: Magnesia Phosphorica.

Is very sensitive to stimuli; becomes more worked up with any change in the environment or too much stimulation: Kali Phosphoricum. (For the patient who is chronically sensitive to change, or as a follow-up to Kali Phos: Natrum Phosphoricum.)

Is very sensitive to noise when upset: Kali Muriaticum, which works well when combined with Kali Phosphoricum for patients who are startled easily by noise. Combine or alternate with Magnesia Phosphorica for patients who are awakened very easily by the slightest noise.

Is very sensitive to music when upset: Natrum Muriaticum is the indicated remedy. Note that Natrum Mur patients are, in general, sensitive to music. They may be made happy or sad by it, but will be deeply moved by it, as it is almost medicinal to them. For patients whose emotional distress is aggravated by music of any sort, think of Natrum Sulphuricum.

Is upset and wants to be comforted: Kali Phosphoricum and/or Natrum Phosphoricum are the leading remedies.

Is upset and does not want to be comforted: Natrum Muriaticum is the indicated remedy.

Neurasthenia

Finally, for patients who suffer from the somewhat antiquated diagnosis of *neurasthenia*, a chronic condition involving both physical and emotional symptoms that usually has its roots in emotionally traumatic experiences, consider the following remedies. Note that the neurasthenic patient often suffers from frequent headaches, even migraines; feels an ongoing sense of weight, fatigue (with equal parts emotional and physical exhaustion), and irritability; and faces the future with feelings of both hopelessness and dread. This combination of symptoms, given both their severity and their vagueness, can make the neurasthenic patient particularly hard to treat.

The remedies associated with this condition are the phosphorus-based remedies, all of which share the same innate state of oversensitivity, plus one other—Natrum Muriaticum, which is the remedy known on the emotional level for its combination of retention and denial, which together are the basis of long-term emotional distress. These remedies are Kali Phosphoricum, Ferrum Phosphoricum, Magnesia Phosphorica, Calcarea Phosphorica, Natrum Muriaticum, and Natrum Phosphoricum.

Note that Mag Phos and Natrum Mur are especially helpful in cases that involve headache.

Kali Phosphoricum

Kali Phos is considered to be a specific remedy for neurasthenic patients and should always be used, either to begin the case before moving on to other remedies or in alternation or combination with other remedies to help bring a sense of emotional balance to the patient.

Ferrum Phosphoricum

Ferrum Phosphoricum is also helpful for beginning the treatment of the chronically upset patient. It is often given in the early stages of treatment, along with Kali Phos or on its own, before other remedies are given in follow-up. Think of this as an acute remedy for what is always a chronic condition. It can promote the beginning of healing but cannot sustain the cure.

Magnesia Phosphorica

This remedy should be considered for the patient who is emotionally unstable, when this instability is revealed in bursts and spells of temperament. When the patient has sudden moments of rage. When emotional upsets become embodied in physical pain. For the patient who suffers intense physical pain that makes one wonder if his or her emotional upset is due to the pain or if the pain is the physical embodiment of the upset. For the patient who regrets, laments, cries out. Especially for the patient who suffers from hiccoughs in moments of emotional upset.

Calcarea Phosphorica

The patients needing this remedy are often very sensitive to change. Even changes in the weather can bring on both physical and emotional symptoms. Often Calc Phos patients will have deep feelings of abandonment that reach back to early childhood. They can be deeply insecure. This is often a remedy for those who grieve (think of Natrum Muriaticum as well) and for those who feel disappointment.

Natrum Muriaticum and Natrum Phosphoricum

The sodium-based Natrum Phosphoricum and Natrum Muriaticum are both excellent long-term remedies that will bring emotional balance. In most cases, either one or the other remedy will be used, and not the two in combination. Natrum Phos is, of course, useful in young patients, while Natrum Mur can be helpful for older patients, although either remedy may defy such ageist categorization and be of help when the patient's symptoms prove a better match for a specific remedy. In most cases, the emotional symptoms of Natrum Muriaticum will have their basis in grief or in feelings of betrayal that the patient can neither let go of and move past nor accept as the cause of their distress. The emotional symptoms of Natrum Sulphuricum, on the other hand, often have a basis in physical injury, especially in injuries to the head.

PAIN MANAGEMENT

Pain management is, to me, the area in which the cell salts come into their full glory. They are an excellent method of treatment for those who suffer from pain in any part of the body, especially for those who suffer from chronic pain—from rather generalized conditions including arthritis, neuritis, neuralgia, myalgia, and fibromyalgia—as well as ailments like gout and costochondritis that are, generally speaking, specific to individual parts of the body. Many of these medical diagnoses are so generalized that they are nearly meaningless, other than to note that the patient is, often inexplicably, in a great deal of pain, so they are not covered in depth here. When using the cell salts for pain management, it is more important to notice the pattern of the pain: its location; its modalities (what makes the pain feel better or worse); and its cycles of worsening and improving depending upon time of day, amount of time between spells, and seasonal improvements.

> Pain management is, to me, the area in which the cell salts come into their full glory. They are an excellent method of treatment for those who suffer from pain in any part of the body, especially for those who suffer from chronic pain.

As is the pattern in this little guide, the remedies listed for pain management begin with the general group of remedies and then move from general to specific, first by modalities and then, as appropriate, by medical diagnosis.

I likely don't have to say this, since those who use cell salts for pain management are usually those who have already gone to an allopath as well as to an acupuncturist, a chiropractor, and an osteopath, but pain can be an important symptom to any number of underlying serious diseases. For that reason, it should not be ignored or treated in the home. It requires the services of medical professionals, if only to get the diagnosis that will, in essence, tell you there is nothing that medical science can do, beyond suggesting rest, heat, analgesics, or what have you.

Those who are in pain, either acutely, as with a back that is in spasm from overlifting, or who are living lives of chronic pain, in which the shadow of pain blots out the sun (speaking of sun, don't forget to explore the possibility of a vitamin-D deficiency if you are in chronic pain, especially if it is worse in winter), should consider the following remedies.

General Remedies for Pain

When it comes to pain, we are going to keep coming back to two cell salts again and again: Natrum Muriaticum and Magnesia Phosphorica. The way to tell these two remedies apart, and there is a very easy way, is by how movement or motion affects the pain.

The patient who needs Natrum Muriaticum will not want to move about, but will want to lie down flat and rest. He or she will want to go to bed. They usually also want to be left alone, not be bothered, and, especially, not be questioned or soothed. The Natrum Mur who is in pain is short-tempered and is best left to cope with the pain on his or her own terms. Note that pains that respond to Natrum Mur are usually those that are slow coming on and slow to end. In fact, they may seem endless, as they linger and linger and linger. Remember Natrum Mur for all pains associated with a particular weakness or tendency to repeatedly injure a muscle or joint. Those with chronic lower back pain or chronic knee or ankle pain often benefit from Natrum Muriaticum. It is the remedy for truly chronic pain. (Note that Silicea is often used on combination with Natrum Muriaticum in the treatment of chronic pain, as we shall see.)

The patient who needs Magnesia Phosphorica will want to do one of two things. Either he will want to sit up in a chair (the patient will feel that he has to get up out of bed, even if he is very ill, because he cannot bear to lie down flat) and sit very still, or, more commonly, he will need to get up and move about. He may pace the floor in pain the whole night through, resting only by sitting upright before he is driven to his feet again because only motion will soothe his pain. Indeed, he may even dance when he is in pain because the rhythmic motion will help him cope with it. It is important to note that motion does not usually really help the Mag Phos's actual pain. Instead it either helps the patient to cope with the pain, or the severity of the pain itself drives the patient from his resting position and forces him to move about. Note that unlike Natrum Mur, the pains associated with Mag Phos disappear quite suddenly. They tend to come in spells, which can be notable both for their sudden onset and sudden end. Mag Phos is the remedy of choice for those with periodic pain, rather than a remedy for constant and chronic pain.

When it comes to pain—especially acute pain—that involves inflammation (usually muscle pain), we are going to keep coming back to Ferrum Phosphoricum. This is the best remedy, often the first remedy to use, for cases of strains and sprains, when the affected area of the body is red, hot, and swollen. When the injury has just taken place and the pain first begins, Ferrum Phos is the best remedy to open the case. Often it will need to be followed by another remedy, but for the first stage of acute pain, Ferrum Phos is the best possible remedy.

Specific Remedies for Pain

For pain that is truly overwhelming: Natrum Muriaticum, Magnesia Phosphorica, and Kali Muriaticum. Each of these three remedies often relates more to chronic pain than to acute conditions. Natrum Mur can be used for pain in any part of the body, whether it is hard or soft tissue, and can be used for conditions of pain ranging from the mildest to the most extreme. What often suggests Natrum Mur as the remedy of choice is the fact that the patient reacts in the same way no matter the degree of actual pain, which is to say that he or she reacts as if the pain were very severe indeed.

The intolerable pains associated with Magnesia Phosphorica are almost always cramping in nature. They can shift from spot to spot or radiate from one point to another, and shift about without rhyme or reason. They are better from heat and from pressure. The patient, driven mad by his or her pain, will pace about, unable to stop and rest.

The remedy Kali Muriaticum is an excellent general choice for patients whose pain feels like a great wall, that it not only weighs them down but also separates and surrounds them. They feel cut off by their pain. They feel that it defines their lives. It is most associated with dull, achy pains, pains that never stop, that slowly grind down on the patient's strength, happiness, and quality of life.

For cases of chronic pain, Kali Muriaticum will most often have to be given repeatedly, often beginning by dosing every twenty minutes to thirty minutes until improvement begins. In addition to placing the pellets on the tongue, Kali Mur can also be dissolved in water and applied externally to the affected areas (as can all the other pain remedies). Warm or cool applications of moist cloths that have been dipped in the dissolved remedy can offer increased comfort to those in pain.

For the patient who feels no pain, although they face a condition that suggests that they should have great pain: Kali Phosphoricum. You will not see this situation often, but I mention it because it can help us to understand the nature of Kali Phos and the sort of pain medication it is. Kali Phos is indeed an important remedy to those in pain and, along with Ferrum Phos, is often a first remedy in clearing away acute or even chronic pain, but it is as changeable in terms of pain as it is in the emotional states it treats. The pains associated with Kali Phos will not shift, as do those associated with Mag Phos, but they appear suddenly, without warning, and may disappear just as quickly.

Note that, as part of Kali Phos's picture, it will help patients at both ends of the spectrum—those who should be feeling pain but don't, and those who are so sensitive that they are feeling mysterious pains that the rest of us wouldn't feel under similar circumstances. The patient's reaction to the presence of pain seems to have only an on/off switch rather than the usual multiple settings that most patients have.

For aching pain: Calcarea Phosphorica and Kali Muriaticum are the remedies that are most often used. Calcarea Phosphorica is especially useful for aching pains in the limbs or in the shoulders. In joint pain, the ache can make the patient feel as if the joint, especially the ankle, is dislocated. Calcarea Phosphorica has a special affinity for the areas at the top and bottom of the spine: for the back of the neck into the shoulders and the lower part of the back. Think of this as an excellent remedy for those who suffer from lumbago. Think of Calc Phos when stiffness accompanies the achy pain, especially in cases of long-term pain.

Kali Muriaticum, as has been noted, is an excellent general remedy for those in chronic pain. For joint pains, particularly if heat and swelling accompany the ache in the joints. When the ache is accompanied by stiffness. The pain associated with Kali Muriaticum is greatly increased from motion of the affected part. The patient may rest comfortably if he or she does not move. The patient will want to sit or lay very still and not be disturbed (much like the patient needing that other great chloride-based remedy, Natrum Muriaticum). The patient may experience a sensation of chill, most especially in his or her hands and/or feet, during times of pain.

The third remedy to consider for cases of aching pain is Kali Phosphoricum. It is useful when emotional upsets accompany the physical pain. Think of this as a good general remedy for patients who have pain who are also agitated or anxious during spells of pain.

For boring pain: Use Magnesia Phosphorica for pain that seems to bore into the body. Mag Phos, as one of our best remedies for those with pain, speaks to many different types of pain. It is an important remedy to keep in mind for pains that seem to dig in deep in specific small areas of the body, especially if those small spots seem to shift about without rhyme or reason. As always with Mag Phos, these pains will be improved by heat and by pressure placed upon the specific, small affected area.

For bruising pain: Think of Ferrum Phosphoricum as the first remedy for bruising pain, especially in acute cases. In chronic cases, think of Kali Muriaticum or Natrum Muriaticum. If these fail to bring about a cure, add Silicea to either remedy to bring relief.

This is for cases that involve parts of the body that feel sore, that feel as if they are bruised. In fact, they may be used for cases in which physical trauma has occurred and there is real bruising present.

Ferrum Phos is the first remedy if the area is swollen, hot, and red. If the pain has just begun. It is basically a short-term, acute remedy, but it can bring relief in chronic cases if the pain occurs in specific spells that involve a feeling of inflammation.

Kali Muriaticum and Natrum Muriaticum are the two chloride-based remedies that are most commonly associated with a sensation of bruising pain or a chronic sense of a sore ache. (See above for more on aching pains.) While Kali Mur and Natrum Mur may certainly be used in conjunction with each other, I would start by choosing which of the two remedies seem to best fit the overall picture of the patient's pain. I would only try the second remedy, and then only as an individual remedy, if the first totally failed to act. Remember that Silicea can be added to either remedy, either at the same time or alternating with it, to bring about a cure.

For burning pain: Burning pain is one of the instances in which Natrum Muriaticum and Silicea are the two remedies used most often. They may be used individually for cases in which the symptoms suggest a specific remedy, but more often they are used concurrently or in alternation. Remember that either the Natrum Mur or the Silicea patient can feel chilly, even though their sensation of pain is burning in nature.

Two other remedies that share the symptom of burning pains are Calcarea Phosphorica and Kali Sulphuricum.

The Calc Phos patient will experience aching pains that are accompanied by a sensation of weakness in the affected area. This can be especially pronounced if the patient feels pain in his arms or legs. He might feel that his arms cannot lift anything and that his legs are too weak to support his weight. During bouts of pain, the lower limbs may feel numb as well as achy. The patient may also feel that his feet are icy cold during pain.

The Kali Sulph patient, on the other hand, will feel that his pains are, in general, dull and achy and constant. They do not grow better or worse over time, but remain maddeningly constant. The pains will feel better if the patient is in a cool place or in open air. They will be worse if the patient is in a warm room or becomes too warm. Paradoxically, the pain may also be improved by hot applications or by a hot shower.

For cramping pain: Magnesia Phosphorica. It is keynote for this remedy that it works extremely well for cramping pains in any part of the body. For this reason, it is the leading PMS remedy, as well as an excellent remedy for any muscle cramps that are brought on by exercise or exertion.

Calcarea Phosphorica is also useful for cramping pains, particularly when they are located in the forearms, wrists, fingers, and, especially, in the thumb. A sensation of weakness in that area may accompany the pain.

Cramps in the calves or throughout the lower extremities are often helped by Kali Sulphuricum. Since this is a remedy that is most often used in cases of chronic pain, it may have to be repeated fairly often in order to set things right.

In addition to these three remedies, which may be used separately or in tandem, consider Silicea for cases in which cramping pains are chronic. It works especially well as a follow-up remedy for any of the other three in stubborn cases, and pairs especially well with Magnesia Phosphorica in all cases of cramping pains that are better from heat and from pressure but are not completely healed by the use of Mag Phos alone.

For truly gnawing pains, when it feels as if a part of the body is being chewed on by the pain: Kali Sulphuricum and Natrum Sulphuricum (two sulfur-based remedies) are excellent, as is Silicea, which should be used in combination with either of the other two.

Choose Kali Sulphuricum if the pain shifts about in the body and improves when the patient is in a cool place, but is made worse when he or she is too warm or is in a warm, closed room.

Choose Natrum Sulphuricum if the pain is made much worse by exposure to damp or when the patient gets wet. The pains will improve in dry, sunny weather. Damp is a keynote aggravation to the type, the patient will not be made worse by getting cold, only from damp.

Both remedies are important for patients who suffer from rheumatic pains, which are often gnawing in nature. They work well together and may be used in alternation or combination. Both work especially well with Silicea, which can follow or combine well with either remedy.

For pinching pain: Natrum Mur and Silicea. This combination of remedies is excellent for those in pain, especially if the pain is associated with a pinching sensation. Think of a pinching pain in the lower back, which makes the patient want to use his or her hands to support the lower back, makes the patient want to lie down on something firm. This is the remedy combination for that condition. Start with Natrum Mur and use it alone for a day or two. If it fails to clear away the pain, add Silicea, alternating it with the Natrum Mur. Use each remedy up to every two hours, depending upon the severity of the pain, and lessen the dosage as improvement begins.

For shooting pain: Kali Sulphuricum is the remedy of first choice for shooting pains. Magnesia Phosphorica is also useful. These two remedies can seem similar at times, and, for this reason, they are a good combination for those who suffer pain. Both remedies are useful for cases in which the pain wanders or shifts from place to place in the body. In the same way, both remedies are very useful for pains that shoot from spot to spot, for a pain that shoots down the side of the body, for instance, or down the leg, like sciatica. Both remedies share these symptoms and work well together, but generally the Kali Sulph patient will be better from a cool or open atmosphere, while the Mag Phos patient will want heat and pressure applied to the painful area in order to bring relief. Do not overlook the remedy for cases—and you will find them—in which the pattern of the pain follows that of Kali Sulph but the patient is improved by a hot application or shower. Give it and alternate it with Mag Phos, as they work well together in these cases. If the Kali Sulph stays true to the remedy's usual improvement from cold, they do not alternate well, although Kali Sulph may be used as a follow-up remedy for Mag Phos.

Note that Calcarea Phosphorica also should be considered in a limited way for patients with shooting pains. When Calc Phos is useful, the pain will shoot down the forearm into the wrists and hands. Think of this remedy when the pain is in the area between the elbows and fingertips. (The patient can also have pains that shoot down the neck into the shoulder, although this is less common.)

For stabbing pain: Think of Magnesia Phosphorica for pains that are stabbing in nature.

For wandering pains: Magnesia Phosphorica is the remedy of first choice for patients who experience pains that shift from place to place without warning. The remedy is especially indicated if the patient feels the pain in small, specific spots of the body, or if the pain suddenly lifts without warning, just as it shifted from place to place without rhyme or reason.

The other remedy, once again, is Kali Sulphuricum. I would hold it back as a second remedy, or as one to be alternated with Mag Phos later if Mag Phos alone proves insufficient.

While these two remedies are most commonly associated with wandering pains, they are not the only ones that can be useful. Natrum Muriaticum can be helpful for those who have pains that shift from place to place, although this remedy is not often thought of for this purpose. More often, the Natrum Mur will have chronic pain in specific regions of the body that may involve a sense a general weakness in that area or a likelihood of injuring and reinjuring that area very easily. But the Natrum Mur pain can and does shift from place to place in many cases. It can be affected by the weather, and especially by wet weather or by being near the seashore. It can also be affected by the patient's emotional state, and the pains may shift if the patient gets upset.

Natrum Sulphuricum, a sister remedy to Natrum Muriaticum, is another remedy in which the pains may shift from place to place. An extreme sensitivity to damp in any form—the patient can have terrible pain after sitting on damp ground at a picnic—can be your guiding symptom for its use.

Finally, don't overlook Silicea when it comes to traveling or wandering pains. While we tend to think of Silicea for pain that is more all-pervasive, that is blanketlike in the way it covers an area of the body, it can be useful for pain that shifts from place to place as well. Think of this remedy especially for cases in which the sensation of pain seems to weaken the patient, to drain him of his vital force. Also think of this remedy in combination with any of the other listed remedies, or as a follow-up remedy to any of them, if a general sense of exhaustion and/or depletion is present.

Other Pain Issues

For pain that is aggravated by:

Motion: Kali Muriaticum, Natrum Muriaticum, and Ferrum Phosphoricum. Also Calcarea Phosphorica, to a lesser degree. Kali Phosphoricum if the pain is made worse from continuous motion.

Rising up from a prone position: Natrum Muriaticum.

Rising up from a seated position: Kali Phosphoricum.

Exertion: Kali Muriaticum, Magnesia Phosphorica, Ferrum Phosphoricum.

Resting (pain increased after resting or sleeping): Kali Phosphoricum.

Being touched: Magnesia Phosphorica.

Lying on right side: Magnesia Phosphorica.

Lying on left side: Natrum Sulphuricum.

Cold environment or applications: Magnesia Phosphorica, Kali Phosphoricum.

Cold weather: Natrum Muriaticum.

Cold water specifically: Magnesia Phosphorica.

Patient's feet getting cold or damp: Silicea.

Dampness or becoming wet: Natrum Sulphuricum, Calcarea Fluorica.

Being at the seaside: Natrum Muriaticum.

Open air: Silicea.

Drafts: Calcarea Phosphorica, Kali Phosphoricum. Also Magnesia Phosphorica to a lesser degree.

Warm environment or atmosphere: Kali Sulphuricum.

From the warmth of a bed specifically: Kali Muriaticum.

Nighttime: Kali Sulphuricum. (For pain that occurs only at night, think of Magnesia Phosphorica.)

Daytime: Natrum Muriaticum.

Morning: Natrum Muriaticum, Natrum Sulphuricum.

Afternoon: Natrum Phosphoricum. Also Natrum Muriaticum to a lesser degree.

Full moon: Silicea.

Any change in the weather: Calcarea Phosphorica.

A change in the weather from dry to damp: Natrum Sulphuricum.

A change in the weather with a thunderstorm approaching: Natrum Phosphoricum.

Company/attention: Natrum Muriaticum.

Being alone: Kali Phosphoricum, Kali Sulphuricum.

Eating: Calcarea Phosphorica.

For pain that is ameliorated by:

Resting (lying down): Natrum Muriaticum, Calcarea Phosphorica.

Gentle motion: Kali Phosphoricum.

Touch: Calcarea Fluorica.

Pressure: Magnesia Phosphorica.

Cold or cold applications: Ferrum Phosphoricum, Calcarea Fluorica.

Warmth, in general: Magnesia Phosphorica, Silicea.

Heat: Magnesia Phosphorica.

Wrapping up, especially by wrapping the head and/or feet: Silicea.

Changes in the weather from damp to dry: Natrum Sulphuricum.

Moist warm weather in general: Silicea.

Company/attention: Kali Phosphoricum.

Excitement/fun: Kali Phosphoricum.

Eating: Kali Phosphoricum.

Strains and Sprains

As the result of overlifting, overexerting, or physical trauma, strains and sprains are most often simple acute conditions that are self-limiting and, while painful, not serious. To put it simply, strains involve muscles and sprains involve joints, particularly the ligaments and tendons around joints. Both conditions can be helped by cell salts, which will reduce pain and speed healing. These remedies can be taken by mouth and used topically as well.

General Remedies for Sprains

Ferrum Phosphoricum is the first aid remedy for any sprain. Think of it first and use it especially if the affected joint is swollen, hot, and red. Ferrum Phos should be taken by mouth in the 12X potency in these cases and repeated often, every few minutes if need be, until improvement begins. Then it should be repeated only as needed, only as the pain returns.

Along with the Ferrum Phos by mouth, dissolve five tablets of Ferrum Phos and Kali Muriaticum in water (Calcarea Fluorica can also be added to the mixture if you wish—see the section on Calc Fluor for details). Soak a clean cloth in the water and apply the cloth directly to the sprain. Kali Mur and Ferrum Phos will work effectively together, particularly if the sprained area around the joint is swelling. If the sprain is especially painful, or if it prevents the patient from standing, add Magnesia Phosphorica to the mix as well and apply as often as needed. Keep rinsing the cloth in the mixture every few minutes and applying it to the affected area.

Any time an ankle or other joint seems to have been weakened by a sprain, so that it has a tendency to reinjury or seems less capable of lifting, supporting, or performing as it did before, think of Natrum Muriaticum as a good follow-up to the acute remedies. Natrum Muriaticum is always an excellent remedy for chronic pain, as is Silicea. Silicea can be used instead of Natrum Muriaticum if the symptoms of the case point to its use, or in tandem with Natrum Mur when in doubt. Silicea and Natrum Mur always work well together in cases of chronic weakness and pain.

Also, if the patient has injured a joint long ago and the joint has been troublesome ever since, give Natrum Mur to help clear up the trouble.

General Remedies for Strains

The first remedy to consider for all acute strains is, again, Ferrum Phosphoricum. Always think of it first for cases in which the injured area of the body is red, swollen, and hot to the touch. The patient will want ice on the injury. This is the first remedy to think of if a patient has thrown his or her back out from lifting too heavy a weight, or from forgetting to lift with the knees, not the back.

Ferrum Phos will not often complete the cure itself, but it is a good first remedy. Give the patient Calcarea Sulphurica and Kali Muriaticum in combination quickly on its heels, or dissolve Ferrum Phos, Calc Sulph, and Kali Mur in water and apply a cloth soaked in the mixture to the affected area of the body. As always, Calcarea Fluorica can be added to increase the potency of the mixture and to help speed healing because of its special affinity to the elastic tissues of the body.

If it's the back that has been strained, add Natrum Muriaticum into the mix or give Natrum Mur by mouth while applying the others topically. In the first stages of the strain, give Ferrum Phos by mouth, then alternate with Natrum Mur. Move on to Natrum Mur alone as the inflammation resolves itself in all cases of a strained back.

For general strains, use Kali Muriaticum instead, as it is the best general remedy for pain associated with strained muscles. Kali Mur works well with Calc Sulph in these cases. The two remedies have an affinity for each other and will work better together than either will alone.

For strains that seem to have caused permanent damage or that have left the affected area weakened or in chronic stiffness and/or pain, use Natrum Muriaticum and/or Silicea. These two remedies also have an affinity for each other in cases of chronic weakness and pain, when the injured area will want firm support and when the patient feels they cannot "trust" that muscle group as they once could. Natrum Mur and Silicea should be alternated until relief results.

Specific Remedies for Strains

For acute strains that are associated with exercise: Magnesia Phosphorica. The Mag Phos patient often is addicted to exercise, especially to dancing, and will injure himself or herself as a result. Think of Mag Phos if the strained area feels as if it has been worked too hard, exercised too vigorously or too often, especially if the patient feels a sensation of heat in the strained area. If Mag Phos fails to cure on its own, add Calcarea Sulphurica to the mix. Give both remedies by mouth, alternating between them, as often as every few minutes at first, and less often as improvement begins.

If the strained muscle goes into spasm: Magnesia Phosphorica or Ferrum Phosphoricum are the two best remedies. If the area feels hot, is swollen and red, and feels better for ice, give Ferrum Phosphoricum. If the patient feels that heat flow into the area like a lava flow, or if the spasm, although hot, is improved by heat, give Mag Phos. Alternate both when in doubt, or when the patient has no strong preference between hot and cold.

For the final stage of a strain, when the area still feels sore, but the pain is largely gone: Natrum Sulphuricum will usually put things right. Give two or three times a day until improvement begins. Should Natrum Sulph fail to work, add Natrum Mur and alternate the two remedies.

Note: Keep Natrum Sulphuricum in the back of your mind for both strains and sprains that become sources of chronic pain that is worse from damp in any form, especially when the weather is changing from dry to damp. Think of this remedy for all cases of chronic pain in which the patient is worse from damp, better from sunny and dry weather. You can use Natrum Sulph in place of Natrum Mur for these cases and alternate with Silicea just as you would have Natrum Mur. Any number of "trick knees" and achy elbows can be improved by a few doses of Natrum Sulphuricum.

Muscle Pain

Those seeking information on either acute or chronic muscle pain should also see the information above on strains, as many of the remedies listed in this section will complement those listed above.

In general, the major remedies to be considered for the treatment of all forms of muscle pain are Ferrum Phosphoricum, Magnesia Phosphorica, and Kali Phosphoricum. Note that if muscle pain is associated with the presence of acid in the system—

such as a buildup of lactic acid in the muscles after exercise—the remedy of first choice is Natrum Phosphoricum.

But perhaps the most overlooked remedy when it comes to muscle pain, especially chronic muscle pain, and for the overall health of the muscles, is Calcarea Phosphorica. Keep this remedy in mind for all cases of muscle pains, especially those that involve a sensation of weakness in the muscles—the patient will feel as if his or her legs may give out at any moment—or a real atrophying of the muscle tissue. It is especially helpful for those with cramping pains in the neck and shoulders, and for those with pain in the lower back that spreads down into the muscles of the buttocks. (Therefore it is, quite literally, the remedy of first choice for either a pain in the neck or a pain in the ass.) It works well in conjunction with any other of the phosphorus-based remedies listed in this section, and with the calcium-based Calcarea Fluorica (see below).

Safe to say, when it comes to muscle pain, the phosphorus-based remedies are the ones that will be most helpful, but in addition to any or all of these, always consider adding Calcarea Fluorica to the mixture. Calcium fluoride is an important component of all the elastic tissues in the body, so the remedy Calcarea Fluorica is vital to the treatment of muscle pain or pain in ligaments and tendons. It can be used in combination with any of the phosphorus-based remedies listed above, and will make those remedies work more dynamically and speed recovery. Calc Fluor is an important remedy to think of for all cases of muscle pain, in any part of the body. Whatever phosphorus remedies you choose for muscle pain, use them in conjunction with Calc Fluor.

I find that the combination of Calc Fluor and Calcarea Phosphorica is ideal for chronic muscle pain, unless specific symptoms suggest another remedy. Note that topical applications of remedies can be extremely helpful in all cases of muscle pain. Consider dissolving Calcarea Fluorica and Calcarea Phosphorica in warm or cool water, as desired, and then applying it directly to the site of the pain with a moist cloth. Indicated remedies may be taken orally while the topical application helps speed relief.

For any muscle pain that is associated with a sensation of inflammation or of heat: Ferrum Phosphoricum. This is especially true for any acute muscle pain. Ferrum Phosphoricum is the remedy of first choice when the affected muscles are swollen, hot, and red. The pain is worse from any motion. Ferrum Phos is particularly helpful for muscle pains in the neck, the chest (especially the sides of the chest), and the back.

For Muscle Pains Associated with Trembling, Weakness, Numbness

For muscle pains in any part of the body that are accompanied by a sensation of trembling or twitching: Magnesia Phosphorica. Motion is the key to spotting the need for Mag Phos. The patient will want to pace the floor if he can, in spite of his pain.

Look for trembling of the affected parts. Look especially for trembling of the hands and for twitches, like nervous tics, throughout the body.

For any muscle pains that are accompanied by a sensation of weakness in the affected muscles: Kali Phosphoricum. The sensation of physical weakness accompanying pain is keynote to Kali Phos. However, this remedy works especially well with Calcarea Fluorica and the two should be used either in alternation or combination with one another.

For any muscle pain that is accompanied by a sensation of numbness: Calcarea Phosphorica is the indicated remedy. If the pain and numbness are chronic, alternate or combine this with Silicea.

For Muscle Pain in the Neck

As noted above, Calcarea Phosphorica is the single best remedy for the pain in the neck. Think of this remedy for the stiff neck, when muscles are tight and it is hard to move the neck from side to side. Think of this remedy for neck pain that comes on after the patient is in contact with a draft. For neck cramps, especially those that begin on the right side and travel left, or that alternate sides.

For the sensation of a "crick" in the neck: Natrum Phosphoricum. For sudden sensation of a crick in the neck, give Ferrum Phosphoricum.

For a stiff neck: Calcarea Phosphorica is the indicated remedy in acute situations. It may be combined with Kali Sulphuricum, as needed.

For chronic still necks that also involve back pain: Natrum Muriaticum and Silicea in combination are indicated.

If the muscles on the right side of the neck feel tightened or shortened: Kali Sulphuricum.

If the muscles on the left side of the neck feel tightened or shortened: Natrum Muriaticum.

For the sensation of having "slept funny," when neck pain comes on when arising from the bed in the morning: Kali Muriaticum is the indicated remedy.

For Muscle Pain in the Shoulders

The general remedy for muscle pain in the region of the shoulder is Calcarea Phosphorica. It is especially helpful if the muscle pain extends down into the sides and chest or if it extends down the arms. (If it extends down into the sides with a burning sensation, give Ferrum Phosphoricum.)

When the muscles of the neck and shoulders are tight: Calcarea Phosphorica and

Calcarea Sulphurica combined can be very helpful. If the pain has a burning sensation, substitute Ferrum Phosphoricum for the Calc Sulph.

For chronic pain in the back that extends upward into the shoulders: Silicea.

For pain only in the left shoulder: Kali Muriaticum.

For pain only in the right shoulder: Calcarea Phosphorica.

For shoulder pain that is better from motion: Ferrum Phosphorica is the indicated first remedy. Add Kali Phosphoricum if Ferrum Phos alone fails to act.

For shoulder pain that is worse from motion: Natrum Muriaticum is indicated and may be combined with Natrum Muriaticum.

For chronic muscle pain in the region of the shoulder: Natrum Muriaticum in combination with Silicea is indicated.

For Muscle Pain in the Arms

Two remedies most commonly help with muscle pain in the arms. They are Silicea, for the muscles of the upper arm, and Kali Muriaticum, which soothes pain in the muscles of the forearm. Think of Kali Phosphoricum for pain in either part of the arm that is associated with a loss of strength in the arm. Arms that ache also suggest the need for Kali Phos.

For cramping, burning pains in the arm after exercise: Magnesia Phosphorica, which is indicated if the pain is better from pressure (rubbing) and from hot applications.

If the arms feel tired as well as sore and especially if the hands are cold: Natrum Phosphoricum.

For Muscle Pain in the Hands

For pains in the hands while doing detailed work, especially if those pains extend to the wrists: Natrum Phosphoricum. The patient's hands will be cold during spells of pain in most cases needing Natrum Phos. For cases involving pains in the hands in which the hands, especially the palms, are hot, give Ferrum Phosphoricum.

For Muscle Pain in the Back

For acute back pain, especially if associated with strained muscles: Ferrum Phosphoricum. If Ferrum Phos does not clear away the inflammation, add Kali Muriaticum. (See Strains.)

For acute spasms of the muscles of the back: Magnesia Phosphorica, especially if the pain is relieved by heat and by pressure. If the spasm is long-lasting, add Silicea as well.

For general back pain: the combination of Calcarea Phosphorica and Calcarea Fluorica works very well. For chronic back pain, always include Natrum Muriaticum in the treatment, especially if the back pain is made better from lying down on a firm mattress or on the floor. Natrum Muriaticum is especially helpful in cases of chronic back pain. The Natrum Mur pain will have a sensation of weight to it. The patient feels that he or she is dragging about. The patient will seek support and will push his hand against his back to support it, especially when rising up out of a chair.

Other remedies for general back pain include Natrum Sulphuricum, which should not only always be considered for chronic back pain that gets worse in damp weather, but also for general back pain located in the small of the back, or that runs up and down the center of the back near the spine; Natrum Phosphoricum, which works best for pain in the upper and middle part of the back, and for pain in the neck that extends down into the back; and Kali Phosphoricum, when the pain in the back is associated with a sensation of weakness in the muscles.

If back pain extends upward into the neck: Silicea.

If back pain extends around to the chest: Calcarea Phosphorica.

If back pain extends down into the hips or legs: Kali Muriaticum.

If back pain is better from rest: Natrum Muriaticum is indicated.

If back pain is worse from rest: Kali Phosphoricum is the best remedy, but also consider Silicea.

If back pain is better from motion: Calcarea Fluorica in combination with Calcarea Phosphorica is most often indicated. Also consider Kali Sulphuricum.

If back pain is both worse from rest and better from motion: The only remedy in this case will be Kali Phosphoricum.

If back pain is worse with the first motion of getting out of bed in the morning: Natrum Muriaticum is indicated. In stubborn cases, combine with Silicea.

If back pain is worse from walking: Calcarea Phosphorica is indicated, although Kali Phosphoricum should also be considered for patients who feel weakness as well as pain in the back.

If back pain is made better by walking slowly: Silicea.

If back pain is worse when stooping: Natrum Muriaticum and Silicea should be combined.

If back pain is worse when rising up from a stooping or sitting position: Calcarea Phosphorica is the best remedy. In chronic or stubborn cases, bring in Natrum Muriaticum and/or Silicea for complete relief. Note that the patient needing Kali Phosphoricum may also have trouble getting up from a sitting position and will have a sensation of weakness in addition to his or her pain.

If back pain is worse from bending backward: Calcarea Phosphorica.

If back pain is better from bending backward: Natrum Muriaticum and/or Silicea.

If back pain is worse from riding in a vehicle: Calcarea Fluorica is most indicated and may be combined with Calcarea Phosphorica. In stubborn cases, add Silicea for complete relief.

If back pain is worse from moving side to side or by turning either to the left or the right: Natrum Muriaticum.

If back pain is worse from lifting the arms: Natrum Muriaticum.

If back pain is better from pressure: Natrum Muriaticum may be indicated, but in some cases it may be worse from pressure, so don't go on this symptom alone. Magnesia Phosphorica will be useful in back spasms that are better from pressure.

If back pain if better from rubbing: Natrum Muriaticum or Natrum Sulphuricum.

If back pain is worse on the left side of the back: Silicea.

If back pain is worse on the right side of the back: Kali Phosphoricum.

If back pain alternates sides: Calcarea Phosphorica.

For Muscle Pain in the Buttocks

The single best remedy for any pain in the ass is Calcarea Phosphorica. Think of it for all pain in the muscles of the buttocks, especially if the muscles feel "asleep" when the patient sits for any period of time. This is the remedy for lower back pain that extends into the buttocks and for pain in the buttocks when the patient rises up from a sitting position.

For chronic lower back pain that extends into the buttocks: Natrum Muriaticum. This remedy is especially indicated if the pain has a sore, bruised feeling or if the muscles feel tightened.

For Muscle Pain in the Thighs

For general pain or soreness of the muscles of the thighs, use Calcarea Phosphorica. Combine with Calcarea Fluorica if Calc Phos alone fails to give relief. Calc Phos is the best remedy for strained muscles in the inner thighs as well as for sore hamstrings. The pain associated with this remedy leaves the patient walking unsteadily. He may feel as if his legs will give out from under him. In cases combining pain and weakness, give Kali Phosphoricum in addition to Calc Phos.

Note that the pain that extends from the thigh down into the calves and carries with it a sensation of weakness. It shows itself in an uncertain gait that may suggest the need for Natrum Phosphoricum, especially if the feet are icy cold at the time of pain.

For Muscle Pain in the Calves

For general pain in the calf muscles, three remedies are most commonly used: Calcarea Phosphorica, Natrum Phosphorica, and Silicea. Of these, perhaps Calcarea Phosphorica is most important.

Silicea is the leading remedy for cramping pains in the calves or for a feeling of weakness in the muscles. Think of it if the calf muscle feels tired, tightened, or short-ened and if this tightness extends down into the back of the foot.

Calcarea Phosphorica is a good general remedy for calf pain, especially if the pain is shooting in nature, if it comes and goes, strikes like lightning. For aching soreness in the thighs that extends downward into the calves, think of Calc Phos.

Magnesia Phosphorica is the specific remedy for cramps in the calf muscles that are better from pressure (rubbing) and from applications of heat. Cramps may come on from exercising or while dancing.

For Muscle Pain in the Feet

Magnesia Phosphorica is the best remedy for sudden foot cramps. It may be combined with Kali Sulphuricum if Mag Phos alone does not relieve the cramping.

Bone Pain

In general, there are only two remedies to consider when dealing with pains that drive deep into the bones.

The first and dominant remedy for bone pain is Calcarea Phosphorica. The sub-stance calcium phosphate is essential to both the blood and the bones. It is found in the body in both places. For this reason the remedy Calc Phos is important to bone health and bone pain. For general pain in the bones in any part of the body, think of this rem-edy first. The pains associated with Calcarea Phosphorica will tend to be worse at night and better from motion of the affected area.

The second remedy is Natrum Sulphuricum. Think of this remedy when the pain in the bones accompanies illnesses, such as flu, or when the pain is triggered by changes in the weather from dry to damp or when the patient enters a damp environment.

For pain in areas of the body that involve both bone and connective tissue, con-sider the two remedies listed here along with those suggested by the soft tissue pain. All may be considered in the selection of an appropriate remedy or remedies.

Joint Pain

The basic information on the treatment of joint pain (at least in the context of acute pain) is dealt with in the section above on sprains. In this section I will look at the specific remedies that work well with specific joints in the body, and look at the way the cell salts can be used in the treatment of chronic joint pain, either due to injury or to such conditions as rheumatism, arthritis, or gout.

The remedies that will most often be used in the treatment of patients with joint pain include two potassium-based remedies, Kali Muriaticum and Kali Sulphuricum, and three phosphorus-based remedies, Calcarea Phosphorica, Magnesia Phosphorica, and Ferrum Phosphoricum.

In addition to these, Calcarea Fluorica will often be helpful in the resolution of joint pain, especially chronic pain. It will work especially well with Calcarea Phosphorica for those with joint pain, especially for those with pain in the elbows and knees.

For Joint Pain in the Shoulders

Natrum Muriaticum is the most commonly needed remedy for pain in the shoulder joints, especially if the joint audibly cracks when the patient moves, or when the shoulder pain makes it all but impossible for the patient to move his or her arms.

For shoulder pain in which the joint is inflamed, swollen, red, and hot, use Ferrum Phosphoricum. Natrum Mur will work well as a follow-up remedy in these cases.

For generalized pain that runs from the shoulders into the shoulder blades or from the shoulders down to the elbows, or when the pain is shooting or darting in nature, use Calcarea Phosphorica.

For Joint Pain in the Elbows

Pains in the elbows always suggest Calcarea Phosphorica. This remedy is useful for shooting pains in the elbows or for pain in the elbow that extends either up to the shoulder or down to the wrist. If an aching pain starts in the elbow and extends outward in all directions until the patient cannot move his arm, give Calcarea Phosphorica.

If the elbow joint is swollen: Calcarea Fluorica.

If the elbow feels stiff and cracks when moved: Natrum Muriaticum.

For Joint Pain in the Wrists

The general remedy for pain in the wrist joint is Calcarea Phosphorica, especially if the pain is worse from any motion of the wrist, if the pain in the wrist is cramping in nature and extends into the hand, or if only the right wrist has pain.

For wrists so painful that it feels as if the wrists were broken: Silicea. The pain in this case can be so severe that the wrists cannot be moved at all. The patient feels as if the wrist has been broken; as if it has no strength at all, can't be used at all, and cannot be moved even in the slightest. Silicea works best if the pain in the wrist responds and is improved by warmth and to wrapping the affected area.

For joint pain in the wrists if the joint feels hot and swollen and the pain moves upward from the wrist into the forearm: Ferrum Phosphoricum is a helpful remedy.

For Joint Pain in the Fingers

There are two remedies that are commonly used for pain in the joints of the fingers: Natrum Muriaticum and Calcarea Fluorica. Think of using both remedies in tandem when the knuckles crack or when the joints of the fingers have become distorted in shape due to long-term pain associated with arthritis. Natrum Muriaticum is particularly associated with joints that crack and are stiff throughout the body in general. If the joints are painful and swollen, make sure to include Calcarea Fluorica in the mix.

If the finger joints are red, hot, and swollen: Ferrum Phos works particularly well in tandem with Calcarea Phosphorica when painful finger joints have a sensation of heat or of burning associated with the pain. It also works well with Natrum Phosphoricum, which can be used in place of Calc Phos if the patient's symptoms indicate its use.

If stiffness of the joints is the predominant symptom: Natrum Muriaticum and Natrum Sulphuricum should be used, either in alternation or combination.

For Joint Pain in the Hips

Several remedies can be used for those with pain in the hip. The first among these is perhaps the most commonly used remedy for joint pain, Calcarea Phosphorica. Think of Cal Phos as the general remedy for hip pain when there are no specific guiding symptoms.

Along with this remedy, consider Kali Muriaticum, Natrum Muriaticum, and/or Silicea (for chronic cases or if the hip joint feels stiff), and Calcarea Sulphurica (for cases of acute or chronic hip pain, in which a sensation of burning or heat accompanies the pain; you may have to alternate this with Ferrum Phosphoricum). Think of Kali Phosphoricum for simple pain in the hips that also involves a sense of weakness in the joint, as if it would give way.

If walking makes hip pain better: Kali Sulphuricum is the leading remedy. But also consider adding the combination of Calcarea Phosphorica and Calcarea Fluorica to soothe the pain.

If walking or stooping makes hip pain worse: Natrum Muriaticum and/or Silicea should be considered. Most often in these cases using both in tandem will work better than either will alone.

If climbing stairs makes the hip pain worse: Natrum Sulphuricum.

If resting in bed makes the hip feel better: Natrum Muriaticum.

If moving about in bed makes the hip pain worse: Natrum Sulphuricum.

For Joint Pain in the Knees

The first remedy that I think of for pains in the knees is Natrum Muriaticum, especially for patients with chronic knee pain, when the knee is achy, stiff, and cracks when the joint is moved. When getting up from a kneeling position is very difficult, because the knee joint is stiff. Think of Natrum Mur if the patient feels as if the knee is weak, as if it will not support his or her weight. If Natrum Mur alone fails to help soothe the pain, give Silicea along with it.

If the knees are swollen as well as painful: Natrum Muriaticum and/or Silicea. If the swelling is red and hot, and a sensation of heat runs through the knee, give Ferrum Phosphoricum, alone or in alternation with Natrum Mur and/or Silicea.

If a sensation of coldness runs downward from the knee, or if the feet are icy cold while pain lingers: Calcarea Phosphorica is an important remedy for knee pain, especially for these cases.

For stubborn cases of knee pain that do not respond to treatment: Calcarea Phosphorica should be taken internally while Natrum Muriaticum and Silicea are used topically. Or all three may be taken internally, in alternation or combination.

If the knee joint feels worse from motion: Ferrum Phosphoricum.

If the knee joint feels better from motion: Silicea—but only if from gentle, tender motion. If the knee is better from regular motion, use Natrum Sulphuricum.

If the knee joint is worse when the patient walks: Natrum Muriaticum is indicated. If that fails to cure, add Natrum Sulphuricum.

If the knee joint is better when the patient walks: Kali Sulphuricum.

For Joint Pain in the Ankles

There are, in general, four remedies for ankle pain. The most commonly used is Natrum Muriaticum, which is the first remedy to think of for ankle pain that is so bad that the patient cannot put any weight on the ankle at all. For ankles that are chronically weak and have a tendency to turn, always use Natrum Muriaticum as the remedy of first choice. If it fails to cure when used alone, combine it with Natrum Sulphuricum, especially if any motion of the ankle joint changes the circumstances of the pain—for better *or* worse.

Think of Natrum Sulphuricum when motion of a joint is an issue, whether the joint is supporting weight or not.

For acute ankle pain, when the ankle is swollen, hot, and red, use Ferrum Phosphoricum. If the pain is stubborn, add Natrum Muriaticum. Natrum Mur can be taken internally while Ferrum Phos and Natrum Phosphoricum are used topically .

For ankle pain that extends upward into the leg, combine Ferrum Phosphoricum and Natrum Sulphuricum.

Finally, think of Silicea for ankle pain. It works well in combination or alternation with Natrum Muriaticum in joints that are chronically painful and weak or have a tendency to be painful for the slightest cause. For ankles that always seem weak, that feel as if they may give way at any moment, give Silicea.

For Joint Pain in the Toes

The two great remedies for painful joints in the toes are Natrum Muriaticum and Natrum Sulphuricum. They work well in combination. If the cause of joint pain is specific to gout, combine Natrum Sulphuricum with Natrum Phosphoricum (see below).

Rheumatism

Use Ferrum Phosphoricum for all cases of acute rheumatic pains. In acute cases, follow Ferrum Phos with Calcarea Sulphurica if the Ferrum Phos alone does not cure.

Specific Remedies for Rheumatism

If fever accompanies the pain: Natrum Phosphoricum should be added in addition to Ferrum Phos.

If the pain shifts from place to place: Magnesia Phosphorica is the remedy of choice for acute cases, while chronic cases will usually need Kali Sulphuricum.

For chronic cases of rheumatism: Ferrum Phos will be useful in times of inflammation, but other remedies are needed to bring about a cure. Among the most commonly used remedies for the patient with rheumatism are Natrum Phosphoricum, Kali Sulphuricum, Kali Phosphoricum, and Silicea.

For those who suffer from rheumatoid arthritis: Natrum Phosphoricum is the most important remedy, especially when the pain is centered in the joints of the fingers, or when pain is accompanied by a throbbing sensation through the body or by palpitations of the heart. Pains in the knees, ankles, and shins are common with this remedy type. The patient's joints feel sore, their muscles contracted.

For cases of rheumatism in which a sensation of weakness accompanies the pain, or

when periods of pain are followed by physical exhaustion: Kali Phosphoricum. The patient, however, will tend to feel stiff and achy after rest or sleep. Numbness and stiffness accompany the pain. The patient's palms and or/soles of the feet feel itchy and hot during pain.

When trembling accompanies the pain or when the patient's pain is improved from warmth or from wrapping the painful area in blankets or bandages: Silicea is the indicated remedy (Magnesia Phosphorica can also have this symptom, especially in the patient's hands). The patient needing Silicea for his or her pain will be worse from any stimulus, from being jarred or touched, becoming cold or wet, from changes in the environment or the weather, from the full moon. The patient, like the Kali Phosphoricum type, will seem exhausted. But where Kali Phos will be exhausted after a spell of pain, the Silicea is always tired, always exhausted.

For cases in which rheumatic pains alternate with diarrhea or in which a bout of diarrhea brings about sudden ceasing of the rheumatic pain: Always think of Silicea.

When swelling of the affected area is a major feature of the rheumatic state: Kali Muriaticum is the indicated remedy. It combines well with Ferrum Phos, and follows it well if Ferrum Phos is used at the first sign of pain. Kali Muriaticum is useful in all cases of chronic rheumatic pain when any motion makes the pain worse and when swelling is present. Look for the characteristic white coating of the tongue as an indication of the need for Kali Mur in the patient who has rheumatism. Motion is such a strong keynote of the remedy that the patient may feel no pain at all if he or she does not move the affected area.

If the rheumatic pains are worse during hot weather: Always think of Kali Sulphuricum. The pains will be worse if the patient gets overheated or if he or she is in a closed, too-warm room. The patient will seek open air for relief.

If rheumatic pain is combined with asthma, especially if the symptoms alternate: Kali Sulph is also the remedy of choice. Think of Natrum Sulphuricum if the pain is constant and the asthma comes and goes, especially during damp weather. The two remedies may be used in alternation or combination in stubborn cases.

In cases of long-term rheumatism or of rheumatism in older patients: Consider using Natrum Sulphuricum. It will be helpful in all cases of rheumatism in which the pain is worse from changes in the weather from dry to damp or when the patient enters a damp environment. For cases in which the patient can foretell oncoming weather changes due to the onset of pain. For cases of trick knees, and ankles and elbows that become painful when rain is coming. (For those cases in which any change in the weather seems to impact the case, think of Calcarea Phosphorica.)

If Natrum Sulphuricum alone fails to bring about a cure, consider combining it either with Natrum Muriaticum or with Silicea, whichever best matches the symptoms at hand. The Natrum Muriaticum/Natrum Sulphuricum patient likely seeks open air or slow walks for comfort in times of pain, or wants to lie down quietly. The Silicea/Natrum Sulphuricum patient needs to be covered, wrapped tight, to soothe his or her pain.

In cases of stubborn rheumatism or when rheumatic pains return again and again: Always make Natrum Sulphuricum your central remedy.

Arthritis

Like colds, arthritis often requires three stages of treatment to bring about complete relief.

The first stage of treatment involves Ferrum Phosphoricum, which is to be used at the stage when inflammation is present. When affected parts are red, hot, and swollen, and affected parts are worse from any motion.

Note that if Ferrum Phos fails to bring about total relief during stages of inflammation and extreme pain, Magnesia Phosphorica can often soothe the pain. Like Ferrum Phos it will not likely cure the condition, but it will be an asset in times of acute pain, especially if that pain is soothed by hot applications and by rubbing the painful part of the body.

If swelling is a major symptom of the disease state even when inflammation is not present, the remedy to think of is Calcarea Fluorica. This is one of our most important remedies for the treatment of chronic gout—the second stage of treatment. Calcarea Phosphorica should be used either in alternation or combination with Calc Fluor in the treatment of patients with arthritis.

In the third stage—if the arthritis pain is truly stubborn and long-term—consider Natrum Phosphoricum, Natrum Muriaticum, and Silicea as the remedies of best choice. Natrum Mur is the remedy of choice when the affected joints crack and pop when moved and feel stiff as well as painful.

Think of Natrum Phosphoricum when the joints crack and the affected parts feel weak. Look for the characteristic yellow coating on the tongue as an indication of the need for this remedy. This is a great remedy for stubborn old arthritis pain, or pain in elderly patients, whether it is used alone or along with the other two. This remedy is notable in that it will break down lactic acid (or, as we shall see, uric acid) in the system that can cause chronic arthritic or rheumatic pain.

Silicea can be used with either Natrum Mur or Natrum Phos in the treatment of those with stubborn arthritic pain.

Gout/Gouty Arthritis

Gout, also now called "Gouty Arthritis" by some practitioners, requires three remedies to treat.

The first, Ferrum Phosphoricum, is used only acutely during stages in which inflammation is present, usually in a joint of the large toe. The affected area will be red, hot, and swollen, and the skin will be very tender to the touch. Motion will increase pain, as will putting weight on the affected area. Ferrum Phosphoricum will not bring about a cure, but it can soothe an acute attack of gout.

Gout is caused by a buildup of uric acid in the system. Crystals of acid form in joints, usually in the small joints of the body such as the toes, fingers, or elbows. Since gout is caused by an excess of acid, Natrum Phosphoricum is the indicated remedy because it is the remedy of choice for all conditions caused by an excess of acid in the body. One of the roles of sodium phosphate in the body is to keep uric acid from forming crystals. When the body has a deficiency of sodium phosphate, any excess of uric acid is stored as crystals in the joints, which cause the painful bouts of gout, as well as in body fat. Natrum Phosphoricum will help to dissolve the uric acid, making it possible for the body to rid itself of it, mostly through the urine.

This is where the third remedy comes into play. Natrum Sulphuricum, added to the mix, will help the body remove excess uric acid through urination.

The best treatment for chronic gout, therefore, is to first give Natrum Phosphoricum for a few days when no acute inflammation is present. If the Natrum Phos causes an inflammation by overwhelming the system with uric acid, use Ferrum Phosphoricum acutely to clear the inflammation and continue with Natrum Phos. Then alternate Natrum Phos and Natrum Sulphuricum to help the body rid itself of the uric acid. Finally, allow Natrum Sulphuricum to work alone to clear away the remaining uric acid. Once balance is restored to the system, Natrum Sulphuricum alone should suffice to quickly clear away any recurrence of gout.

Treating gout, like treating those with rheumatism or arthritis, is, of course, something that should never be undertaken casually in the home. All require careful treatment and all require that a medical professional take charge of the case. However, in all cases, when they are used appropriately and wisely, the cells salts can offer relief and, ultimately, an actual method of cure for these otherwise stubborn conditions.

Treating pain always requires patience and skill. The more stubborn the pain, the longer the arthritis or rheumatism or gout has been in place, the longer it will take to clear away. Cell salt treatments for those with chronic pain can take many months to complete, although improvement of the condition will usually be seen in only a handful of days.

Neuritis/Neuralgia

Two phosphorus-based remedies are key to general nerve pain. They are Kali Phosphoricum and Magnesia Phosphorica.

Kali Phosphoricum is the first remedy to think of in cases of nerve pain. Think of it for neuralgic pain in any part of the body, especially when the pain is accompanied by a sensation of weakness, when the patient feels as if he cannot get up, cannot lift anything, including his own body weight, and yet the patient's pain is actually decreased if he stands up or moves around slowly and gently. This is a patient whose pain has driven him into a state of hypersensitivity; who cannot bear light, noise, touch, or any other form of stimulation. And yet the Kali Phos patient wants company, wants to feel that he is being taken care of and is loved. The patient's pain will actually get worse if he is left alone to contemplate his pain. He feels better from being distracted and entertained, as long as it does not overexcite him to the point that the pain begins again from overstimulation. (A patient with the opposite emotional reaction, who wants to be alone and is worse from company, suggests the need for Natrum Muriaticum, as does the patient whose pains appear at the same time every day.)

Kali Phos is especially effective for cases in which the pain is accompanied by numbness, and, if the pain extends into the legs, making the patient lame as well. Therefore this is an important remedy for sciatica, as we shall see. Kali Phos pains tend to be right-sided, which is to say they start on the right and move left, or they dominate on the right side of the body. Face pain is common, particularly pain that runs from the teeth into the ear. The patient will experience hearing loss and the sound of ringing or humming in his ears during periods of pain.

Hypersensitivity and exhaustion are the keys to understanding this remedy. Patients are emotionally, mentally, and physically overly sensitive. They seem to feel everything too deeply; everything seems to have a great impact upon them while they are in their state of pain. And their pain weakens them, they will be completely exhausted by their pain once it has passed.

Think of Kali Phos especially for cases in which the nerve pain is deep-seated and has been in place for a long period of time, or especially for cases in which the patient in pain is elderly and/or depleted.

The other most important remedy for patients with nerve pain is Magnesia Phosphorica. Think of it for nerve pain that carries with it the sensation of constriction, as if a band were tightening around the affected area. This is also the remedy to think of if the pains move about quickly, strike quickly and end just as quickly, without warning. For sudden pains in the head, or in any part of the body, that have a spasmodic character, pains in which the nerve endings themselves seem to be frayed.

It is keynote to the type that the pains will come on suddenly, will be improved by pressure—the patient may rub or press the pained area, or may bend over double to reduce the pain—and by warmth (most of the time the patient will specifically seek dry warmth for pain relief, and will not seek out, for example, a hot shower). The patient will want hot applications placed against the painful area and will press hard on them. This is such an important aspect of the remedy that pains that are improved by cold counterindicate the use of the remedy.

In general, the patient needing this remedy will have pain at night and will feel better during the day. (Again, Natrum Mur plays counterpoint, and the patient needing that remedy will often feel better at night and worse during the day.)

Like the Kali Phos patient, the patient needing Mag Phos will tend to have pains on the right side of his or her body.

This is an excellent acute remedy because it helps pains upon their sudden appearance. Think of another fast-acting phosphorus-based remedy, Ferrum Phosphoricum, as an alternative acute remedy in cases of acute nerve pain in any part of the body. Think of Ferrum Phos for cases in which inflammation in present, if the affected area is hot, red, and swollen. Think of Ferrum Phos for cases in which the patient's pain is soothed by cold, just as the Mag Phos's pain is improved by warmth. These are our two best acute remedies for those with pain. They may be given internally or used topically, as the need arises.

Another phosphorus-based remedy that is an excellent general remedy for those suffering from nerve pain is Calcarea Phosphorica. Think of this remedy in cases of pain that feel like bolts of lightning running along the paths of nerves. Think of this remedy when a sensation of cold accompanies the sensation of pain, when the pain feels cold and numb. The patient may have tics and twitches accompanying his or her pain. (The Magnesia Phosphorica patient will also have this, especially hand twitches.) Calc Phos is the remedy to think of for generalized pain that follows this pattern that comes on at night or during changes in the weather.

Mag Phos is generally considered an acute remedy for those with nerve pain, while Kali Phos is considered the chronic remedy for the same sort of pain. Therefore, these two remedies are seldom combined in the treatment of nerve pain. Calc Phos, however, combines or alternates well with either of them, should the pattern of pain match the remedy's action.

Calcarea Sulphurica is another remedy for the middle stage of nerve pain, when it has moved beyond the stage of being a simple acute situation, but has not yet become a part of the patient's daily life. Calc Phos and Calc Sulph combine well (as they seem to always do) in the treatment of patients in this middle range.

The other very general remedy for this stage, at which the pains are becoming chronic, is Kali Sulphuricum, another sulfur-based remedy. Its use will often be indicated by the fact that it runs counter to most other remedy types. Patients needing Kali Sulph are improved in fresh, cool air and worse from warmth.

Consider adding Natrum Sulphuricum for truly stubborn cases of nerve pain that do not yield to Kali Phos alone, especially if the pain increases when the patient comes into contact with dampness in any form in their environment. Or Silicea, if the patient is elderly and/or feeble. The Silicea patient will want to be covered, wrapped up, and especially will want his head covered in order to stay warm.

Specific Remedies for Nerve Pain

If the patient is better from motion: Kali Phosphoricum.

If the patient is neither better nor worse from motion, but is driven to pacing by the pain: Magnesia Phosphorica.

If the patient is worse from motion: Natrum Muriaticum.

If the patient is better from dry heat: Magnesia Phosphorica.

If the patient is worse from heat in general: Ferrum Phosphoricum, Kali Phosphoricum, Kali Sulphuricum.

If the patient is worse in a warm, stuffy room: Kali Phosphoricum, Kali Sulphuricum.

If the patient is better from cold and cool, open air: Kali Sulphuricum.

If the patient is worse from cold and cool, open air: Magnesia Phosphorica.

If the patient is worse at the seashore: Natrum Muriaticum.

If the patient is worse from damp, or from weather changes from dry to damp: Natrum Sulphuricum.

If the patient is worse from any change in the weather: Calcarea Phosphorica.

If the patient is worse in the winter, in cold weather: Natrum Muriaticum.

If the patient is worse in spring, when the snow melts: Natrum Sulphuricum.

If the patient is worse at the time of the full moon: Silicea.

If the patient is worse during the day: Natrum Muriaticum, Ferrum Phosphoricum.

If the patient is worse at night: Kali Phosphoricum, Magnesia Phosphorica.

If the pain is accompanied by a flow of saliva or tears: Natrum Muriaticum.

If the pain is accompanied by twitches or tics: Magnesia Phosphorica, Calcarea Phosphorica.

Sciatica

Consider all the general remedies for those with nerve pain listed above. In addition to these, the basic remedy for those who suffer from sciatica is Calcarea Sulphurica. The other remedy that may or may not be combined with Cal Sulph is Silicea. Think of Kali Phos as the remedy of first choice, and Silicea for cases of long-term or stubborn sciatica. Begin by giving Kali Phos alone to see what improvement results. Add or alternate with another remedy as the pattern of pain is revealed.

Kali Phos pain usually will extend down the back of the leg, from the thigh to the knee, and will carry with it a sensation of stiffness and a feeling of weakness in the affected leg or legs. The patient will not want to get up because of the pain, and rising up from a bed or chair will be very difficult, but the pain will be improved by gentle motion if the patient walks about a bit.

As is common in all forms of nerve pain, Magnesia Phosphorica will tend to play acute remedy to Kali Phos's chronic remedy in cases of sciatica. Think of Mag Phos alone or combined with Ferrum Phos for cases of sciatica that come on very quickly or recur from time to time. When the pain is improved by heat, think of Mag Phos. When the pain is improved by cold, think of Ferrum Phos.

Calcarea Phosphorica is an important general remedy for those with sciatica, especially if the pain comes back with changes in the weather, such as a change from wet to dry or dry to wet, or from cold to warm or warm to cold. The change itself will bring on the pain. In cases helped by Calc Phos, the pain begins in the hip joint and travels down the leg. The patient will feel a tingling or numbness in the leg in addition to the pain.

Another remedy for those with sciatica involving the hip joint is Natrum Muriaticum. In these cases, pain will dominate between hip and knee. The patient will want to stay still and stay off his or her leg during times of pain, will be worse from motion. The pain is worse during the daytime, better at night.

For cases of sciatica (or any nerve pain, for that matter) in which the patient has a history of gout, give Natrum Sulphuricum, even if the patient's pain does not specifically follow the pattern of sensitivity to damp. Natrum Sulphuricum may be used alone or as a follow-up to the indicated remedy.

Finally, the remedy to bring in for cases of stubborn sciatica is Silicea, as usual. Think of Silicea when the pain extends from the hip all the way down the legs, when the thigh, and especially the calf muscles, feel drawn tight and shortened during periods of pain. For cases of sciatica in elderly patients.

AILMENTS OF DIGESTION AND ELIMINATION

The cells salts were created with the concept of deficiency in mind and were seen as a means of adding nourishment to the entire body—from the smallest cells to the organs and systems to the body as a whole. So it may seem obvious that these remedies can be highly effective for cases of malabsorption and indigestion, ranging from simple acute heartburn to chronic irritable bowel syndrome (IBS) and Crohn's disease.

The term "indigestion" as used here is something of an umbrella term for myriad conditions of the area of the body, from mouth to anus, through which food is taken in, digested, and, once the digestion process is finished, eliminated. Thus, the term covers many aspects of life and touches on many of the body's systems. It covers ailments from simple to complex, acute to chronic. As always, the information in this section moves from general to specific, beginning with the most basic and commonly used remedies for those patients with any form of illness having to do with digestion and elimination.

Considering the Tongue

As the digestive system begins in the mouth, the tongue is a good indicator for the remedy needed to set things right when indigestion is an issue. This is especially true in chronic cases, but even in simple acute indigestion, the color of the tongue can lead you directly to the needed remedy, especially in cases that are indistinct in terms of other symptoms. In other words, always try to find out all of the information you can and try to assemble as complete a picture of the patient's health as you can, but when things are not clear—when there are no particularly guiding symptoms—look to the tongue to guide you. If you have been given enough information to form an opinion as to the needed remedy or remedies in a case, look at the tongue as well, as a confirmation that your decision is correct.

> While it is not an absolute indicator of a needed remedy, the appearance of a patient's tongue, especially when that patient is suffering from any form of indigestion, can at least help you rule out certain remedies and consider others.

While it is not an absolute indicator of a needed remedy, the appearance of a patient's tongue, especially when that patient is suffering from any form of indigestion, can at least help you rule out certain remedies and consider others. The patient needing a specific cell salt will have a tongue that meets one of the following descriptions:

Calcarea Fluorica

The Calc Fluor patient will have a tongue that is cracked, whether the cracked areas are painful or not. Always think of this remedy first for a tongue that is cracked or swollen, no matter the color of the tongue or whether or not it is coated.

Calcarea Phosphorica

The patient will typically have a tongue with a white coating. While the tongue may also be swollen, this is not as outstanding a feature here as it is with Calc Fluor. Consider this remedy whether the white coating is thin or thick like a carpet. Consider this remedy for those who have pimples or bumps on their tongues (also Natrum Muriaticum).

Calcarea Sulphurica

The patient will have a tongue that is coated yellow. Often the coating will only be at the base, the back part of the tongue. The patient may complain of a sour or acidic taste on his or her tongue.

Ferrum Phosphoricum

This is the remedy to consider when the tongue is dark red and swollen.

Kali Muriaticum

Think of this remedy when you see a tongue with a white coating. The tongue may or may not be dry, but don't be surprised if the coating is sometimes slimy. With Kali Mur, it is the color that matters. The coating may be pure white or darkish, a gray-white color.

Kali Phosphoricum

This is the first remedy to think of when you see a brown tongue, or if the tongue is brownish-yellow. It is also the first remedy to think of when you see a really dry tongue. The tongue may be so dry that it sticks to the roof of the mouth. This will, of course, be especially true in the morning when the patient first awakens. Note that while the center of the tongue may be coated yellow, the sides may be red and the patient may say that the reddened portions are painful, irritated.

Kali Sulphuricum

The Kali Sulph patient tends to have a tongue that ranges from white to yellow, usually somewhere in between, with a coating that is whitish-yellow or a very pale yellow. The patient may feel that their sense of taste is impaired in general.

Magnesia Phosphorica

This patient has a tongue that is a bright, shiny yellow.

Natrum Muriaticum

The Natrum Mur patient will usually have a very wet tongue and a moist mouth. Look for saliva, even bubbles of froth, on the tongue. The tongue is coated in a thick, clear coating, like raw egg white. This is a clean, wet tongue. Even though his tongue is moist, the patient will say that his mouth feels dry, and he will be very thirsty. The patient will sometimes have the sensation of a hair on his tongue (Silicea will sometimes share this sensation).

Natrum Phosphoricum

This patient will also share the sensation of a hair on the tip of the tongue. The Natrum Phos tongue is divided between the tip and the base. The base (the back of the tongue) is coated yellow, sometimes with a whitish tinge, but more often a deep golden yellow. The tip of the tongue is inflamed, reddened, and feels acidic. As this is the remedy for patients with too much acid in their systems, their entire digestive tracts, beginning with the tongue, will feel acid. The base of the tongue is moist, the tip dry.

Natrum Sulphuricum

This remedy, along with Kali Phos, has a brown tongue. But where Kali Phos has a brownish-yellow tongue, the Natrum Sulph will have a tongue that is coated brownish-green or even green. The tongue may also have a greenish-gray coating. The tongue may or may not have a triangular red patch at the tip. The patient may complain of a bitter taste in their mouth.

Silicea

Silicea has a swollen tongue, so that you will see teeth marks on the side edges of the tongue, especially at the base of the tongue. Also think of Silicea for patients who have ulcers on their tongues, especially on the tip, or who have a swollen tongue and ulcers on the sides of their gums or interior cheeks.

Yellow Tongues

For yellow tongues in general, consider: Natrum Phosphoricum, Kali Sulphuricum, and Calcarea Sulphurica.

If the tongue is yellow at the base: Calcarea Sulphurica.

If the tongue has a thick bright yellow coat: Natrum Phosphoricum.

If the tongue has a pale yellow or whitish-yellow coating: Kali Sulphuricum.

If the tongue has a slimy yellow coating: Kali Sulphuricum.

If the tongue is very dark yellow, or brownish-yellow: Kali Phosphoricum.

Brown Tongues

For brown tongues in general, consider Kali Phosphoricum, and Natrum Sulphuricum.

If the tongue is brownish-yellow: Kali Phosphoricum.

If the tongue is brownish-green: Natrum Sulphuricum.

White Tongues

For white tongues in general, consider Kali Muriaticum, Calcarea Phosphorica.

If the tongue is white to darkish white-grey: Kali Muriaticum.

If the tongue has a general white coating, whether the coating is thick or thin: Calcarea Phosphorica.

Gray Tongues

For gray tongues in general, consider Natrum Sulphuricum, Kali Muriaticum.

For tongues that are grayish-white: Kali Muriaticum.

For tongues that are grayish-green: Natrum Sulphuricum.

Red Tongues *

For red tongues in general, consider Ferrum Phosphoricum, Magnesia Phosphorica, Natrum Sulphuricum, and Natrum Phosphoricum.

If the whole tongue is red: Ferrum Phosphoricum, Magnesia Phosphorica.

If the whole tongue is bright red: Magnesia Phosphorica.

If the whole tongue is dark red: Ferrum Phosphoricum.

If the tongue is only red in part: Natrum Sulphuricum, Natrum Phosphoricum.

If the Tongue Is Clean

Consider Natrum Muriaticum, Ferrum Phosphoricum, and Magnesia Phosphorica.

If the tongue is clean during times of inflammation: Ferrum Phosphoricum, Magnesia Phosphorica.

If the tongue is clean and moist or has a clear, slimy coating: Natrum Muriaticum.

If the Tongue Is Moist

Consider Natrum Muriaticum, and Natrum Phosphoricum.

---

* Note that, unlike the other colors, the color red refers to the tongue itself and not to a coating on the tongue. Both Magnesia Phosphorica and Ferrum Phosphoricum present what is in essence a clean tongue, albeit one that is colored red.

If the Tongue Is Dry

Consider Kali Muriaticum and Kali Phosphoricum.

If the Tongue Is Swollen

Consider Calcarea Fluorica, Silicea, Calcarea Phosphorica, Kali Muriaticum, and Ferrum Phosphoricum.

If the Tongue Is Slimy

Consider Kali Muriaticum, Kali Sulphuricum, Kali Phosphoricum, Natrum Muriaticum, and Natrum Sulphuricum.

General Remedies for Indigestion

There are three basic remedies for indigestion, two of which are equally indicated for both chronic and for acute cases of indigestion. The third is most often used only in chronic cases.

Calcarea Phosphorica

The first remedy is Calcarea Phosphorica. This is the basic, core remedy for those with indigestion, whether it is chronic or acute, and whether it involves nausea, pain or, especially, bloating. Any case of indigestion that is accompanied by bloating should suggest Calc Phos.

In chronic cases, always give Calc Phos an hour after each meal, as it will help the patient digest his or her food properly and will help to avoid the bloating, gas, and general discomfort that is common to the remedy type. When heartburn, flatulence, bloating, and belching occur after eating, think of Calc Phos. Think of it especially for those cases in which the patient feels that he or she must eat, cases in which the patient has stomach pain if he does not eat and feels much better, in the short term, from eating. But discomfort begins to build two to three hours after eating, so the patient feels that he is in a quandary as to which is worse: the pain he has from an empty stomach, or the fullness and bloating he experiences after eating. Typical Calc Phos patients are hungry, ravenous; they want to eat, even though they know that they likely will suffer after eating. They tend to overeat and to eat the wrong things. They crave ice-cold drinks and ice cream, even though they may vomit them up once they have become warm in their stomachs. They crave ham, bacon, smoked meats. They like meat, salty things, and sweet things. They crave cold things as well. They can seem to crave only the things they cannot digest and live lives of chronic discomfort as a result.

Think of Calc Phos for the patient who feels a weight in his stomach after eating, who has to lean back and loosen his belt because of the bloat that the meal causes.

These patients are worse both from eating and from not eating. They are better from belching, and, initially, from eating, until the process of digestion causes discomfort. Calc Phos needs to be taken an hour after each meal to turn things around. This is a remedy that will help from the very first dose, but which will work better and better as time passes and as the cell salt helps the body digest its food and helps the patient learn to eat foods that are more easily digested.

Also think of Calc Phos is acute situations, when bloating, heartburn, and general discomfort come on from overeating during holidays, or two to three hours after any meal. It is the general remedy for those with bloating as Natrum Phosphoricum is the general remedy for acid indigestion.

Natrum Phosphoricum

Natrum Phos is the second remedy to consider for those with indigestion. The next time you are considering reaching for an antacid, reach for Natrum Phosphoricum instead. Think of this remedy for any case of indigestion in which the pain is limited to only one spot in the abdomen. Think of it for any case of acid indigestion, when acid rises in the back of the throat, or when the patient experiences sour or acid vomiting. Typically, as with Calcarea Phosphorica, the pains associated with Natrum Phos will come on two hours after eating. But instead of featuring bloating, they feature acid burning. Flatulence may accompany the acid indigestion, and the gas will have a particularly foul smell.

Silicea

Silicea is the third remedy for acid indigestion. It most often relates only to chronic cases, and in those cases it may be used along with either of the two remedies listed above. Think of Silicea especially for patients who are very young or very old, who are depleted, weakened, and have imperfect digestion. Think of this remedy first for cases in which the stomach is distended during indigestion. Think of this remedy for cases in which the patient cannot eat when the food arrives, although he is very hungry. When nausea prevents him eating, or when he cannot stand the sight or smell of cooked food, especially meat. Think of this remedy also for cases in which the patient vomits immediately after eating. This is the remedy for children with failure to thrive, for babies who vomit up their own mother's milk.

The picture that we all have seen of the starving child with thin legs and arms and an extended stomach is the portrait of the seriously undernourished Silicea patient. More commonly, these patients will not show the signs of starvation so clearly, but Silicea types, especially the young or elderly Silicea types, will have underdeveloped or withered arms and legs and distended stomachs. They are chronically chilly and will want to be kept warm. They will insist that they are very hungry, yet will eat little.

Think of this remedy for cases of chronic malabsorption of food, in which the patient does not seem able to digest the simplest thing, or for cases in which the patient experiences heartburn, pain, and terrible nausea after eating.

Silicea should not be given after meals, because the symptoms caused by eating are nearly instantaneous and this is a slow-working remedy. It should, instead, be given twice a day, first thing in the morning and last thing at night. It may take some days to see improvement, but continue giving the remedy until the patient's digestion is built back up and he is able to eat and enjoy his food and fully digest what he has eaten. With depleted patients the remedy may have to be given for weeks or months to be fully effective.

Note that any or all of these three remedies can be used in alternation or combination with any of the other cell salts when treating patients who are experiencing symptoms related to indigestion.

Stomachache

The first remedy to think of for cases of simple stomachache is, again, Calcarea Phosphorica. Other remedies for the condition are Natrum Muriaticum, which can be used for acute or chronic cases, Natrum Phosphoricum, Calcarea Sulphurica, and Ferrum Phosphoricum, for acute cases. As always for stubborn, chronic conditions, think of Silicea as well. It will blend well with any other remedy, with the exception of Ferrum Phosphoricum, for the treatment of stomachache.

This is the basic group of remedies that we will consider for stomachache.

Ferrum Phosphoricum

The acute cases that are cured by Ferrum Phosphoricum often accompany flu or some other acute condition. The patient will have a flushed, red, hot face and a sense of sudden pain in the stomach, which may also be accompanied by a sense of heat. The Ferrum Phos patient in digestive distress typically is very thirsty for cold water. He may vomit whatever he eats, especially meat and/or dairy. He may vomit blood. He also will tend to have acid reflux, which will bring up the flavor of the food he has eaten.

Calcarea Sulphurica

Think of Calcarea Sulphurica for the patient who is hungry, who craves stimulants, such as caffeinated drinks, but does not handle them well and feels shaky after drinking them. This patient feels nausea and vertigo along with the pain in the stomach. This is a raw, burning pain, a throbbing in the stomach. Calc Sulph is an excellent acute or chronic remedy and may be combined very well with others as needed, especially with our core remedy Calcarea Phosphorica.

Calcarea Phosphorica

As noted above, Calc Phos is perhaps our best all-around remedy for indigestion in any form, from stomachache to bloating, belching, and flatulence. This is the remedy to think of for the malaise that comes on from overeating and from eating those things that disagree, especially from eating dairy. This is the remedy for the dyspeptic, for the day after Christmas, or for Thanksgiving night. Taken an hour after a meal, it will help the patient digest the meal and avoid the bloating and discomfort that would otherwise lie ahead. Calc Phos should be part of any treatment for those with stomachache.

Natrum Muriaticum

Natrum Muriaticum is similar to Calc Phos and combines or alternates very well with it for the treatment of the patient with a stomachache. Like Calc Phos, the Natrum Muriaticum patient often eats himself into his stomachache. This is a remedy of extreme hunger, of overeating. This is also a remedy with a great thirst. No other patient will be as thirsty for cold water. These patients also tend to crave salty things (the remedy is made from table salt, after all). They crave bitter tastes as well, and tend to avoid sweets. They will either crave or be totally adverse to bread and other baked goods, although my experience is that they tend to crave carbohydrates. This is the stomachache that carries with it a sense of weight in the stomach, in the whole body. Contrast these symptoms with Calc Phos's sense of bloating. In this case, patients feel as if they have a lead weight in their stomachs. They may belch, and the belching will carry a sour taste up into their mouths. This is the remedy for those with offensive breath after eating. For those who have a sinking sensation that accompanies their stomachache; for those who will want to lie down after eating.

Natrum Phosphoricum

Natrum Phosphoricum should be considered whenever a stomachache comes on from an excess of acid in the patient's system. When the patient feels sour, acidic, and feels the stomach pain in one specific spot. When he can point to one spot and say, "Right here. Here is where it hurts." For that case, think of Natrum Phosphoricum. This remedy is also useful for patients with acid reflux, with burning and a sour taste rising up into the mouth. Typically, the stomachache will come on within two hours after eating.

Specific Remedies for Stomachache

For the stomachache that comes on two to three hours after eating: Calcarea Phosphorica, Natrum Phosphoricum.

For the stomachache that begins while the patient is still eating: Calcarea Phosphorica.

For the stomachache that is better for eating: Kali Phosphoricum, Magnesia Phosphorica, Natrum Sulphuricum, Silicea.

For the stomachache that is better at first from eating, but worse two hours later: Calcarea Phosphorica.

For the stomachache that comes on after lunch: Calcarea Sulphurica.

For the stomachache that comes on at night, when the patient has gone to bed: Natrum Sulphuricum.

For the stomachache that is better from belching: Calcarea Phosphorica.

For the stomachache that is worse from belching: Silicea.

For the stomachache after overeating: Calcarea Phosphorica, Natrum Muriaticum.

For the stomachache after eating bread: Natrum Muriaticum.

For the stomachache after eating dairy: Calcarea Phosphorica.

For the stomachache after eating fatty foods: Kali Muriaticum, Natrum Phosphoricum.

For the stomachache after drinking alcohol: Natrum Sulphuricum.

For the stomachache after drinking hot drinks: Kali Muriaticum.

For the stomachache that is worse from drinking cold drinks: Calcarea Phosphorica, Magnesia Phosphorica.

For the stomachache that is better from drinking cold drinks: Ferrum Phosphoricum, Calcarea Sulphurica.

For a stomachache with a burning sensation: Calcarea Phosphorica, Natrum Muriaticum, Silicea, Kali Muriaticum, Ferrum Phosphoricum, Kali Phosphoricum, Natrum Sulphuricum.

For a stomachache that is accompanied by flashes of heat in the stomach: Ferrum Phosphoricum, Natrum Muriaticum, Natrum Phosphoricum, Natrum Sulphuricum.

If flashes of heat extend upward into the chest and throat: Natrum Muriaticum, Ferrum Phosphoricum.

If the patient's face is hot and flushed: Ferrum Phosphoricum.

For a stomachache with a bloating sensation: Calcarea Phosphorica, Natrum Muriaticum, Natrum Sulphuricum, Ferrum Phosphoricum, Kali Phosphoricum, Kali Sulphuricum, Calcarea Sulphurica.

For the sensation of bloating in which the clothes feel tight: Natrum Muriaticum, Calcarea Phosphorica.

For the sensation of bloating in which tight clothing is intolerable: Natrum Muriaticum.

For a stomachache with the sensation of weight: Natrum Muriaticum, Silicea, Natrum Sulphuricum, Kali Sulphuricum.

For a stomachache that is worse from any sort of touch or motion: Natrum Muriaticum.

For a stomachache that is better if the patient yawns: Natrum Muriaticum.

For a stomachache caused by strong emotion, especially fear: Kali Phosphoricum.

Heartburn

There are two major remedies for those with heartburn: one for sudden, severe heartburn and the other for more chronic cases.

For acute cases of sudden heartburn, in which the pain is intense and the patient suddenly feels as if he or she will vomit, the remedy is Ferrum Phosphoricum.

For general cases of heartburn, always consider the remedy Natrum Phosphoricum. It is the remedy of first choice for all cases of acid reflux or acid indigestion. It will seldom fail to cure cases of indigestion in which heartburn is the most pronounced symptom. It works for both acute and chronic cases. Even the most stubborn cases of acid indigestion will yield to Natrum Phos.

If heartburn is accompanied by either belching or flatulence, combine Natrum Phos with Calcarea Phosphorica, giving Natrum Phos an hour before meals and Calcarea Phosphorica an hour after. This combination of remedies, given three times a day for a period of a few days or even weeks, in potencies as low as 3X or as high as 12X will bring relief to even the most stubborn case of chronic heartburn.

See the section on "Stomachache" for more information.

Nausea

For specific cases of nausea, consider this small group of remedies: Natrum Muriaticum, Calcarea Phosphorica, and Silicea.

But note that as nausea is a very general symptom, every cell salt may be considered, if the symptoms of the case match the patient's own. Look at the tongue for an indicator of the correct remedy or remedies. And consider adding other cell salt remedies to our group of three, as specific conditions merit.

Natrum Muriaticum

Think of Natrum Muriaticum for cases in which a patient feels nauseous immediately after eating, no matter how little he or she eats. Note that Natrum Muriaticum is the major remedy to consider for all cases of morning sickness in pregnancy, and you will get the idea. The Natrum Mur patient may become nauseous at the smell or just the thought of food. When nausea is the pronounced symptom associated with a given patient's indigestion, give Natrum Muriaticum. When nausea and general indigestion are present, combine or alternate Natrum Muriaticum with Calcarea Phosphorica to complete the cure.

Calcarea Phosphorica

As perhaps our most general remedy for all conditions relating to digestion or lack of same, Calcarea Phosphorica is an important remedy to consider for all cases involving nausea. Consider it for all cases of nausea that come on two to three hours after eating in general and specifically from eating cold things or drinking cold drinks, which lead to feelings of nausea and to vomiting, headache, and diarrhea once they warm in the patient's stomach. Think of this remedy for the patient who becomes nauseous after eating even small amounts of food.

Silicea

This is the remedy to consider for cases in which the patient becomes nauseous at the very thought of food, or especially upon smelling food being cooked. He or she has feelings of terrible nausea especially when smelling meat being prepared, or when thinking of actually eating meat or other warm foods.

Specific Remedies for Nausea

For nausea first thing in the morning when the patient is just getting up: Ferrum Phosphoricum.

For nausea that is, in general, worse in the morning: Natrum Muriaticum.

For nausea during breakfast, or that prevents the patient from eating breakfast: Natrum Muriaticum.

For nausea after breakfast: Calcarea Phosphorica.

For nausea that is worse from coffee, even the smell of coffee: Natrum Muriaticum, Calcarea Phosphorica.

For nausea in the afternoon: Silicea.

For nausea that comes on at 4:00 P.M. in the afternoon: Calcarea Phosphorica.

For nausea after large meals (lunch or dinner): Natrum Muriaticum, Natrum Sulphuricum, Silicea, Kali Phosphoricum, Kali Sulphuricum.

For nausea in the evening: Natrum Muriaticum.

For nausea in the nighttime, while the patient is in bed: Natrum Sulphuricum.

For nausea that wakes the patient during the night: Ferrum Phosphoricum.

For nausea that is better from resting: Natrum Muriaticum.

For nausea that is better if the patient lies on his or her stomach: Natrum Muriaticum.

For nausea that is better from walking in the open air: Calcarea Sulphurica.

For nausea that is worse from walking in the open air: Natrum Muriaticum, Silicea.

For nausea that is worse from entering a warm room: Calcarea Sulphurica.

For nausea that is better from entering a warm room or from wrapping up: Silicea.

For sudden, acute nausea: Ferrum Phosphoricum.

For long-term, chronic nausea: Natrum Muriaticum, Natrum Sulphuricum, Silicea.

Vomiting

Since the specific treatments for the patient who is vomiting often involve studying the matter that has been vomited, most of us tend to want to take a more general approach to treatment. In all cases of treatment of the patient who is vomiting, you may combine a small group of remedies and give them all at once to settle the case. Once the vomiting has ceased, you can take a more specific case, to select the most appropriate remedy for the treatment of the patient as a whole being.

But for the moment in which you are dealing with a patient who is vomiting, I suggest that you combine Ferrum Phosphoricum, Natrum Muriaticum, and Kali Muriaticum, a few pellets of each, in about a quarter of a glass of room temperature water. The patient should sip the water as he or she is able, taking a sip every couple of minutes at first and then less often as symptoms begin to fade. Even after the vomiting has stopped, I would suggest that you continue to give sips of this mixture every few hours for another day or two, until the patient feels fully recovered.

If this mixture does not help the patient to fully recover, or if the substances vomited contain a great deal of undigested food, add Calcarea Fluorica to the mixture.

Before treating, note whether the vomiting seems to be a simple acute case, such as a twenty-four-hour flu or a case of tainted food. If so, all well and good. But if the symptoms linger or are severe, a trip to the emergency room may be called for. In any case, any patient who does not feel fully himself or herself after a few hours deserves to have his or her case fully taken and the right remedy or remedies given. Make sure to study both the things vomited up (blood, undigested food, and lumps of mucus are particularly telling) and the patient's tongue for indications of the needed remedy.

If you feel you have enough information to treat with an individual remedy or two remedies in combination or alternation, consider the following remedies.

Ferrum Phosphoricum

Ferrum Phos is the indicated remedy for sudden, surprising vomiting that is accompanied by a severe pain the stomach. For vomiting when the patient has a hot, flushed face, or pain and vomiting right after eating.

Natrum Muriaticum

Natrum Mur is indicated when the vomiting is preceded by a gathering of a good deal of saliva in the patient's mouth. When vomiting is preceded by a sour taste or by bad breath.

Kali Muriaticum

Kali Mur should be considered when vomiting comes from food poisoning, when food disagrees with the patient who otherwise has been well. When vomiting is preceded by or accompanied by flatulence.

Calcarea Fluorica

Cal Flour should be considered for cases in which the vomit mostly consists of undigested food (Ferrum Phos may also have this symptom), and for cases in which vomiting is proceeded by hiccoughs.

Specific Remedies for Vomiting

If vomit contains undigested food: Calcarea Fluorica, Ferrum Phosphoricum, Calcarea Phosphorica.

If vomit contains blood: Ferrum Phosphoricum, Kali Muriaticum.

If blood is bright red: Ferrum Phosphoricum.

If blood is dark red, or clotted: Kali Muriaticum.

If vomit contains mucus: Natrum Muriaticum, Kali Muriaticum, Natrum Sulphuricum.

If mucus is watery: Natrum Muriaticum.

If mucus is thick but clear: Natrum Muriaticum.

If mucus is thick and white: Kali Muriaticum.

If mucus is greenish: Natrum Sulphuricum.

If mucus is thick and stringy: Natrum Sulphuricum.

If the patient vomits water: Natrum Muriaticum, Kali Phosphoricum.

If the patient vomits greenish water: Natrum Sulphuricum, Kali Phosphoricum.

Flatulence

There is no better remedy for those who suffer from intestinal gas than Calcarea Phosphorica. No matter what other remedy or remedies are given, give Calc Phos, first and foremost.

The other remedy for flatulence, especially when it combines with belching after eating, is Magnesia Phosphorica, which we have not encountered much in the study of remedies for indigestion. That makes it especially valuable for cases in which flatulence or belching are the most pronounced symptoms. For cases in which flatulence comes on after eating, think of Magnesia Phosphorica if bloating, pressure, and indigestion are not as pronounced as they are in cases requiring Calc Phos. For cases in which the gas itself is the major symptom, give Mag Phos. For acute cases of gas, give Mag Phos first and follow up with Calc Phos if the Mag Phos alone fails to act. For cases of chronic flatulence after eating, give Calcarea Phosphorica.

Specific Remedies for Flatulence

If the gas is particularly noisy: Kali Phosphoricum.

If the gas is particularly offensive: Natrum Sulphuricum.

If the flatulence is chronic and stubborn: Combine Calcarea Phosphorica and Kali Muriaticum.

Belching

When belching is the issue, the phosphorus-based remedies are the cure.

Calcarea Phosphorica

Think of Calcarea Phosphorica as the best general remedy for cases of indigestion in which the patient typically feels bloated and gassy, and belches after eating, particularly after eating dinner. Think of this remedy for the patient who loosens his pants after eating a heavy dinner, leans back, and belches. Who enjoys the sensation of the belch and feels better for it.

Magnesia Phosphorica

This is also an excellent remedy for those who are belching. It is particularly helpful for cases in which belching and passing gas occur at the same time.

Specific Remedies for Belching

If the belching tastes acidic or bitter: Natrum Phosphoricum.

If the belching has a burning taste: Magnesia Phosphorica.

If the belching has no taste: Magnesia Phosphorica.

If the belching brings up the flavor of food that has recently been eaten: Ferrum Phosphoricum.

If the belching tastes sour: Calcarea Phosphorica, Kali Phosphoricum, Natrum Phosphoricum.

Bad Breath

There are four remedies to consider for bad breath. They are Natrum Muriaticum, Kali Phosphoricum, Natrum Phosphoricum, and Natrum Sulphuricum. Of these, Natrum Muriaticum and Kali Phosphoricum are more commonly used. Patients needing either Natrum Sulphuricum or Natrum Phosphoricum have truly fetid breath, the smell of which indicates a deeper illness. This is often caused by the presence of toxins, especially an overabundance of acids such as uric acid in the patient's system, and the two remedies will be needed in combination, with Natrum Phos being given first and then alternated with Natrum Sulph later on to clear away the toxins and restore better smelling breath.

For cases of what would be considered "normal" bad breath, Natrum Muriaticum is the first remedy to consider. Think of this for breath that smells bad after eating, for breath that is stale, and for patients whose breath always seems to smell bad.

Kali Phosphoricum is useful for cases in which emotional upsets lead to stomach upsets and bad breath, indigestion, and hiccoughs are the result.

As both patients will be thirsty, dyspeptic, and irritable, it may be hard to determine which remedy to use. In these cases, alternate both to bring about positive results.

Hiccoughs

Only four cell salts help with cases of hiccoughs.

The first and most general remedy, Magnesia Phosphorica, can be considered specific to hiccoughs, and treats them as the muscle spasms they are. For all cases of hiccoughs, think of Mag Phos first, especially if the hiccoughs are accompanied by flatulence.

The second remedy to consider is for hiccoughs that suddenly come on after a patient laughs, is scared, or experiences any other profound emotion. For these cases, give Kali Phosphoricum.

When either of these remedies fails to cure, add Natrum Muriaticum, either in combination or alternation with the first remedy.

Finally, give Calcarea Fluorica for cases of really stubborn hiccoughs, or cases in which the hiccoughs are so intense that they make the patient feel as if he or she will vomit. For these cases, dissolve the Calc Fluor in lukewarm water and have the patient sip it, every few minutes at first until improvement begins, and then less often until the hiccoughs are gone.

Diarrhea

The most important remedies for those with diarrhea include Natrum Muriaticum, Natrum Phosphoricum, Natrum Sulphuricum and Silicea. All of these relate to chronic cases especially. In acute cases, the choice will often be between Ferrum Phosphoricum and Magnesia Phosphorica. Other remedies that should be considered are Kali Phosphoricum, Calcarea Sulphuricum, and Kali Muriaticum.

Calcarea Phosphorica

Because Calcarea Phosphorica is our general remedy for all forms of indigestion includ-ing diarrhea, it must always be considered, especially for cases in which a patient has chronic diarrhea or in which diarrhea alternates with constipation (Natrum Muri-aticum is the other important remedy for this), as in cases of chronic irritable bowel syndrome. This is also the first remedy to consider for teething children with diarrhea. Think of this remedy for all cases in which the stool is noisy, if it passes with a good deal of sputtering. The patient will feel that the passing stool is hot and burning. The rec-tum will feel irritated by the diarrhea.

Ferrum Phosphoricum and Magnesia Phosphorica

Acute cases of diarrhea, often associated with flu or other acute diseases, usually will respond to either Ferrum Phosphoricum or Magnesia Phosphorica. In both cases, the bout of diarrhea will be quite sudden. In cases that respond to Mag Phos, the diarrhea is usually preceded by cramps in the abdomen that force the patient to bend over double to find relief.

In cases of stomach flu, when the patient has both diarrhea and vomiting, the rem-edy is most often Ferrum Phosphoricum, although Magnesia Phosphorica may be called for instead. Often the only way to quickly tell the two types apart is by the temperature of cloth they want placed on their heads or stomachs to bring relief. The patient who wants a cold cloth needs Ferrum Phosphoricum. The patient who clutches a hot cloth to his or her stomach to put pressure on the area needs Magnesia Phosphorica.

Both of these remedy types will have acute cases of diarrhea that come suddenly, with pain and that come in spells or waves. They will have moments in which they feel better before the bout begins again. Both have diarrhea that is forcefully expelled, that is watery, and that causes them to cry out in pain both just before and during the bout.

Kali Phosphoricum

Kali Phos is the remedy to think of in acute cases, when diarrhea comes on after strong emotions, especially after the patient experiences fear, often the fear of public speaking. The Kali Phos patient will pass a stool that is particularly foul smelling, making this the general remedy for patients with diarrhea who pass a cadaverous stool. It is also the first remedy to think of for cases of diarrhea that are very noisy as well, when the patient loudly passes gas while passing the loose stool. The discharge is painful. The patient will typically feel a burning in the rectum while passing stool.

Natrum Muriaticum

Natrum Mur is the first remedy to consider for cases of stubborn or chronic diarrhea, especially in very young patients. Typically, the patient will pass a loose stool that contains thick, clear mucus, or that is comprised of large amounts of water. This is the first remedy to think of for cases of chronic diarrhea that are painless to pass. It is also the first remedy to think of for cases of diarrhea that come on after the patient has eaten fruits or vegetables that contain a large amount of liquid, such as watermelon.

Silicea

Silicea is another remedy (with Natrum Muriaticum) to consider for chronic cases of diarrhea in young patients. Especially for cases of failure to thrive in which the young child seems incapable of digesting even the simplest foods, which pass out of the body undigested in the loose stool. Like Kali Phosphoricum, this patient is also known for having particularly foul smelling stools. Look for the patient to have sweat on his or her whole head both while and after passing the stool. The patient will want his or her head wrapped and will feel cold and weak after the diarrhea has passed. This is the first remedy to consider for cases of chronic diarrhea in young patients who have distended stomachs.

Natrum Sulphuricum

If the patient is elderly and the case of diarrhea is long-term and stubborn, the remedy is Natrum Sulphuricum. Think of this remedy for cases in which the patient has to rise up and move about before the sudden urge to pass stool. For cases in which you can hear fluid sloshing around inside the patient's stomach before the sudden bout of diarrhea. This is the remedy when the stool is loose, liquid, and green. For diarrhea that gushes out.

Natrum Phosphoricum

Natrum Phos is the remedy of choice for cases of chronic diarrhea that are accompanied by vomiting. When the stool is loose but hard to expel, when the patient has to strain to pass the stool that then shoots out. The stool is jellylike, yellow or yellow-green. Think of this remedy especially for the patient who chronically has constipation, but who, from time to time, experiences a sudden bout of diarrhea that relieves the constipation and expels the built-up toxins from the body. These stools are sour smelling.

Calcarea Sulphurica

Think of Calcarea Sulphurica for all cases in which the diarrhea is bloody. This is especially true if the diarrhea comes on during any dramatic change in weather.

Kali Muriaticum

Think of Kali Muriaticum for cases in which diarrhea comes on after eating rich or fatty foods, after eating baked goods, cookies, cakes, pies, and such. For cases in which the diarrhea is the characteristic white color associated with the remedy and when the patient's tongue is coated white. The stool may be slimy or bloody (in which case, alternate or combine with Calc Sulph).

Specific Remedies for Diarrhea

For cases of diarrhea in young patients: Natrum Muriaticum, Silicea, Calcarea Phosphorica, Calcarea Sulphuricum.

For cases of diarrhea in old patients: Natrum Sulphuricum.

For cases of diarrhea in the very early morning that wake the patient: Kali Phosphoricum.

For cases of diarrhea in the morning: Natrum Sulphuricum, Ferrum Phosphoricum, Silicea.

For cases of diarrhea in the morning that drive the patient out of bed: Natrum Sulphuricum, Silicea.

For cases of diarrhea in the morning that occur only after the patient is up and about for some time: Natrum Muriaticum.

For cases of diarrhea in the afternoon: Ferrum Phosphoricum.

For cases of diarrhea that occur in the daytime: Natrum Muriaticum, Kali Muriaticum, Natrum Sulphuricum.

For cases of diarrhea that occur at night: Magnesia Phosphorica, Kali Phosphoricum, Kali Muriaticum, Ferrum Phosphoricum, Natrum Sulphuricum, Silicea.

For cases of diarrhea that occur when the patient has gone to bed at night: Natrum Sulphuricum.

For cases of diarrhea that occur late in the night, waking the patient: Kali Muriaticum.

For cases of diarrhea that are painless: Natrum Muriaticum, Silicea, Natrum Sulphuricum.

For cases of diarrhea that are preceded by cramping pains: Magnesia Phosphorica.

For cases of diarrhea that are accompanied by cramping pains in the calves: Kali Phosphoricum, Magnesia Phosphorica.

For cases of diarrhea that are preceded by a pain in the groin: Natrum Sulphuricum.

For cases of diarrhea that are preceded by sounds of gurgling: Natrum Muriaticum, Natrum Sulphuricum.

For cases of diarrhea in hot weather: Natrum Muriaticum, Ferrum Phosphoricum, Natrum Phosphoricum.

For cases of diarrhea during cold weather: Natrum Sulphuricum.

For cases of diarrhea during a change in the weather: Calcarea Sulphurica.

For cases of diarrhea during damp weather: Natrum Sulphuricum.

For cases in which diarrhea alternates with constipation: Natrum Muriaticum, Calcarea Phosphorica.

Constipation

The general remedies for constipation are Natrum Muriaticum and Silicea. They work especially well for chronic cases, and may be used together with good results. For chronic cases of constipation in which the patient experiences a sudden bout of diarrhea from time to time, consider the remedy Natrum Phosphoricum.

As Calcarea Phosphorica is perhaps our most important cell salt remedy for all aspects of indigestion, it will come into play for cases of constipation as well, especially for cases in elderly patients (also Natrum Sulphuricum). Think of this remedy if the bowel movement is accompanied by a sensation of weakness or vertigo.

Natrum Muriaticum

For patients with constipation, Natrum Muriaticum is the most important remedy. It is especially suited to overweight patients with sluggish metabolisms. For patients who have both constipation and hemorrhoids. For cases in which the stool is small and hard to pass and when the stool may be bloody. For cases in which the stool is small and dry, when it seems that the constipation is caused by a lack of fluid in the body.

Silicea

Since Silicea is the remedy for malnutrition and its consequences, it should come as no surprise that it is an important remedy for those with constipation, especially chronic constipation. Silicea has the keynote symptom that the stool seems to recede after having been partially expelled from the body. Think of this for the most stubborn cases of constipation, in which days go by without a bowel movement, in which the body seems to have lost the ability to pass a stool.

Natrum Sulphuricum

For very bloody bowel movements, think of Natrum Sulphuricum, especially if the stool is streaked with blood. As always with this remedy, the stool will be greenish in color. It will be soft, but very hard to pass. This is a painful bowel movement. And this is, again, a remedy for patients with stubborn constipation.

Kali Phosphoricum

Kali Phos is a very important remedy for those with constipation, although it is one that you will likely seldom use. Think of this remedy in cases of the most stubborn constipation, in which the patient has no desire or urge to have a bowel movement at all. What bowel movements there are will be scanty and small, and very dark in color.

Specific Remedies for Constipation

For constipation accompanied by headache: Natrum Muriaticum, Calcarea Phosphorica.

For constipation that requires much straining: Silicea.

For constipation in which there is much urging, without result: Natrum Muriaticum, Silicea.

For constipation in which bowel movement is insufficient or unsatisfactory: Natrum Muriaticum.

For constipation in which the stool is soft, and yet hard to pass: Natrum Sulphuricum, Silicea.

For constipation in which the stool is very small and hard: Natrum Muriaticum, Silicea.

For constipation during pregnancy: Natrum Sulphuricum.

For constipation when traveling: Silicea.

For constipation every other day: Natrum Muriaticum.

For chronic constipation: Natrum Muriaticum, Silicea, Natrum Phosphoricum.

For chronic constipation in which, from time to time, there is a sudden bout of diarrhea: Natrum Phosphoricum.

For constipation that alternates with diarrhea: Calcarea Phosphorica, Natrum Muriaticum.

For the most extreme cases of constipation, in which there is no desire at all for a bowel movement: Kali Phosphoricum.

Hemorrhoids

The simplest treatment for those with hemorrhoids involves simply taking all four of the most commonly needed remedies used for those with hemorrhoids, dissolving them in lukewarm water, and applying the water directly to the affected area, as this method may be much more pleasant and successful than trying to decide on the exact right remedy. Certainly remedies can be taken internally, as always, in addition to the topical application.

The most commonly needed remedies for hemorrhoids are Ferrum Phosphoricum, Calcarea Fluorica, Natrum Muriaticum, and Kali Sulphuricum.

Calcarea Phosphorica

In cases of chronic hemorrhoids, the remedy is always Calcarea Phosphorica, which may or may not be used in combination with the other remedies listed for topical applications in chronic cases. In these cases, Calcarea Phosphorica should also be taken by mouth even if the topical application is used.

Natrum Muriaticum

The most general, basic remedy for those with hemorrhoids is Natrum Muriaticum. It is especially indicated in patients who suffer both from constipation and hemorrhoids. It can be taken in combination or alternation with Calc Phos to bring about a cure. In cases calling for Natrum Mur, the hemorrhoids will smart, will hurt, and may also bleed a little during and after a bowel movement.

Specific Remedies for Hemorrhoids

For cases in which hemorrhoids bleed: Ferrum Phosphoricum.

For cases of external hemorrhoids: Kali Sulphuricum.

For cases in which the hemorrhoids are swollen and hard: Calcrea Fluorica.

For cases in which hemorrhoids itch: Kali Phosphoricum.

For cases in which hemorrhoids sting: Natrum Muriaticum.

For cases in which hemorrhoids burn: Ferrum Phosphoricum.

For cases in which hemorrhoids are worse from warmth or heat: Kali Sulphuricum.

For cases of hemorrhoids in a constipated patient: Natrum Muriaticum.

For chronic cases: Calcarea Phosphorica.

CONDITIONS OF THE SKIN, HAIR, AND NAILS

Since the cell salts are the building blocks of the hard and soft tissues of the body, it stands to reason that yet another use for these remedies is to sustain the health of these cells. In this section we consider the cells of the skin, which is the largest organ of the body. The remedies listed here are those that will maintain the health of the skin and the hair and nails as well.

General Remedies for the Skin

No matter the issue, the three major remedies for anything having to do with the skin are Silicea, Kali Sulphuricum, and Natrum Muriaticum. The other cell salts that are used in treatment of those with skin conditions include Calcarea Phosphorica, Calcarea Sulphurica, Kali Phosphoricum, and Ferrum Phosphoricum. Of the twelve biochemical remedies, these seven are those that are most often used in conditions relating directly to the health of the skin.

Silicea

Perhaps the single most important remedy when it comes to the health of the skin is Silicea. It is, perhaps, the most important when considering the health of the skin, the hair, and the nails as a whole. No other remedy will soothe or heal the skin as quickly or as well as Silicea. No other remedy will both allow for the expulsion of foreign materials from the skin and the reabsorbing of scar tissue as Silicea. No other remedy is as wide or deep in its healing action when it comes to the skin, the hair, and the nails. It is the first remedy to consider for all cases in which any or all—the skin, the hair and the nails—look sickly or weak. The list of skin conditions for which Silicea is a suggested remedy goes on and on: for itching and/or burning; for rashes, blotches, and discolorations; for ulcers and boils; for wounds to the skin that do not heal; for nodes; for carbuncles; for felons; for acne and pustules of all sorts; for abscesses; for keloids; for swollen glands; for bursa; and, finally, as mentioned earlier, for splinters and other foreign objects in the skin.

And yet, as with so many other conditions, Silicea often works best for skin conditions when it is used in conjunction with other remedies, most often with Natrum Muriaticum, especially in chronic or stubborn cases.

Natrum Muriaticum

Natrum Muriaticum, along with Silicea, is one of our most commonly used homeopathic remedies in addition to being a cell salt, so it stands to reason that these two polycrests would have as much impact upon the health of the cells of the skin as they do for the cells in the other organs of the body.

Like Silicea, Natrum Mur has myriad uses in terms of skin conditions. Think of it for cases of dandruff, for eczema, for warts, for blisters that are filled with clear liquid, even for herpes and for insect bites. Think of this as a great remedy for chapped or dry skin, especially for dry skin in winter. Keynote to this remedy is the fact that the lips crack down the middle.

Kali Sulphuricum

The other great remedy for the skin is Kali Sulphuricum. It is our great remedy for eczema, for psoriasis, and for dandruff. It is vital to all conditions that involve the scaling or flaking of the skin. Kali Sulph promotes the falling off of crusts, flakes, and even scabs, and helps in the formation on new, healthy skin. Further, it is an important remedy for all cases in which the skin fails to perform an important function: it promotes sweating as a means of detoxifying the body through the skin. This is also the remedy of first choice for any and all eruptive acute diseases of the skin, like measles or chicken pox, and for any condition that involves scabbing.

Calcarea Phosphorica

Like Silicea, Calc Phos is a good general remedy for the skin, just as it is for the digestive tract. Calc Phos should be considered the remedy of choice, or among the remedies used, for all cases involving dry skin, or skin that is prematurely wrinkled or has lost its elasticity. It is an excellent remedy for discolorations of the skin, especially those that are copper colored, such as freckles. Because its actions are generalized, Calc Phos, like Silicea, should be considered a remedy that works well in concert with others, rather than as a cure in and of itself. It works well in alternation or combination with Calcarea Sulphurica and the other phosphorus-based remedies. As Calc Phos (rather like Silicea, once again) helps the human body to better digest food and utilize its nutrients, it is a powerful healing tool not only for the digestive organs, but also for the skin, hair, and nails.

Calcarea Sulphurica

Calcarea Sulphurica is used most often for skin conditions involving infection and the formation of pus. Calc Sulph works to decrease pus and reabsorb it into the body. It is useful, therefore, in the earlier stages of infection for such conditions as whitlows, before or just as pus is forming. Use Calc Sulph for all cuts or wounds that do not heal, that continue to be infected. This is also the remedy to think of for burns or scalds that do not heal, but instead fester.

Note that Calc Sulph and Silicea are not used together in skin conditions because of their opposing actions. Silicea is used for the later stages of infection, when the pus must be forced out of the body. It encourages a gathering of matter, which results in the bursting of abscesses and the subsequent healing of the wound. Calc Sulph, on the other hand, heals in the opposite manner by discouraging the formation of pus. It is best used in earlier stages of infection or for infections that do not heal.

Ferrum Phosphoricum

Ferrum Phos is the remedy to think of for the first stage of a skin condition, when the symptoms have just begun. Think of Ferrum Phos in all cases of mechanical injury to the skin, especially when the skin is inflamed and/or swollen at the site of the injury. Think of Ferrum Phos as the remedy to hurry for at the first stage of eruptive diseases of the skin as well, for example, during the first hours of the onset of measles or chicken pox. Think of Ferrum Phos in all cases of conditions affecting the skin in which fever is also present. Like Kali Sulphuricum, Ferrum Phos will tend to bring on a sweat as a means of detoxifying the body. Think of this remedy for cases of fever in which the skin is hot and dry.

Kali Phosphoricum

This is another remedy whose actions on the skin are generalized, rather than specific. Yet it is a remedy to consider for such things as skin that is wrinkled, that has lost its elasticity and luster. Also for conditions that affect the normal sense of touch—for skin that itches, skin that tingles, for skin that is chaffed, for skin that is so sensitive that it cannot bear to feel cloth against it. This is also the remedy for myriad conditions including abscesses, carbuncles, and pustules of all sorts, most especially if their presence is accompanied by a bad smell. This is the remedy for body odor, for skin that smells bad.

Dry Skin

The two general remedies for dry skin are Kali Sulphuricum and Calcarea Phosphorica, which work very well together.

Kali Sulphuricum

Kali Sulph is usually the first remedy to think about, as this is the remedy for general dryness and flaking or scaling of the skin. This is the remedy when the skin is inactive, when it is not removing toxins from the system as it should. Think of Kali Sulph for patients who do not sweat enough—the use of Kali Sulph promotes detoxification through sweat and will, therefore, naturally put an end to dry skin.

Calcarea Phosphorica

Calc Phos is a cell salt that is more generalized in its action than in Kali Sulph. It should be considered for any chronic skin conditions, just as it is for chronic digestive disorders. Calc Phos soothes the skin. More important, Calc Phos triggers the growth of soft tissues throughout the body. Therefore, it promotes the growth of healthy skin cells, and its use will help make skin in general fresher and moister. It is essential to all those who suffer from dry skin, or from skin that seems older than the patient's real age.

Natrum Muriaticum

The other remedy to consider for dry skin is Natrum Muriaticum. It is especially important to the skin of the hands. Patients needing Natrum Mur chronically have dry hands and lips (this is, as we shall see, the most important remedy for cracked lips, and one of the major remedies for chapped or cracked skin in general). Patients with palms that are dry and leathery should use Natrum Muriaticum to end the dryness, either alone or in alternation with Calcarea Phosphorica.

Also, add Natrum Mur into the mix for patients with dry skin on any part of the body if the skin is extremely dry or if the dry skin is very stubborn and the other remedies fail to cure. For chronic cases of dry skin.

Chapped Skin

Four cells salts work well for patients with chapped or cracked skin. All of these remedies work best if taken orally, although irritated skin can also be treated topically by dissolving pellets of Natrum Muriaticum, Calcarea Fluorica, and Calcarea Sulphurica in cool water and applying that mixture directly to the skin with a moist cloth. Natrum Muriaticum and Silicea can also be taken internally while they are applied topically. (For general information on the remedies, see above.)

The two general remedies used specifically for cases of chapped skin are Calcarea Fluorica (which is important in that it is naturally found in the elastic tissues of the skin and in connective tissue) and Calcarea Sulphurica. For simple cases of chapped or cracked skin, especially in winter, the two remedies can be given in alternation or combination. In stubborn cases, especially those occurring in winter, add Natrum Muriaticum.

Silicea is the remedy to think of for truly stubborn cases of cracked skin. When the skin itself seems unhealthy, when it is sore, sensitive, and tender to the touch of fabric. In these cases, add Silicea to the mix. (Note that in cases of very sensitive skin, Silicea given in alternation with Kali Phosphoricum will usually set things right.)

Specific Remedies for Chapped Skin

For chapped lips: Use Natrum Muriaticum, especially if the bottom lip is cracked. This is the best remedy for cases of chapped lips in winter.

For chapped hands: Again, use Natrum Muriaticum for hands that are chapped and dry. Calcarea Fluorica can be added in combination or alternation for stubborn cases of chapped hands.

For chapped or rough feet: If the skin of the feet becomes chapped or cracked, if it is dry and rough, give Natrum Muriaticum, especially if the skin between the toes is cracked. In stubborn cases, use Natrum Mur with Calcarea Fluorica.

Itchy Skin

Skin that itches, especially if the itching is chronic, usually benefits from a combination of topical and internal doses of the cell salts. The chief remedies for this condition include Kali Phosphoricum, Calcarea Phosphorica, Calcarea Fluorica, and Kali Sulphuricum. Natrum Muriaticum and/or Silicea can be added in very stubborn cases.

Cases of simple skin itch can often be soothed by Kali Phosphoricum alone. It can be used topically and given internally at the same time. If this alone fails to soothe the skin, combine Kali Phos with Calcarea Phosphorica, Calcarea Fluorica, and Kali Sulphuricum. Take a few pellets of each and dissolve them in either cool or warm water, as the patient chooses. Apply the mixture with a moist cloth as needed. Give the remedy Kali Phos internally at the same time.

Specific Remedies for Itchy Skin

For itching that results in skin that is irritated, red, and painful: Dissolve pellets of Kali Phosphoricum and Calcarea Phosphorica in water and apply the mix topically to the affected area. If the affected area is swollen, give Ferrum Phosphoricum by mouth while continuing topical applications.

For itching that is accompanied by burning: Kali Phosphoricum and Calcarea Phosphorica are indicated. They can be used topically and/or taken orally, as desired.

If burning is pronounced, and the skin red and swollen: Ferrum Phosphoricum should be given internally while Kali Phosphoricum is applied topically.

For itching that is accompanied by a sensation of tenderness or numbness: Kali Phosphoricum is the remedy of first choice. If it fails to work, add Silicea.

For itching of the soles of the feet and/or the palms of the hands: Combine Kali Phosphoricum with Calcarea Sulphurica.

For itching on the legs only: Kali Phosphoricum and Kali Muriaticum.

For itching of the eyelids: Natrum Muriaticum should be taken orally.

Wrinkles

While Calcarea Fluorica has not been written about much in these pages, especially in comparison with other cell salts, it comes into its own and earns its place among the twelve remedies for its ability to smooth our wrinkles, especially those that come before their time. Calcarea Fluorica is the most important remedy when it comes to the elastic tissues of the body, and therefore it is the most important remedy for restoring elasticity to the skin. For all cases in which the patient's skin is wrinkled, give Calcarea Fluorica. Give it especially for patients who have crow's feet or laugh lines on their faces.

Other remedies come into play for skin that is weathered, withered, and wrinkled. They are Calcarea Phosphorica, Kali Phosphoricum, Kali Sulphuricum and Silicea.

In cases of wrinkled skin, the indicated remedies can be dissolved in water and applied directly to the skin. Calcarea Fluorica and Calcarea Phosphorica should be taken orally as well. Give Calc Fluor an hour before and Calc Phos an hour after meals. The remedies must be used for some period of time, often weeks, before benefits become apparent. If the desired results are not obtained add Silicea into the mix, giving it first thing in the morning and last thing before bed.

Calcarea Phosphorica

As Calcarea Phosphorica soothes the entire system, it also helps forestall the aging process. It should be included in the treatment of wrinkles.

Kali Phosphoricum

This remedy is important because it is indicated for all patients whose bodies are deficient in potassium phosphate and who therefore tend to show the deficiency in their skin—in skin that looks weather-beaten and prematurely aged.

Kali Sulphuricum

Another general remedy to fight against wrinkling of the skin is Kali Sulphuricum, which can restore moisture to skin that seems weathered and dry. It is especially helpful to elderly patients whose skin has lost its natural moisture and texture.

Silicea

The general remedy for skin that looks old before its time, that has many fine wrinkles all over the face, especially if the patient's arms and legs are very thin and lacking muscle tone, is Silicea. Silicea can be added to any of the other remedies being used to tone the skin and will add strength to the elasticity that Calc Flour restores.

Eczema

Eczema can present itself in a variety of symptoms. It can be acute or chronic. The inflammation of the skin can involve lesions that are either moist or dry, and there can be itching and burning of the affected areas of the skin. Because of these varying symptoms there are several cell salts that can be used to treat the condition. Note that, in all cases of eczema, whether acute or chronic, the tongue is a very important indicator of the needed remedy or remedies and should be checked as part of case taking.

Most often the remedies used are the sulfur-based Calcarea Sulphurica and/or Kali Sulphuricum (which is sometimes considered the single most important remedy for those with eczema), as well as Calcarea Phosphorica, Natrum Muriaticum, Calcarea Fluorica, and Silicea. Natrum Muriaticum and Silicea are most often considered for chronic cases of eczema and can be used in combination with other remedies that have failed to bring about a cure, although they were well chosen and indicated.

Natrum Phosphoricum

May be especially called for in cases of eczema in which there are yellow scabs or a yellow discharge. While it is not a cell salt that is commonly used in the treatment of skin conditions and is more often thought of as a remedy for those with conditions caused by an overabundance of acid in their system, it can be helpful in cases of eczema in which the scales or scabs are golden yellow and the discharge a milky yellow. Also note that a watery yellow discharge may indicate the need for Natrum Sulphuricum.

Specific Remedies for Eczema

For cases of dry eczema: Calcarea Sulphurica.

For cases of moist eczema: Kali Sulphuricum.

For cases of eczema in which the scales or scabs are white: Natrum Muriaticum, Calcarea Phosphorica, Kali Muriaticum.

For cases of eczema in which the scales or scabs are yellow: Natrum Phosphoricum, Calcarea Sulphurica, Kali Sulphuricum.

If the discharges are yellow: Kali Sulphuricum, Natrum Phosphoricum, Natrum Sulphuricum, Calcarea Sulphurica.

If discharges are watery: Natrum Muriaticum, Silicea, Kali Phosphoricum.

If discharges are bloody: Kali Phosphoricum.

For cases of eczema in which the skin is thickened and/or cracked: Calcarea Fluorica.

When eczema occurs on the scalp: Natrum Muriaticum, Silicea.

When eczema occurs behind the ears: Natrum Muriaticum.

When eczema occurs in the eyebrows: Natrum Muriaticum.

When eczema occurs in the joints of the body: Natrum Muriaticum.

Psoriasis

Psoriasis is, of course, always a chronic condition, one that involves the formation of patches of inflamed white or silver-white scales on the skin, especially on the scalp, chest, elbows, and knees. The most commonly used remedies for those suffering from psoriasis are Natrum Muriaticum, Calcarea Phosphorica, and Kali Muriaticum. If the condition is primarily on the scalp, the remedy is Natrum Muriaticum, which can be applied topically as well as taken orally.

In most cases of psoriasis, give the remedy Calcarea Phosphorica by mouth, one hour after each meal. Dissolve Natrum Muriaticum and Kali Muriaticum in cool or warm water, as the patient prefers, and apply the mix directly to the affected area with a moist cloth. Use as needed, applying less often as the condition improves. Continue giving Calc Phos for a period of days after symptoms have cleared.

Psoriasis can be stubborn. The cells salts may have to be used for a period of weeks before improvement is complete. For especially stubborn cases, Kali Sulphuricum may also be added to the topical mixture.

Hives/Rash

Hives is sort of a generic term for a general rash, what is called *urticaria* in homeopathic literature. It is generally characterized by redness and by the presence of small raised bumps, which may itch and/or burn. The bumps may or may not be fluid-filled.

As the diagnosis of a simple rash is very general, the condition suggests several potential remedies among the cell salts. Remedies include three sodium-based remedies, Natrum Phosphoricum, Natrum Sulphuricum, and Natrum Muriaticum; two potassium-based remedies, Kali Phosphoricum and Kali Sulphuricum; and an acute remedy, Ferrum Phosphoricum, which should be kept in mind when inflammation and/or fever are present.

Note that, in all cases of hives or of general rashes, a mixture of remedies can be topically applied. Dissolve a few pellets of Natrum Muriaticum, Natrum Phosphoricum, and Kali Sulphuricum in cool or lukewarm water and moisten a clean cloth in the water. Apply the mixture as needed. If inflammation or fever is present, give Ferrum Phosphoricum orally along with topical applications of the mixed remedies. If fever is not present, give the best-indicated remedy orally.

In all cases of hives or rashes, the tongue acts as an excellent indicator of the appropriate remedy. Make sure to look at the patient's tongue as part of the case taking.

Specific Remedies for Hives/Rashes

For dry rashes, especially if the skin is scaly: Kali Sulphuricum.

For moist rashes, in which the discharge is milky: Natrum Phosphoricum.

For moist rashes, in which the discharge is watery: Natrum Muriaticum.

For rashes when the skin is painful: Natrum Muriaticum.

For rashes when the skin is irritated, sensitive: Kali Phosphoricum.

If the rash is bright red and swollen: Ferrum Phosphoricum.

If rash is red and blotchy, like measles: Kali Sulphuricum.

If the rash is rose-colored: Natrum Phosphoricum.

For rashes that itch: Natrum Phosphoricum, Natrum Muriaticum.

For rashes that feel like insect bites: Natrum Phosphoricum, Natrum Muriaticum.

Poison Ivy

Only two cell salts, Natrum Muriaticum and Kali Sulphuricum, work for cases of poison ivy. For best results use them both, and use them topically only. Taking the remedy by mouth will help to cure the rash, but may do so by spreading it first as the poison is expelled from the body through the skin. So the rash will grow worse before it gets better.

For poison ivy, dissolve Natrum Muriaticum and Kali Sulphuricum, in 3X or 6X potency, in cool or lukewarm water and apply the mixture topically with a clean cloth. Apply as needed, being very careful not to spread the rash. Kali Sulph especially will help with the itch of the rash while Natrum Muriaticum will help dry it up and clear it away.

This is the best treatment for this condition among the cell salts. The general homeopathic pharmacy offers alternatives, including the remedy Rhus Toxicodendron, which is made from the poison ivy plant.

Acne

The cell salts work wonders for cases of acne. They are among the most effective treatments available.

Silicea

If the skin of the patient looks unhealthy, especially in adolescent patients whose skin
looks dirty and greasy, make Silicea part of the treatment. Unlike other conditions in
which Silicea is saved for last and used if the other remedies fail to act, for cases of acne
in young patients, give Silicea first and see the effects.

Calcarea Phosphorica and Calcarea Sulphurica

During adolescence, boys will need a different remedy for acne than girls. Usually, after
Silicea, you should follow up Silicea with Calcarea Sulphurica with boys and Calcarea
Phosphorica with girls. If the first selection fails to cure, try the other remedy, as Calc
Sulph and Calc Phos are the two best general remedies for patients with acne, espe-
cially when used in combination or following Silicea.

For especially stubborn cases, add Kali Muriaticum into the mix.

Specific Remedies for Acne

In cases of acne in adult patients: Give Silicea. If that remedy fails to clear, combine
with Natrum Muriaticum, especially if the skin seems unclean and unhealthy.

In stubborn cases: Combine Calcarea Sulphurica, Calcarea Phosphorica, Kali Muriaticum, and Silicea and dissolve in water. Apply with a moist towel to the affected area.

Abscesses/Boils

The four remedies that are generally associated with the appearance of abscesses or
boils are Ferrum Phosphoricum, Calcarea Sulphurica, Kali Muriaticum, and Silicea. As
always, the use of Calcarea Sulphurica and Silicea together is discouraged since the
functions of the two remedies are opposite—Calc Sulph discourages the formation of
pus, while Silicea encourages it.

A good general treatment is to dissolve Kali Muriaticum in water for use as a topical application. Another indicated remedy can be given by mouth at the same time.

With either abscesses or boils, the choice of appropriate treatment will have a good
deal to do with the stage of the abscess at the time of treatment.

Specific Remedies for Abscesses/Boils

For the first stage of an abscess, when the skin is beginning to swell and the boil or

abscess is beginning to form: Ferrum Phosphoricum. (Ferrum Phos is especially indicated if the forming abscess is very painful.)

For the second stage, when an abscess has formed but has not yet formed pus: Calcarea Sulphurica. (Note that Kali Muriaticum, given in the stage just following Ferrum Phosphoricum, may help clear away the abscess.)

To ripen an abscess in the third stage, one that has formed pus, to promote discharge of pus and clear away the abscess: Silicea.

For a ripened, long-standing abscess that has failed to heal: Calcarea Sulphurica.

For chronic cases: Silicea. (Note that in chronic cases it sometimes helps to combine Silicea with Calcarea Phosphorica. Check the patient's tongue as an indicator.)

For abscesses of the gums: Calcarea Fluorica, Calcarea Sulphurica. (Dissolve in water and swish around in the mouth for best results.)

Warts and Growths

For warts in general, and for growths of soft tissue such as skin tags, treat topically with a mixture of Natrum Muriaticum, Natrum Sulphuricum (which is excellent at shrinking warts until they fade away), and Kali Muriaticum dissolved in water and applied directly to the growth. In stubborn cases, add Silicea into the mix.

As Kali Muriaticum is the general remedy, take it orally while using the mixture topically. Note that Kali Muriaticum is especially helpful for warts on the hands. If it fails to cure, add Natrum Muriaticum to the oral dosage and continue to apply the topical mixture.

General Remedies for the Hair

The key remedy for the hair is Silicea. Silicea maintains the strength and luster of the hair and will help make it fuller and stronger. It also helps patients retain what hair they have and stops hair loss. Further, it is a natural conditioner, restoring beauty to hair that has become limp, thin, and damaged due to malabsorption of food and lack of nourishment to the cells of the body. No matter what other remedy or remedies are given, if the health of the hair is in question, Silicea is the remedy.

The other general remedies for the hair are Kali Sulphuricum, Calcarea Fluorica, Kali Sulphuricum, and Natrum Muriaticum.

Hair Loss

If male pattern baldness is the issue, the remedy to include along with Silicea is Kali Sulphuricum. Kali Sulph is said to inspire the regrowth of hair that has been lost to hormonal changes associated with aging. It works best in combination with Silicea and better still if used as an adjunct to traditional constitutional homeopathic treatment.

If the patient's hair is just beginning to thin, consider using Calcarea Fluorica as the remedy of choice. Again, use it in conjunction with Silicea or combined with Silicea and Calcarea Phosphorica. While Kali Sulphuricum can help restore hair once it has been lost, Calc Fluor can help the patient retain the hair he or she still has and prevent further loss. Calcarea Phosphorica will help the body absorb what nutrients it can from food, nourishing the body and encouraging hair growth.

For those patients whose hair is actually falling out, Kali Sulph should be alternated with Calcarea Phosphorica. This is especially true for all cases in which hair loss can be associated with acute diseases, especially with fevers. Alternate Calc Phos and Kali Sulph, each three times daily, Kali Sulph one hour before meals and Calc Phos one hour after. Treatment will be slow and the remedies may have to be taken for weeks or months before improvement begins.

For male patients who are experiencing bald patches in their beards, the remedy is Natrum Muriaticum. Again, treatment in this case will be long and slow. I suggest that Natrum Mur be given along with Silicea to improve the quality of the skin and to encourage new hair growth.

Dandruff

There are two remedies that are most closely associated with dandruff. They are Natrum Muriaticum and Kali Sulphuricum. Usually the choice between the remedies is determined by the color of the flakes themselves.

Kali Sulphuricum is the remedy we think of first for cases of flaking skin, and as dandruff is, after all, flaking skin on the scalp, Kali Sulphuricum is the first remedy to consider. Typically, however (although not always), the dandruff that Kali Sulph will clear away has yellowish flakes, not white. If the flakes are pure white, the indicated remedy is Natrum Muriaticum. In either case, when the problem is dandruff, I would have both remedies in hand and ready to use. Start with the remedy of best choice, based on the color of the flakes, and be ready to alternate with the other remedy if that remedy does not clear away the problem. As with all skin, hair, and nail conditions, it may take some time, weeks or months, to totally get rid of the dandruff, so be patient. If these remedies together fail to work, add Silicea into the mix to assist the action of the other remedies.

Note that the remedies can be dissolved in water and the water can be applied directly to the scalp. Wet the head with the dissolved remedies and let it dry. Do not rinse the head, just leave the remedies on the scalp to assist healing. The remedies may be used topically and taken orally at the same time or the topical application may suffice.

General Remedies for Nails

The major remedies for the nails are Silicea, Calcarea Phosphorica, Calcarea Fluorica, Kali Muriaticum, and Natrum Muriaticum.

The general remedy is Silicea—always Silicea. If the patient has brittle nails, Silicea. If the patient has weak nails, Silicea. If nails split, Silicea. For patients who have white spots on their nails, give Silicea. If the patient has nails that are crumbly, that can be peeled back, Silicea.

For patients whose nails grow very slowly, combine or alternate Kali Sulphuricum and Silicea, just as you would for baldness. Give Kali Sulphuricum to start, and if it does not cure, add Silicea to assist in the healing process.

For nails that are thickened, Silicea is still the major remedy, although it may have to be used in concert with Calcarea Fluorica in these cases. Natrum Muriaticum is indicated for nails that grow soft and thick. And as for so many other conditions, it may be used in combination with Silicea.

Hangnails

The two remedies for hangnails are Natrum Muriaticum and Silicea. Silicea is important because it speaks to the general health of the nails, while Natrum Muriaticum is important because it is associated with a chronic dryness of the tissue of the skin, hair, and nails, especially the tissue of the skin surrounding the fingernails. Therefore the best treatment for those with hangnails is the use of both remedies, in combination or alternation.

Ingrown Toenails

Think of Silicea first for ingrown toenails, but if they are inflamed, the best first remedy is Ferrum Phosphoricum for the inflammation. Then add the Silicea for the health and strength of the nail. Calcarea Fluorica and Kali Sulphuricum may also both be used in cases of chronic ingrown nails. Silicea, Calc Flour and Kali Sulph can be dissolved in warm water and applied to the toe topically via a warm cloth that has been soaked in the solution. When inflammation is present, apply the remedies topically while taking Ferrum Phos orally.

Whitlows/Felons

Whitlows (also called felons) are small but very painful infections of the area at the tip of the fingers adjacent to the fingernails, in the corner of the nails. The inflammation can make it all but impossible to perform delicate tasks with the hands, such as typing at a computer keyboard.

For those with inflammation present, Natrum Sulphuricum is an excellent remedy if the pus formed is greenish in color. Silicea may be added to this remedy to help draw out the pus and heal the site of the infection. Silicea is also the remedy to use in the long-term to keep whitlows from forming.

If the inflammation is just beginning, give the patient Calcarea Sulphurica to help prevent the formation of pus. Note that Calc Sulph and Silicea should not be given together for this condition since they perform opposite functions. Silicea forces pus out of the body, encouraging the infection to grow and burst, thus ending it. Calc Sulph helps prevent the formation of pus in the first place, healing the infection by absorbing the pus. Therefore if the whitlow is already formed and pus is present, give Silicea and Natrum Sulphuricum to clear it away. If the inflammation is just beginning, give Calc Sulph to heal it at this earlier stage.

ACUTE AILMENTS

Since there are only twelve cell salts, the cost of having a full kit of the remedies on hand in the home is low, especially relative to the amount of good that these remedies can do for treating common complaints and acute conditions. The cell salts offer a simple system of treatment for colds and flu, and for childhood ailments ranging from chicken pox to measles to earaches. Depending upon the severity of the illness, they can completely resolve an acute condition or provide a stopgap that can be used until the patient can be taken for professional medical care.

It is important to note, once again, that the cell salts should not be used in place of appropriate professional medical care and those using them should never work above their level of expertise. This having been said, the cell salts are an excellent alternative to the many over-the-counter medicines available. These are often of far less value in treating these same conditions and can have a suppressive impact upon the patient's immune system, leaving the patient worse off than they were before the over-the-counter treatment was begun.

Note that the categories in this section are somewhat vague and general. This is because it can be difficult to identify the exact line between illnesses like colds and flu. For this reason, I strongly suggest that the most effective way to use the cell salts in the home is to always start by looking at the patient's tongue and then by carefully considering the symptoms exhibited. If the overall symptoms match and the tongue, the expectoration, the cough, the aches and pains, the patterns of onset, aggravation, and improvement all match a given remedy or remedies, then improvement will result, regardless of whether the strict diagnosis of the condition is a cold, the croup, bronchitis, or asthma. In all cases of acute conditions, I encourage readers to allow for overlap and refer not only to the pages dedicated to a given specific diagnosis, but also to those on all related topics. For example, the fact that information dedicated to the tongue is found under the general category of digestive disorders does not mean that the tongue and its symptoms are not helpful for determining the appropriate remedy to give to a patient with a sore throat. Keep in mind that the cell salts, like all homeopathic remedies, are given based on the totality of symptoms. They will be far less effective if the user looks only at a specific complaint without taking into account the patient's whole being.

Fever

When it comes to cells salts and fevers, there can be a bit of a knee-jerk reaction when we immediately reach for Ferrum Phosphoricum. Indeed, for any sort of inflammation, especially for fevers, Ferrum Phos is the leading cell salt remedy. However, there are others that can be useful as well. For fevers, the cell salt remedies are Ferrum Phosphoricum, Kali Muriaticum, Kali Phosphoricum, Kali Sulphuricum, Natrum Muriaticum, and Silicea.

Ferrum Phosphoricum

Ferrum Phosphoricum is the first remedy to think of for all fevers. It is the most useful remedy for fever, to the point that it might be considered the specific remedy of choice. However, Ferrum Phosphoricum is especially indicated for fevers that carry with them a quickened pulse and dry skin. Especially the skin of the face and head, and the hands, throat and chest tend to be red, hot, and dry. (If there is sweat associated with the remedy, it appears in the middle of the night.) This is a remedy of heat during fever (some patients needing Ferrum Phos, however, may feel chill in the afternoon hours). The patient will feel a sense of heat internally as well. Will want cold things, cold drinks and applications, to find relief. Think of this remedy when nausea and/or vomiting accompany the fever.

Kali Muriaticum

In terms of fever, Kali Muriaticum is in some ways the total opposite of Ferrum Phosphoricum. No matter how high the fever, the patient is cold and cannot stand the slightest chill or any movement of air. He or she seeks heat, will want to be bundled up tight, or to hug the fireplace to feel warm. The tongue, as always, can be helpful in identifying the need for Kali Mur. Look for the patient's tongue to have the characteristic thick white or gray-white coating during fever. The fever may also be accompanied by constipation.

Kali Phosphoricum

Kali Phosphoricum can resemble Ferrum Phosphoricum in patients with fevers. As two phosphorus-based remedy types, both have increased pulses, but the Ferrum Phos patient will have a fast pulse while the Kali Phos will have a pulse that is both rapid and irregular. The Kali Phos patient often will further identify himself by his behavior. This is a patient who is highly agitated during fever, who is restless, worried, afraid, and who demands much attention. (Note that the opposite will sometimes be the case as well. In these cases the Kali Phos patient can be very depressed and quiet. What the patient will not be is within the range of his expected, normal behavior—he will either be much more demanding than usual or much more withdrawn.) This is an excellent remedy for high fevers, for erratic fevers. When in doubt as to whether Kali Phos or Ferrum Phos is the right remedy, consider the patient's sense of temperature. The Ferrum Phos is almost always hot, while the Kali Phos may be cold or may alternate wildly between feeling hot and feeling chilly. This may be the best symptom to guide you in the choice of your remedy.

Kali Sulphuricum

Like Ferrum Phos patients, Kali Sulphs will feel heated during fever and will seek cool air, moving air, open air. They will feel much worse in closed rooms and warm places, and will kick off their covers. What will help you choose between this remedy and Ferrum Phos is that the Kali Sulph patient sweats a great deal during fever, while the Ferrum Phos has skin that is red, hot, and dry. Typically, the patient needing this remedy will have a fever that is worse at night; that begins in the evening and grows worse until midnight, and then drops off. Kali Sulph repeats well in fever cases and should be given often to promote sweating until the fever breaks.

Natrum Muriaticum

Natrum Muriaticum is often used in alternation or combination with other cell salts in the treatment of fevers. This is a good remedy, especially for those who are chilly during fever. Natrum Mur carries the characteristic symptom that the patient, while chilly, will still be very thirsty for cold water. The patient will have great chill and great thirst at the same time. This is also a remedy to think of when the patient is very sweaty, especially for the patient with night sweats. Think of this remedy for cases of fever in which the sensation of chilliness is worse in the morning, especially in the early morning.

Silicea

Think of Silicea for cases of fever in which the patient is very chilly, and is exhausted and depleted by the fever. When the patient's feet are hot, but the rest of him is cold. When the patient is very sensitive to cool air and wants to stay bundled up, especially wants to cover his head, in an attempt to stay warm. Chills run through these fevers, as can delirium. Think of this remedy for all fevers that accompany wasting diseases, for long-term fever states involving night sweats that are accompanied by exhaustion and chills. Think of Silicea for fevers in which the patient's head is very sweaty. In which the patient feels heat and burning in his feet, when the feet sweat and are very smelly.

Specific Remedies for Fevers

For fevers that are worse in the morning: Natrum Muriaticum, Kali Muriaticum.

For fevers that are worse in the morning and again at late afternoon: Kali Muriaticum.

For fevers that are worse at noon: Kali Muriaticum, Silicea.

For fevers that are worse in the afternoon: Natrum Muriaticum, Kali Muriaticum, Silicea.

For fevers that are worse in the evening: Silicea.

For fevers that are worse at night: Ferrum Phosphoricum, Kali Sulphuricum.

For fevers that are worse at night while the patient sleeps: Silicea, Natrum Muriaticum.

For fevers with an internal sensation of heat: Ferrum Phosphoricum.

For fevers with an internal sensation of chills: Silicea, Natrum Muriaticum, Kali Phosphoricum.

If the patient uncovering ameliorates symptoms: Natrum Muriaticum, Kali Sulphuricum.

For fevers that alternate between heat and chills: Kali Phosphoricum, Silicea.

For fevers without sweat: Ferrum Phosphoricum, Silicea (dry except for head and feet), Kali Phosphoricum.

For fevers with sweat: Natrum Muriaticum, Kali Sulphuricum.

For fevers with sweat during daytime: Natrum Muriaticum.

For fevers with night sweats: Ferrum Phosphoricum, Natrum Muriaticum, Silicea.

For fevers with sweat only on the head and/or feet: Silicea.

For fevers accompanying chicken pox: Ferrum Phosphoricum, Natrum Muriaticum, Silicea, Kali Muriaticum.

For fevers accompanying flu: Ferrum Phosphoricum, Silicea.

For fevers accompanying measles: Ferrum Phosphoricum, Silicea, Kali Sulphuricum, Kali Muriaticum.

For high fever (especially in very young patients): Ferrum Phosphoricum.

For fevers that are erratic, bouncing up and down: Kali Phosphoricum.

Colds/Hay Fever

Colds and hay fever are given under the same heading because, in terms of treatment with cell salts, it is not really important whether symptoms were caused by the presence of a virus or an allergen. Treatment is primarily based upon the patient's symptoms—as long as the symptoms of the patient match those of the remedy, improvement will result.

Note, however, that I have included the remedies for hay fever here only as a stop-gap. Allergies, even seasonal allergies, are always the product of a chronic state of ill health and should be treated by a medical professional. Therefore, although the remedies for hay fever may effectively curb all symptoms in a given season, they should be considered more of a bandaid than a cure.

Whether you are treating a patient with a cold or with seasonal allergies, you will have to gather the same information. The quality and color of the nasal discharge will be of importance, as will the other symptoms that are part of the illness. Are the patient's eyes affected? Is the patient feeling hot or cold? Is there fever? What is the patient's mood? Is the patient sneezing? The answers to all these questions and others will assist you in the selection of an appropriate remedy.

Remember, colds have three distinct stages and will often take three different remedies to clear away. Sometimes a fourth remedy will be a good idea as a follow-up remedy for the period of recovery after the cold or, especially, flu.

The first stage is the onset of the cold. This is the stage at which the patient first feels that he or she is getting sick: the stage from the first chill, the first flush, to the beginning of the flow of mucus. The speed of onset of symptoms will indicate an appropriate remedy, as will the presence or absence of fever.

The second stage of a cold is the stage involving a flow of clear mucus.

The third stage is the stage in which the mucus becomes colored, either yellow or green, and becomes thicker.

Some colds stay in the head, others may move into the chest or ears. Some will also involve a sore throat.

When looking for the appropriate remedy for a cold or for seasonal allergies, begin with the symptoms that you are seeing in the moment of case taking. Begin with the stage in which you find the patient and follow these symptoms as they shift, making changes in prescription as needed. The right remedies will help the cold (or seasonal allergies) end more quickly and will help support the patient's healing process so the patient will not become as ill as he or she might have otherwise. Given the right remedies, the patient will still move through the stages of a cold—that is the process by which he or she will get well—but will move through them both faster and more easily.

In the same way, the right remedies for hay fever will keep the patient from suffering during a given pollen season as they might have in previous years, will lighten the load of the allergic response. With time and appropriate treatment, the patient may find that they have no allergic response at all in future seasons, just as the patient who receives appropriate homeopathic constitutional treatment may find that the number of colds they get in a year becomes lower and lower as their vital force is strengthened.

The cell salt remedies most commonly used in the treatment for those with colds or seasonal allergies include Ferrum Phosphoricum, Natrum Muriaticum, Calcarea Phosphorica, Magnesia Phosphorica, Kali Muriaticum, Kali Sulphuricum, Calcarea Sulphurica, and, to a lesser degree, Kali Phosphoricum (which is more of a cough remedy than a cold remedy), Natrum Sulphuricum (which is more of a remedy for those with chronic sinus conditions than a cold remedy), and Silicea (which is an excellent remedy for colds that linger and linger or for patients whose systems have been run down by the cold).

Ferrum Phosphoricum

Ferrum Phosphoricum is the remedy that we most associate with the first stage of a cold. Think of this remedy just as the cold is beginning, when there is the first itch or ache in the nasal passages or the sinuses. When the sense of congestion is just beginning. And especially for the first hint of fever associated with a cold. If Ferrum Phosphoricum is given in time, it is possible to avoid the cold altogether. For symptoms that come on quickly, with a sensation of heat, think of Ferrum Phosphoricum. When the flow begins, the mucus will be watery and frothy.

Natrum Muriaticum

Natrum Muriaticum should be considered for the cold that starts with sneezing. The Natrum Muriaticum patient will have fits of sneezing. This is the first remedy to think of for the traditional head cold, when the patient's nose is completely blocked, when the patient's sense of smell is gone, and his or her sense of taste is diminished. This is perhaps the best general remedy that we have for colds, for flu, and for allergies that linger, when the patient feels depleted and miserable in his or her symptoms and wants to lie down and be left alone. Think of this remedy first when the symptoms of the cold center around the nose, when the nose runs fluently, constantly, when sneezing comes in bouts, and when there is no postnasal drip at all. The mucus will be clear and watery most of the time, although it may also have the consistency of raw egg white.

Calcarea Phosphorica

Like Natrum Muriaticum, Calc Phos (which is often used in conjunction with Natrum Mur in treatment of those with colds) can be considered a great general remedy for an acute cold, and a leading remedy for those who are chronically given to colds or allergies. This is the remedy to remember to give regularly as cold season is approaching to those patients who are given to catching colds, or to those who have seasonal allergies in the weeks before the allergy season. This is our best preventive remedy for these conditions. Like Natrum Mur, Calc Phos is for the traditional head cold centered in the nose. Again, like Natrum Mur, the patient will be given to sneezing—although the Natrum Mur patient will have more fervent bouts of sneezing—and will have an acute or chronic discharge that is clear and watery or with the consistency of raw egg white. The Calc Phos tends to have the specific symptom of having a cold nose—particularly the tip of the nose will be icy cold. As good a general remedy as Calc Phos is and as excellent as it is as a preventive, it seldom will act alone in the treatment of a cold or hay fever. It is best used in alternation or combination with other remedies, especially Natrum Muriaticum, and will help other remedies act more strongly and quickly. It is an excellent ancillary remedy for the treatment of colds and allergies, especially during the period of onset. This is the remedy to keep on hand between colds and allergy seasons as a preventive.

Magnesia Phosphorica

Magnesia Phosphorica is useful in the second stage of a cold if it follows a specific symptom pattern. Think of this remedy for colds in which the patient's nose is sometimes dry and clear and sometimes has spells in which there are sudden bouts of wild sneezing and a gushing of mucus from the nose. This makes Mag Phos a particularly helpful remedy for those who suffer from seasonal allergies and whose symptoms follow this pattern—never constant, but instead, sudden coming and going, sudden fits of sneezing, sudden discharge of copious amounts of mucus.

Kali Muriaticum

It is easy to spot when Kali Muriaticum is the indicated remedy. Consider this remedy for the second or third stage of a cold in which the nasal discharge is white and opaque. The patient's tongue will also be coated white or whitish-gray. Consider this remedy for colds or seasonal allergies in which the symptoms include postnasal drip and a sensation of pressure in the ears. When both the nose and ears are clogged. Think of this remedy for the cold that does not involve much nasal discharge, when most discharge goes down the back of the throat. When discharges are thick, making the patient struggle to swallow them.

Kali Sulphuricum

Kali Sulphuricum is an excellent remedy for the third and final stage of a cold. The discharges associated with the need for this remedy are yellow to yellow-green, thick, and slimy. When the patient feels that his nose is completely stopped up, and when there is not a great deal of discharge. When the patient snores all night and breathes through his mouth and feels worse when in a warm or closed room. When the patient feels as if he cannot inhale enough air to breathe freely. This is not only an excellent remedy for the final phase of a cold, but it is also a great remedy for those with chronic sinus issues, from sinusitis to chronic allergies, especially for cases in which the sense of smell is gone and the patient feels the need for open or moving air in order to breathe. He or she may use an electric fan to stir the air in order to sleep. Think of this remedy not only for all patients in the final stage of a cold, but also for all patients with chronic sinus conditions and nasal allergies.

Calcarea Sulphurica

Calcarea Sulphurica is the remedy of choice for the third stage of a head cold in which the discharge has changed from clear to yellow and, especially, for cases in which the yellow discharge is streaked with blood or cases in which the nose has become so irritated by constant sneezing and blowing that it bleeds. It follows both Natrum Muriaticum and Calcarea Phosphorica particularly well. All head colds that are accompanied by nosebleeds suggest Calcarea Sulphurica.

Kali Phosphoricum

Kali Phosphoricum is indicated for colds that involve coughing (see Cough) and that have the characteristic yellow discharge associated with the third stage of a cold. Kali Phos patients will also typically feel that the cold has moved into their chests in addition to their heads, and will experience both nosebleeds and postnasal drip. Use the characteristic foul-smelling breath as an indication of the need for this remedy.

Natrum Sulphuricum

Natrum Sulphuricum is indicated if the nasal discharge is green and thick and profuse. Think of this remedy for cases of chronic sinus conditions as well, especially those that are made worse by any change in the weather from dry to damp, or from a damp environment in general.

Silicea

Silicea is, as usual, more a remedy for chronic conditions than it is for simple acute ailments like a cold. However, it is sometimes used during the last stage of a cold, when the patient has very little nasal discharge, and when the patient has to work hard at blowing his nose to clear it. This is the patient who snuffles and blows and blows his nose, with no result, who hawks and hacks with little result. Whose nose is chronically dry and blocked. This is, therefore, the remedy to keep in mind for long-term sinus conditions and for colds that drag on and on when the patient never seems to get completely well. This is also the remedy to use after a cold or flu when the patient does not seem fully recovered, when he is struggling to get back his strength. It is especially helpful for very young and very old patients who have had their health compromised by a cold, flu, or seasonal allergy. Think of Silicea especially for allergies in which itching of the nose and at the back of the throat are the dominant symptoms.

Specific Remedies for Colds

For the first stage of a cold (from onset until mucus flows): Ferrum Phosphoricum, Magnesia Phosphorica, Natrum Muriaticum.

For the second stage of a cold (when mucus is clear): Natrum Muriaticum, Calcarea Phosphorica, Magnesia Phosphorica, Kali Muriaticum.

For the third stage of a cold (when the mucus is colored): Kali Muriaticum, Kali Sulphuricum, Calcarea Sulphurica, Kali Phosphoricum, Natrum Sulphuricum, Silicea.

As a preventive, to avoid a cold or hay fever before onset: Calcarea Phosphorica.

As an aid to healing after the cold has finished, to help the patient get his strength back: Silicea.

Remedies for Specific Discharges

Thick: Calcarea Sulphurica, Kali Muriaticum, Kali Sulphuricum, Kali Phosphoricum.

Watery: Natrum Muriaticum, Kali Sulphuricum

Like raw egg white: Natrum Muriaticum, Calcarea Phosphorica.

Slimy: Kali Sulphuricum.

Streaked with blood: Calcarea Sulphurica.

Acrid: Natrum Sulphuricum.

Yellow: Kali Phosphoricum, Calcarea Sulphurica, Kali Sulphuricum, Natrum Phosphoricum.

Green: Natrum Sulphuricum, Kali Sulphuricum.

White: Kali Muriaticum.

If the discharge is smelly: Kali Phosphoricum, Silicea.

If the discharge comes from only one nostril at any given time: Calcrea Sulphurica.

If discharge is always on the left: Kali Sulphuricum.

If discharge is always on the right: Calcarea Sulphurica.

If the discharge alternates suddenly from dry to copious: Magnesia Phosphorica.

For colds in which there is little discharge, but in which the sinuses are blocked and pressurized: Kali Muriaticum, Natrum Sulphuricum, Kali Sulphuricum.

Remedies for Sneezing

For constant sneezing, accompanied by fluent nasal discharge: Natrum Muriaticum.

For constant sneezing that has no discharge, or when discharge is very difficult: Silicea.

For sudden violent bouts of sneezing: Magnesia Phosphorica.

For sneezing in general: Natrum Muriaticum, Silicea, Magnesia Phosphorica, Kali Phosphoricum, Kali Sulphuricum.

For the patient who feels the need to sneeze but cannot; when a sneeze is "trapped": Calcarea Fluorica.

Specific Remedies for Modalities

For the patient whose symptoms are worse in a warm room: Calcarea Sulphurica.

For the patient whose symptoms are worse in a cold room: Calcarea Phosphorica.

For the patient whose symptoms are worse in the daytime: Natrum Muriaticum.

For the patient whose symptoms are worse at night: Natrum Sulphuricum.

Coughs

Out of the dozen cell salts, a total of eleven are useful in treating patients with coughs. Only Natrum Phosphoricum is not used in these cases. The two most common remedies used in the treatment of acute coughs are Ferrum Phosphoricum and Kali Muriaticum.

Ferrum Phosphoricum

Think of Ferrum Phosphoricum for coughs that are sudden, short, and leave the patient feeling sore, especially in his or her throat and chest. Think of this remedy especially for coughs that also involve a sensation of tickling in the throat that can be truly maddening (Silicea will also have this symptom). This can be a spasmodic cough, can involve fits of coughing, but it is always a dry cough. There is no expectoration at all associated with this cough, no matter how violent it is. Even if the patient has mucus in his chest, he will be unable to bring up anything by coughing. In some cases, the patient will suddenly, after long bouts of coughing, bring up expectorate that is blood-streaked or primarily blood. Consider this remedy for cases that suddenly worsen, when bronchitis or pneumonia suddenly seems near. This is an excellent remedy to remember for croupy children, if fever accompanies coughing fits. This is an important remedy for whooping cough if the bout of coughing leads to vomiting of undigested food. On a less serious note, think of this as a good remedy for those who have lost their voices from overuse, from yelling or singing or public speaking.

Kali Muriaticum

Kali Muriaticum is the remedy to think of when you hear a particularly loud cough, when you hear a cough that comes from the abdomen, as opposed to the chest or throat. This is a deep, loud cough. These coughs can come in spells that leave the patient holding his throat or abdomen to support himself through the spell. This is a major remedy for whooping cough, so it should come as no surprise that the cough can leave the muscles of the abdomen feeling sore, and that the patient can be left exhausted and gasping or wheezing for breath at the end of a spell of coughing. As always, a thick white coating on the tongue indicates that the cough can be helped by Kali Mur.

Calcarea Fluorica

Calcarea Fluorica is the indicated remedy for cases of coughs that are tickling in nature. For coughs that seem to be caused by a hair on the back of the throat. For shallow, tickling coughs that are associated with a dry throat and with a hoarse voice. This is a good remedy for patients who have lost their voices. In a chronic setting, it is also a good remedy for patients with asthma. If there is any expectoration, it is in the form of small, hard, yellow lumps that are brought up only with great difficulty. Look for the patient to be worse from lying down, to feel as if he or she is suffocating when lying down flat.

Calcarea Phosphorica

Calcarea Phosphorica is an excellent remedy for very young patients with coughs that bring up thick expectoration, like raw egg white. Think of this remedy for colds that have gone into the chest, when the patient's chest is sore to the touch. When the patient needs to clear his throat constantly or when he continually hacks to bring up phlegm. Think of this remedy for patients who experience suffocative fits of coughing, but who are better from lying down flat. For patients who sigh when they are not coughing, for stubborn coughs that will not go away, for whooping cough.

Calcarea Sulphurica

Calcarea Sulphurica is a good remedy to keep in mind for cases in which the cough is deep, for cases of bronchitis or pneumonia. Think of this remedy when the patient has pain that covers his or her chest, when the patient feels a burning down deep inside the chest, when the patient complains of a sensation of weight on the chest. This is a great remedy to keep in mind for croupy children. It follows Kali Muriaticum for cases of cough, or alternates quite well with it for coughs that are painful and deep. The expectoration will be lumpy and yellow or yellowish-white.

Kali Phosphoricum

Think of Kali Phosphoricum for cases of coughing and loss of voice, especially if both are related to hay fever. For the cough that irritates the throat, causes hoarseness. For coughing fits that leave the patient exhausted—think of this remedy for whooping cough if the young patient is needy, emotionally upset, restless. A general irritation accompanies the cough, on both the physical and the emotional level. The patient's chest and throat hurt every time he or she coughs. The patient may be left exhausted, pale, and weak from coughing.

Kali Sulphuricum

Kali Sulphuricum is an excellent remedy for acute coughs and for chronic coughs associated with bronchial asthma. Think of this remedy first if the expectoration is green or greenish-yellow and slimy. Any time the expectoration is slimy, think of Kali Sulph. Think of Kali Sulph if the cough comes on during warm weather or if the patient is worse when in a warm or closed room; when the patient seeks cool, open air to alleviate his or her cough. This remedy is useful for all coughs, from shallow, acute coughs to whooping cough to pneumonia, when the symptoms follow the pattern of aggravation from warmth and yellowish and slimy expectoration.

Magnesia Phosphorica

Magnesia Phosphorica is indicated in coughs that are spasmodic, that may be associated with hay fever, that have a shrill or high-pitched tone, as they involve spasms that are sudden and violent. This is a cough without expectoration, a cough that hurts the patient all the way down into the abdomen and causes greater pain on the right side of the body than on the left. The patient feels a sensation of constriction in his throat and chest, and is worse from motion during coughing fits. Look for the patient to want to sit very still to avoid coughing. He will not want to lie down flat due to a feeling of suffocation. He fears that he will cough if he moves, so he will want to sit still and not speak.

Natrum Muriaticum

Natrum Muriaticum is as important to coughs as it is to most other conditions. Think of this remedy first for general cases in which the cough is moist, when it brings up a great deal of expectorant that is clear, watery, and foaming. For coughs that involve a sensation of tickling down in the chest, that seem to radiate out from behind the breast bone. This is an excellent remedy for coughs that are acute and coughs that are chronic. For coughs that are deep and serious and for irritating little coughs that go on night and day for extended periods of time after a cold has ended. If the cold is gone but a little cough remains, think of Natrum Mur, especially if the cough is worse during the daytime. Think of Natrum Muriaticum for coughs that appear along with headaches, for coughs that make tears roll down the patient's cheeks.

Natrum Sulphuricum

Natrum Sulphuricum is the remedy for deep, serious coughs, for coughs that are chronic and deep. For coughs that bring up thick, green, ropy expectorant . For coughs that come from deep in the patient's chest. When the patient complains that his or her chest feels empty, sore, when the patient needs to hold his or her chest when coughing, think of Natrum Sulph. The patient has pains that pierce straight through the chest, pains that are worse on the left side of the chest. This is an important remedy for bron-chitis and an important remedy for asthma, especially when the cough, bronchitis, or asthma carries with it the keynote symptom of the remedy type: the patient is worse in damp weather, when the weather is changing from dry to damp, or from being in a damp environment.

Silicea

The patient who needs Silicea seldom has a simple little cough that is associated with a cold or the flu. The Silicea patient has a cough that is most often associated with great debility, with night sweats, with wasting diseases, or illnesses that have greatly weak-ened him. This can be the remedy for the patient who is very ill with pneumonia or with emphysema. In less serious cases, it can be used for patients with irritating coughs that come on every time the patient lies down, that are the result of a sensation of a hair on the tongue or the result of drinking cold water. But Silicea is seldom the remedy in cases of acute cough. Instead, think of this remedy for coughs that are a sign that the body has failed to fully heal after an illness (Natrum Mur shares this symptom and works well with Silicea to clear away remaining issues), or for cases in which the cough is the tip of the iceberg in terms of the patient's symptoms.

Specific Remedies for Coughs

For acute coughs: Calcarea Phosphorica, Calcarea Fluorica, Calcarea Sulphurica, Magnesia Phosphorica, Ferrum Phosphoricum, Kali Muriaticum, Kali Phosphoricum, Kali Sulphuricum, Natrum Muriaticum.

For chronic coughs: Calcarea Phosphorica, Kali Sulphuricum, Silicea, Natrum Muri-aticum, Natrum Sulphuricum.

For dry coughs: Ferrum Phosphoricum, Kali Muriaticum, Magnesia Phosphorica, Calcarea Fluorica.

For loose coughs (with mucus rattling around in the chest): Natrum Muriaticum, Kali Sulphuricum, Silicea, Ferrum Phosphoricum.

For moist coughs (with much expectorant): Ferrum Phosphoricum, Natrum Muriaticum, Calcarea Phosphorica, Kali Phosphoricum, Silicea, Kali Muriaticum, Calcarea Sulphurica.

If expectorant is bloody: Ferrum Phosphoricum.

If expectorant is watery: Natrum Muriaticum.

If expectorant is thin (watery) and greenish: Kali Sulphuricum.

If expectorant is thick: Natrum Sulphuricum, Kali Phosphoricum, Silicea, Kali Muriaticum, Calcarea Fluorica, Calcarea Phosphorica.

If expectorant is thick and ropy: Natrum Sulphuricum.

If expectorant is thick and lumpy: Calcarea Fluorica, Silicea.

If expectorant is thick and slimy: Kali Sulphuricum.

If expectorant is thick and clear, like raw egg white: Calcarea Phosphoricum.

If expectorant is yellow: Kali Phosphoricum, Kali Sulphuricum, Calcarea Sulphurica, Calcarea Phosphorica, Calcarea Fluorica, Silicea.

If expectorant is yellow/green: Kali Sulphuricum.

If expectorant is green: Natrum Sulphuricum, Silicea.

If expectorant is white or milky: Kali Muriaticum, Calcarea Phosphorica.

If expectorant is colorless (transparent): Natrum Muriaticum, Calcarea Phosphorica.

If expectorant is offensive or disgusting: Kali Sulphuricum, Kali Phosphoricum, Kali Muriaticum, Calcarea Sulphurica, Natrum Sulphuricum, Silicea.

If expectorant is easily brought up: Natrum Muriaticum, Calcarea Phosphorica.

If expectorant is difficult to cough up: Kali Muriaticum, Calcarea Fluorica, Calcarea Sulphurica.

If the patient hacks and hawks constantly to try to clear the throat and bring up expectorant: Calcarea Phosphorica, Kali Phosphoricum, Kali Muriaticum, Natrum Sulphuricum.

If there is a great deal of expectorant: Kali Sulphuricum, Natrum Muriaticum, Silicea.

If there is a great deal of expectorant first thing every morning: Calcarea Fluorica.

If there is no expectorant at all, no matter how much the patient coughs: Ferrum Phosphoricum, Magnesia Phosphorica.

For tickling, shallow coughs: Kali Phosphoricum, Silicea, Ferrum Phosphoricum, Calcarea Fluorica.

For deep coughs: Magnesia Phosphorica, Natrum Sulphuricum, Calcarea Sulphurica, Kali Muriaticum.

For loud coughs: Kali Muriaticum.

For coughs that come in short spells: Ferrum Phosphoricum, Calcarea Phosphorica, Kali Phosphoricum, Kali Muriaticum.

If the short spells are very painful: Ferrum Phosphoricum, Calcarea Phosphorica.

If the short spells leave the patient exhausted: Kali Phosphoricum, Kali Muriaticum.

For coughs that come in spasms: Magnesia Phosphorica, Kali Muriaticum.

For whooping cough: Magnesia Phosphorica, Ferrum Phosphoricum, Kali Phosphoricum, Kali Sulphuricum, Kali Muriaticum, Calcarea Phosphorica.

If spasms of coughing make patient vomit: Ferrum Phosphoricum.

For constant coughing: Calcarea Phosphorica, Natrum Muriaticum, Silicea.

For coughs associated with headaches: Natrum Muriaticum.

For coughs associated with night sweats: Silicea, Natrum Muriaticum.

For coughs associated with involuntary urination: Natrum Muriaticum, Ferrum Phosphoricum.

For coughs associated with a flow of tears down the face: Natrum Muriaticum.

For coughs associated with a nose bleed: Natrum Muriaticum.

For coughs associated with fever: Ferrum Phosphoricum.

For coughs associated with vomiting: Ferrum Phosphoricum.

For coughs associated with chronic respiratory illness: Kali Phosphoricum, Calcarea Phosphorica, Natrum Muriaticum, Natrum Sulphuricum, Silicea.

For coughs that are worse when the patient lies down flat: Calcarea Phosphorica.

For coughs that are worse from any motion: Magnesia Phosphorica.

For coughs that are worse in a warm room: Kali Sulphuricum.

For coughs that are worse in cool or open air: Silicea.

If the patient is better in cool or open air: Kali Sulphuricum.

For coughs that hurt in the throat: Ferrum Phosphoricum, Calcarea Fluorica, Magnesia Phosphorica, Kali Phosphoricum, Silicea.

For coughs that hurt in the chest: Ferrum Phosphoricum, Natrum Muriaticum, Natrum Sulphuricum, Kali Phosphoricum, Calcarea Sulphurica, Calcarea Phosphorica.

For coughs that hurt in the abdomen: Magnesia Phosphorica.

For coughs in very young patients: Ferrum Phosphoricum, Calcarea Phosphorica, Kali Muriaticum, Silicea.

For coughs in very old patients: Natrum Muriaticum, Kali Muriaticum, Natrum Sulphuricum, Silicea.

Sore Throats/Laryngitis

The most common two all-around remedies for patients with sore throats are the same as for coughs: Ferrum Phosphoricum and Kali Muriaticum. Other remedies commonly used in the treatment of patients with sore throats include Natrum Muriaticum, Calcarea Phosphorica, Calcarea Sulphurica, Calcarea Fluorica, Magnesia Phosphorica, Silicea, Natrum Phosphoricum, and Natrum Sulphuricum.

Note that all cases of sore throat, whether it is accompanied by laryngitis or not, can be improved by dissolving the selected remedy or remedies in warm or cool water, as desired by the patient. Have the patient sip the water, even gargle it at the back of the throat, if possible before swallowing it down. This topical and internal use of the remedy will enhance its ability to bring about a cure.

Note also that it is important to look at the patient's tongue as an indicator of the needed remedy or remedies in all cases involving sore throats.

Ferrum Phosphoricum

As always, Ferrum Phos is a good remedy to think of for the first stage of a sore throat, when the pain is just beginning. It is a good general remedy for acute sore throats, most notably those that come on as a part of the overall symptom picture associated with a viral infection, such as fever, sneezing, coughing, and so on. Think of this remedy first for all cases of sore throats in which the throat is dry. Think of Ferrum Phos when the throat is red, swollen, and inflamed. When the patient complains of burning pains in the throat or when the patient totally loses his or her voice. Think of this remedy for cases of laryngitis, whether they are caused by an infection or by overuse of the voice from speaking, singing, or yelling, as long as the symptoms follow the pattern of redness, swelling, and burning pain with a dry throat. As always, the symptoms associated with Ferrum Phos are worse at night. Look for the patient to lose his or her voice as evening descends. Note that, for cases

of swollen glands or tonsils, Ferrum Phos will have to be alternated with Kali Muriaticum to bring full relief.

Kali Muriaticum

Kali Muriaticum is as good a general remedy for sore throats as it is for coughs. This
makes good sense, as the pain associated with coughing that is treated by this remedy
tends to hurt into the throat. As always, the color white is important in the selection
of Kali Mur. It will be most useful for cases in which the patient's tongue has the white
or gray-white coating associated with the need for this remedy. It is also suggested by
the presence of any white patches or ulcers at the back of the throat. The Kali Mur
patient typically hacks, hawks, and coughs to try to clear the throat and bring up
expectorant, which is white and lumpy and hard to cough up. The patient has trouble
swallowing, swallowing is very painful in general, so he does not wish to swallow anything and his mouth and throat are dry. This remedy alternates extremely well with
Ferrum Phosphoricum, and together they complete each other's work to bring relief
from inflammation, coughs, colds, and sore throats. Alternate them whenever the sore
throat and cough is accompanied by swelling of the glands at the sides of the throat
and/or by swollen tonsils.

Calcarea Phosphorica

Calcarea Phosphorica is a good general remedy for those with sore throats, especially
when laryngitis is the main symptom. It can be used as needed with any of the other
remedies listed. Think of this remedy first for cases of sore throat that come on from
overuse or from stressing the voice. Calc Phos is also the first remedy to think of for
cases of laryngitis in which there is no pain, but in which the patient has lost his or her
voice completely.

Kali Phosphoricum

Kali Phosphoricum is the remedy to think of for acute sore throats that feel better from
swallowing. The patient's throat is very dry and he or she swallows constantly to control the discomfort. Think of this remedy for sore throats that occur at the same time as
coughs, when the coughs come in short fits or attacks. When the coughs hurt into the
patient's throat.

Magnesia Phosphorica

Magnesia Phosphorica is a good remedy for acute sore throats that feel inflamed and are
worse from swallowing, especially if the pain of swallowing makes it very difficult to eat.
The throat hurts more from swallowing food, and the patient eats very hurriedly, with

the tendency to either choke on the food or to develop hiccoughs that accompany the throat pain.

Calcarea Fluorica

Calcarea Fluorica is often indicated when acute sore throats develop into chronic complaints. The patient needing Calc Fluor will typically have a great deal of mucus at the back of the throat, and will cough to bring it up. The mucus is difficult to bring up and comes up in lumps. The patient's cough intensifies his or her sore throat. The sore throat typically feels better from warm beverages. The patient will want to drink warm things and, especially, sip tea, and will not want to eat. Look for the Calc Fluor patient to cough up a great deal of mucus first thing every morning.

Natrum Muriaticum

Natrum Muriaticum is our general remedy for chronic sore throats. Like Calcarea Phosphorica, it is not so much associated with specific symptoms as it is notable for its use for ill-defined cases. Consider Natrum Mur for any long-term sore throat. It is especially indicated for sore throats associated with smoking, for sore throats in which the mouth and throat are coated with a clear film of mucus. When the patient is thirsty for cold things and feels that his or her throat is dry, even if it is not. For patients who complain of the sensation of a plug in their throats, who feel that their throats are constricted or swollen. Consider this remedy for all cases in which the throat is indeed swollen, either externally or internally.

Natrum Phosphoricum and Natrum Sulphuricum

Natrum Phosphoricum and Natrum Sulphuricum are both remedies to consider when the sore throat is the result of a more serious infection, most often an infection of the tonsils (Silicea, which is less commonly used as a remedy for sore throats, also will have this symptom). With patients needing Natrum Phos, the back of the throat and the area of the tonsils will be coated with yellow, thick mucus. With patients needing Natrum Sulph, the mucus will be thick and green. Like the Natrum Mur patient, the Natrum Sulph patient will often complain of the sensation of a plug in his or her throat and a feeling of constriction. Finally, Natrum Phos is indicated when the sore throat feels better if the patient swallows solid food.

Silicea

As always, the need for Silicea suggests either that the condition being treated is chronic in nature or that a chronic weakness and predisposition toward illness underlies the acute condition. Think of Silicea for all cases of tonsillitis and for all cases in which chronic sore throats are accompanied by chronic swelling of glands. Think of this remedy first for periodic severe sort throats, the condition that classic homeopaths refer to as *quinsy*. Think of Silicea first (and Natrum Mur second, and possibly both in concert) for cases of chronic sore throats that occur in patients with enlarged thyroids.

Specific Remedies for Sore Throat

For sore throats accompanied by inflammation (redness) of the internal throat: Ferrum Phosphoricum, Calcarea Phosphorica, Calcarea Sulphurica, Kali Muriaticum, Kali Phosphoricum, Natrum Muriaticum, Natrum Phosphoricum, Natrum Sulphuricum.

If the inflammation is acute: Ferrum Phosphoricum, Kali Muriaticum, Calcarea Phosphorica.

If the inflammation is chronic: Natrum Muriaticum, Natrum Sulphuricum, Natrum Phosphoricum, Silicea.

For sore throats accompanied by mucus in the throat: Natrum Muriaticum, Kali Sulphuricum, Natrum Phosphoricum, Natrum Sulphuricum, Calcarea Phosphorica, Calcarea Sulphurica, Kali Phosphoricum, Kali Muriaticum.

If mucus is thick: Natrum Muriaticum, Kali Muriaticum, Natrum Phosphoricum, Natrum Sulphuricum, Silicea.

If mucus is watery: Natrum Muriaticum.

If mucus is colorless and somewhat thick, like raw egg white: Natrum Muriaticum, Calcarea Phosphorica, Natrum Sulphuricum.

If mucus is yellow: Natrum Phosphoricum, Calcarea Sulphurica, Silicea.

If mucus is green: Natrum Sulphuricum, Silicea.

If mucus is white: Kali Muriaticum, Natrum Muriaticum, Natrum Phosphoricum.

If mucus is frothy or foamy: Natrum Muriaticum, Silicea.

If mucus smells offensive: Natrum Muriaticum, Silicea.

For sore throats accompanied by swelling of the internal throat: Natrum Muriaticum, Silicea, Calcarea Phosphorica, Calcarea Sulphurica, Kali Muriaticum, Kali Phosphoricum, Kali Sulphuricum.

For pain accompanied by a sense of choking or constriction of the throat: Natrum Muriaticum, Natrum Sulphuricum, Magnesia Phosphorica, Kali Sulphuricum, Kali Phosphoricum.

If the sense of choking or constriction only comes on when the patient swallows: Natrum Muriaticum, Natrum Sulphuricum, Magnesia Phosphorica.

If the sense of constriction is worse when or from drinking: Natrum Muriaticum

If the sense of constriction is better from drinking: Calcarea Fluorica.

If the sense of constriction comes on whenever the patient clears his or her throat: Calcarea Phosphorica.

For raw pain, with or without laryngitis: Ferrum Phosphoricum, Kali Muriaticum, Calcarea Phosphorica, Kali Phosphoricum, Kali Sulphuricum, Natrum Muriaticum, Silicea.

For burning pain: Calcarea Phosphorica, Calcarea Sulphurica, Ferrum Phosphoricum.

For scratching pain: Calcarea Phosphorica, Calcarea Sulphurica, Kali Phosphoricum, Kali Muriaticum, Silicea.

For sore throats that feel as if there is a lump or a ball in the throat: Natrum Muriaticum, Silicea, Ferrum Phosphoricum, Kali Phosphoricum, Kali Sulphuricum, Natrum Phosphoricum, Calcarea Sulphurica.

If the sensation of a lump occurs only on swallowing: Natrum Muriaticum, Natrum Sulphuricum, Silicea.

If the sensation of a lump occurs only on one side of the throat: Silicea.

If the sensation of a lump keeps the patient from speaking: Natrum Phosphoricum.

For sore throats that feel as if there is a splinter in the throat: Natrum Muriaticum, Silicea.

If the sensation of a splinter comes on only when the patient swallows: Silicea.

For pain with itching in the throat: Calcarea Sulphurica.

For pain that extends into the ears: Kali Muriaticum.

For sore throats in which the throat feels dry: Natrum Muriaticum, Calcarea Phosphorica, Calcarea Sulphurica, Kali Muriaticum, Kali Sulphuricum, Natrum Phosphoricum, Natrum Sulphuricum, Silicea.

For dry sore throats with great thirst: Natrum Muriaticum.

For dry sore throats without thirst: Natrum Sulphuricum.

For sore throats that are worse from swallowing: Kali Muriaticum, Kali Phosphoricum, Calcarea Phosphorica, Natrum Muriaticum, Silicea.

If the pain is worse from empty swallowing: Calcarea Phosphorica.

If the pain is better from swallowing solids: Natrum Phosphoricum.

For sore throats that are better for warm liquids: Calcarea Fluorica, Silicea.

For sore throats that are better if the patient is warm: Silicea.

For sore throats that are worse if the patient is warm: Kali Sulphuricum.

For sore throats that are better for cool liquids: Natrum Muriaticum.

For sore throats that are better if the patient is cool: Kali Muriaticum, Kali Sulphuricum.

For sore throats that are worse if the patient is cool: Calcarea Phosphorica, Natrum Muriaticum, Silicea.

For laryngitis, in general: Calcarea Phosphorica, Ferrum Phosphoricum, Kali Muriaticum, Kali Phosphoricum, Natrum Muriaticum, Calcarea Fluorica.

For laryngitis that is accompanied by a dry throat and mouth: Calcarea Fluorica.

For painless laryngitis: Calcarea Phosphorica.

Influenza

In this section on influenza, I describe the body aches and pains associated with flu but not the digestive complaints that may accompany those pains or the sore throat, nasal discharge, or cough that may accompany the onset of influenza. For a comprehensive diagnosis I strongly suggest that the reader refer to the other sections of this book that deal specifically with those complaints. Match that information with the information in this section to find the best possible remedy or remedies.

Our most important remedies for the body aches associated with influenza are Natrum Sulphuricum, Ferrum Phosphoricum, Magnesia Phosphorica, Calcarea Phosphorica, Kali Muriaticum, Kali Phosphoricum, and Natrum Muriaticum.

Natrum Sulphuricum

If there is one remedy that is most associated with flu, it is Natrum Sulphuricum. Think of this remedy for all cases of flu in which the body aches, in which the patient feels both digestive distress with great thirst and pains in the limbs, especially pains in the lower limbs from the hips to the knees. Think of Natrum Sulph for patients with flu who have swollen glands, a sense of burning and coldness in their digestive tract, with aching and cutting pains in the chest and throughout the abdomen. For digestive distress that is associated with headache, with nausea, and with vomiting. The distress associated with this remedy is greatly aggravated during wet or damp weather, when the weather is changing from dry to damp, and when the patient is in contact with a damp environment. This is a chilly patient with a sensation of heat in the abdomen, and with heat and burning in the feet, especially in the soles of the feet. This is a patient with a deep, croupy cough and green, ropy expectoration.

Ferrum Phosphoricum

Think of Ferrum Phos for the first stage of the flu, when the symptoms are just beginning, especially if those symptoms include fever. Think of this remedy for all cases that involve fever, especially when the face and head are red, dry, and hot. When the patient has a rapid pulse. When the onset of symptoms is sudden. Think of this remedy when cough is a major symptom of the ailment, and may be so violent that coughing ends in vomiting. Think of this remedy for cases of body ache that are aggravated by any motion, in which the patient must lie perfectly still to avoid pain.

Perhaps the best and most effective treatment for influenza is to catch it early and treat it by alternating Ferrum Phos and Natrum Sulph every half hour until improvement begins. This combination of remedies is effective for the vast majority of cases of flu. Should it fail to act, add that other great general remedy for colds and coughs, Kali Muriaticum, into the mix. Give the Kali Mur and Ferrum Phos together and alternate it with Natrum Sulph.

Magnesia Phosphorica

Since it is a major remedy for pain, always think of Mag Phos for cases of flu, especially when body aches are the dominant symptom. Think of this remedy for aches and pains that are relieved by heat and by pressure. When the patient wants a hot water bottle and presses it hard against the affected areas. Think of this remedy especially when spasms are the key to understanding the condition: when everything comes on sudden and spasmodically—body aches, coughs, cramps associated with digestive distress that force the patient to bend over at the waist to get relief. This is an excellent remedy for bouts of flu that involve hiccoughs, belches, and flatulence, in which the symptoms appear and disappear suddenly, in which aches and pains move from place to place in the body without warning. For cases of body aches in which the patient is forced to get up out of bed and pace the floor to calm the pain, or in which the patient gets up out of bed and sits in a chair, sitting very tall and very still to quiet the pain and keep from coughing.

Calcarea Phosphorica

Calcarea Phosphorica is not a remedy that is specific to influenza, It is, instead, a remedy that should always be used either as a preventive, and given regularly from the beginning of the flu season or after the patient has suffered through the flu to make sure that he or she is fully cured and back to full strength. Calc Phos is a great general tonic and an excellent general remedy for colds, coughs, and particularly digestive disorders, so it is effective for the flu as well. It can be used in combination or alternation with any of the other remedies listed here to boost their effectiveness and help the patient recover more quickly. It can work especially well with Kali Phosphoricum, Kali Muriaticum, and Natrum Muriaticum in cases of flu.

Kali Muriaticum

Kali Muriaticum is always a good choice as a general remedy for those with influenza when the dominant symptoms are body aches and pains, especially those centered in the limbs and those that cause the patient to walk unsteadily or awkwardly. Look for the characteristic white coating of the tongue, as well as white discharges, as key indicators of the need for this remedy. It combines well with the other remedies listed here, especially with Calcarea Phosphorica for cases of malaise that lingers, in which the patient does not seem sick enough to be in any great danger but is in great discomfort, with a headache and body aches accompanying the general symptoms of flu.

Kali Phosphoricum

Kali Phosphoricum should be kept in mind for flu that involves muscle aches, especially when the muscles visibly twitch and jump during the pain (Magnesia Phosphorica also has this trembling and twitching, especially of the hands). Think of Kali Phos for cases of flu in which weakness is a key symptom, if the patient is truly exhausted and depleted by his or her illness. For this reason, Kali Phos and Calcarea Phosphorica work well together in treating those with flu, especially if Calc Phos is given as a follow-up to Kali Phos. Think of this remedy for patients who are somewhat demanding, who want to be taken care of, who wish for company and a little excitement, but who tire very easily. For patients who are sensitive to everything: to music, to light, to noise, to changes in temperature and weather. These are thirsty patients, with dry mouths. They crave cold water. They are given to body aches that leave them feeling bruised, that leave them feeling stiff. Their aches and pains are better from gentle motion, but are worse on first motion, so Kali Phos patients will have to be coaxed into getting out of bed.

Natrum Muriaticum

Think of this remedy when the flu lingers, when the patient does not respond to other treatment. Add this remedy to any other when the remedy of best choice does not bring about a cure. Think of this remedy for the patient who has taken to his or her bed with the flu, who feels nauseous, exhausted, irritated, and wants to be left alone. Natrum Mur combines especially well with Natrum Sulphuricum for cases of flu. It should be given in combination or alternation with Natrum Sulph after the first, feverish stage has passed (when Natrum Sulph should be alternated with Ferrum Phosphoricum). This is a thirsty patient, who will want cold water even if he or she is chilly. This is a patient who will likely have headaches and body aches accompanying the flu, who will want to get into bed, but who will likely feel better when uncovered, even if he or she is chilly. This is a patient from whom all discharges are watery, from mucus to phlegm to diarrhea. Watery discharges gush and are plentiful.

Specific Remedies for Flu

For the first stage of the flu, especially if fever is present: Ferrum Phosphoricum, Natrum Sulphuricum. Note that these two remedies work very well in alternation or if given at the same time. Should the two fail to work, add Kali Muriaticum into the mix. For very stubborn cases, combine Ferrum Phos, Natrum Sulph, Kali Mur, and Natrum Muriaticum. Dissolve a few pellets of each in warm or cool water, as the patient desires. Have the patient sip the water every few minutes until improvement begins.

For cases of flu in which fever dominates: Ferrum Phosphoricum.

For cases of flu in which cold symptoms dominate: Kali Muriaticum.

For cases of flu in which body aches dominate: Magnesia Phosphorica, Natrum Sulphuricum, Kali Muriaticum.

If the aches and pains are spasmodic: Magnesia Phosphorica.

If the aches and pains shift from place to place: Magnesia Phosphorica.

For cases of flu in which exhaustion dominates: Kali Phosphoricum.

For cases of flu in which digestive symptoms dominate: Natrum Sulphuricum.

For cases of flu in which the patient is not violently ill, but is depleted: Calcarea Phosphorica, Kali Muriaticum.

For cases of flu that linger or if the patient does not fully recover: Natrum Muriaticum, Calcarea Phosphorica.

For cases of flu in very young patients: Ferrum Phosphoricum, Natrum Sulphuricum, Kali Muriaticum. Combine Ferrum Phos and Natrum Sulph in warm water and place on the infant's lips. If this fails to bring an improvement, add Kali Mur into the mix and give every few minutes while watching for improvement.

For cases of flu in elderly patients: Natrum Sulphuricum, Natrum Muriaticum. Give these remedies in alternation or combination. If they fail to bring relief, add Calcarea Phosphorica into the mix. In stubborn or lingering cases, add Silicea.

Earaches

The same two remedies that were most important for colds, coughs, and the like also dominate for earaches and ear infections: Ferrum Phosphoricum and Kali Muriaticum will be the remedies of first choice. However, several other cell salts will be useful for these conditions, as they are for other acute ailments, particularly those associated with childhood. These remedies are Kali Phosphoricum, Calcarea Phosphorica, Magnesia Phosphorica, Natrum Muriaticum, Calcarea Sulphurica, Kali Sulphuricum, Natrum Phosphoricum, Natrum Sulphuricum, and Silicea.

Ferrum Phosphoricum

Ferrum Phosphoricum is an important, vital remedy, especially in the early stages of an earache or ear infection. Think of Ferrum Phosphoricum for the inflammatory stage of ear infection, in which the patient suffers from a burning and throbbing pain. When the external ear is red, hot, and swollen. Think of Ferrum Phos for all earaches that come on from contact with cold, especially a cold wind, that come on after the patient has gotten wet and cold, and for those that appear as part of the general symptoms of a cold or any other upper respiratory infection. Think of this remedy for colds that settle into the ears. Think of it for patients, especially children, who are given to one earache after another. The Ferrum Phos patient feels a throbbing or cutting pain in the ear that radiates deep into the head, into the jaw. The pain pulses and burns. There is a sensation of heat to the internal and the external ear, which burns bright or deep red. The patient has difficulty hearing out of the affected ear or ears, hears whizzing, popping, and cracking in the ear. Think of Ferrum Phosphoricum first for earaches that appear suddenly, especially those that appear in the night. Think of this remedy for earaches, especially chronic earaches, in skinny children, in debilitated children, in children who tend toward respiratory distress. Think of this remedy first and foremost for cases of sudden earaches that are associated with heat, burning, and redness, and that do not produce pus.

Kali Muriaticum

Kali Muriaticum can be used along with or, more often, following Ferrum Phos for cases in which an earache is developing into a middle-ear or inner-ear infection, when the eustachian tubes are becoming involved, when they, along with the throat and the glands under the jaw, are becoming swollen. Think of Kali Mur when the patient hears a cracking sound in the affected ear every time he or she swallows. When swallowing is difficult because of the ear and throat pain. Swelling, even swelling of both the internal and the external ear, is keynote to this remedy, as is the characteristic white or gray-white coating of the tongue. This is our best remedy for middle-ear infections, especially when they are associated with the formation of pus—which, of course, is of the characteristic color white. The patient's ear feels stuffed, swollen. Note that this remedy is right-sided, and for this reason it is used more often for earaches in the right ear than in the left, although it can be used in either case if the symptoms follow. If a simple earache is deepening into an ear infection, alternate Ferrum Phos with Kali Mur. Continue with Kali Mur alone as the inflammatory stage fades, or add other indicated remedies, most notably Calcarea Phosphorica, which works well with Kali Mur in cases of ear infection, especially chronic ear infections in young patients.

Kali Phosphoricum

While Ferrum Phosphoricum is the remedy most closely associated with earaches in young patients, Kali Phos is suggested as a remedy for earaches in elderly patients. Think of this remedy for older patients who are hard of hearing, who have buzzing, ringing, cracking, and other noises in their heads that dull their sense of hearing, and yet are sensitive to noise. These are patients who cannot bear loud or sudden noises. Think of this remedy for long-term, stubborn earaches and deafness that are accompanied by an itching sensation in the ear that drives the patient nearly crazy. For cases of earache or dullness of hearing in exhausted, nervous patients, young and old, who seem to be depleted from the effort of dealing with the discomfort. Look for any discharge to be watery or even brownish, and to smell awful. The patient may have a strong odor emanating from him, may smell rather like his discharges. Note that, if Kali Phosphoricum alone fails to quiet the buzzing and cracking in the patient's ears, it can be followed by Magnesia Phosphorica with good result.

Calcarea Phosphorica

This remedy is often used as a general tonic or as a remedy that can be added to the mix of remedies to boost the overall effect. Calc Phos will most typically be used in this manner for cases of earache, and works particularly well with Kali Mur for cases that Kali Mur fails to cure on its own. However, Calc Phos has a set of specific symptoms that most clearly suggest its use and you will find, from time to time, that it can be used as a cure all by itself. Think of Calc Phos when the external ear feels cold during the earache or ear infection. This is a rather strange little keynote of the remedy. Just as Calc Phos, when it is needed for a cold, will have the symptom of the tip of the nose being cold, here the outer ear will be cold instead of red, hot, and swollen as is more common in infections. This is a true ache—the inside of the ear, the bones around the ear, even the jaw and the teeth just plain hurt, with a cold, aching pain. Calc Phos can be used on its own if the symptoms match or can, especially in treating middle or inner ear infections, be used in alternation or combination with other remedies. It can also be extremely helpful for patients with chronic ear pain and/or chronically swollen glands. Also, think of this remedy as a preventive. Give it after an earache or infection has cleared to keep it from returning.

Magnesia Phosphorica

Magnesia Phosphorica is always a follow-up or adjunct remedy in cases of ear pain, but it can be very helpful. In general ear pain or infection, it is used along with Kali Muriaticum, with which it blends very well, especially if the patient is being driven mad by the pain, if he or she paces the floor in pain. Consider Mag Phos if the patient finds relief from ear pain by applying hot compresses against the ear and pressing them hard against the ear. If the pain in the ear shoots, shifts, and is improved by heat and by pressure. If the patient cannot stay in bed because of the pain and either walks the floor or sits up tall and still because motion aggravates, even though the patient is driven to move by the pain. The patient will not want to talk and hears the echo of his or her own voice inside the pained ear when speaking. The Mag Phos patient will have distorted hearing, will hear many different cracks, buzzes, and other sounds in the ear, but will be sensitive to noise and will have hearing that is, if anything, magnified by the pain. This remedy follows Kali Phosphoricum very well, especially for cases that have distorted hearing as the major symptom.

Natrum Muriaticum

Natrum Muriaticum is helpful for cases of simple earache that occur along with a cold or flu. Look at the Natrum Mur patient's tongue and face for indicators of the need for the remedy. The tongue may be clean or coated with a transparent mucus lining. The mouth will be filled with water, very moist, with foam and froth. Yet these are thirsty patients, and even though they tend to be on the chilly side when ill, they want cold water, which soothes them. The earaches associated with Natrum Mur involve itching of the whole interior of the ear, with accompanying burning pains. The patient complains of stitching pains in the ear, down into the eustachian tubes. There may be copious discharge from the ear that is clear to whitish, watery to the consistency of raw egg white.

Calcarea Sulphurica

The keynote symptom associated with Calcarea Sulphurica is, first and foremost, a discharge from the ear that is either yellow or mixed yellow pus and blood. Any discharge from the ear that contains blood indicates the need for Calc Sulph. The internal ears and the glands below the jaw will be swollen. The area of the glands and behind the ears and jaw will be very sensitive, even painful. The patient will be deaf in the pained ear, will hear only a roaring sound in his or her ear.

Kali Sulphuricum

Think of this remedy as a follow-up to Ferrum Phosphoricum if Kali Muriaticum has failed to act. It can be used on its own or in combination or alternation with Kali Mur. Think of this remedy after the initial inflammation has passed if the discharge from the ear moves from being watery and clear to yellow and finally to being thick and yellow or yellow-green. This is the best remedy for middle ear infections that have reached the stage in which the discharge is thick, in which the internal ear is swollen, and the pain extends from the ear to the glands below the jaw and into the lower jaw itself. When the pain extends into the eustachian tubes. When the pain is sharp and cutting in nature, so that the patient cries out in pain. Check the patient's tongue for an indication of the use of Kali Sulph. The tongue will be coated yellow. The patient will also be worse in a warm room. The patient's sense of deafness accompanying the pain will increase, as will the pain itself, if the patient becomes too warm. The patient will seek cool air for relief.

Natrum Phosphoricum

The best indicator for the need of Natrum Phosphoricum is that the patient will have one ear that is red and hot and swollen while the other ear will be quite normal. Check the patient's tongue for an indication of the remedy—the characteristic yellow tongue, which may be a bright, golden yellow. Typically, the affected ear will have a discharge of the same color and will have dried scabs of yellow matter on the external part of the ear.

Natrum Sulphuricum

Think of Natrum Sulphuricum for intense ear infections that have reached a stage at which the pain is intolerable, especially in damp weather or damp environments. Think of it for patients with chronic ear pain that always comes on when the weather is changing from dry to damp. For patients who have such ringing in their ears that they feel as if they are standing in a cathedral just before church services begin. There is the sound of bells ringing in the patient's ears that blots out all other sounds. The pain is pulsing, pushing, as if there were a physical ball or plug in the ear that is trying to push its way out. The ear is pressured down into the eustachian tube. If there is discharge from the ear—there usually is not, as any discharge would improve the symptoms and the sensation of pressure—it will be green or yellow-green.

Silicea

Silicea is really an excellent remedy for earaches and ear infections, especially in patients who are either very young or very old. It is useful both in acute and chronic cases of ear pain. Silicea often follows Ferrum Phosphoricum very well for cases of ear pain and the two remedies, with Ferrum Phos given first followed by Silicea, can solve many stubborn earaches and infections. Use Ferrum Phos to clear away the initial inflammation associated with the ear pain, and Silicea to bring forth any discharge that needs to be cleansed from the ear and to open the ear and soothe pain. Think of Silicea specifically for the patient who has an ear that is closed, with hearing dulled by ear pain or infection, but who suddenly experiences a brief opening of the ear. The ear will crack open (with a loud, explosive sound that causes him to jump that only he can hear) when the patient sneezes, yawns, laughs, or for no apparent reason. This as a general remedy for all ear infections that involve swelling of the internal ear and pain that extends down into the eustachian tube. Think of it as an adjunct to other remedies for cases of general ear pain that extends into the bones around the ear, especially into the jaw, and for cases in which the discharge from the ear is scanty, thin, and very smelly. Think of Silicea particularly for cases of ear pain that are chronic, that return again and again, especially for cases that have often been treated with antibiotics, only to return again and again. Think of it for chronic earaches in skinny or sickly children or elders. Silicea follows Calc Phos very well in cases of stubborn ear pain in skinny children or sickly elders, and can act—as does Calcarea Phosphorica—as a general tonic, improving not only their ear pain, but also the whole of their being. Because of this, Silicea works well in concert with Calcarea Phosphorica and may be considered to be the deeper version of that remedy for cases of earaches.

Specific Remedies for Earaches

For earaches in general: Kali Muriaticum, Ferrum Phosphoricum, Calcarea Phosphorica, Natrum Muriaticum, Kali Sulphuricum, Magnesia Phosphorica, Natrum Sulphuricum, Silicea.

For earaches in which the external ear feels hot: Ferrum Phosphoricum.

For earaches in which the external ear feels cold: Calcarea Phosphorica.

For earaches with sharp pain in the ear itself: Ferrum Phosphoricum, Magnesia Phosphorica.

For earaches with sharp pain under the ear: Kali Sulphuricum.

For earaches with sharp pain behind the ear: Calcarea Sulphurica.

For earaches with burning pain: Ferrum Phosphoricum, Natrum Muriaticum, Natrum Phosphoricum.

For earaches with throbbing pain: Ferrum Phosphoricum, Silicea.

For earaches with aching pain: Calcarea Phosphorica.

For earaches with cutting pain: Kali Sulphuricum, Ferrum Phosphoricum.

For earaches with shooting/radiating pain: Ferrum Phosphoricum, Magnesia Phosphorica, Calcarea Phosphorica, Kali Sulphuricum, Calcarea Sulphurica, Silicea, Natrum Muriaticum.

If the pain shifts and shoots from place to place: Magnesia Phosphorica.

If the pain is inconsistent, starts and stops: Magnesia Phosphorica, Natrum Muriaticum.

If pain radiates out in all directions: Ferrum Phosphoricum.

If the pain radiates into the bones around the ear: Calcarea Phosphorica, Calcarea Sulphurica, Silicea.

If the pain radiates into the jaw: Kali Sulphuricum, Calcarea Sulphurica.

If the pain radiates into the neck: Natrum Muriaticum, Silicea.

If the pain radiates into the shoulder: Natrum Muriaticum.

If the pain radiates back behind the ear: Calcarea Sulphurica.

If the pain radiates above the ear: Natrum Muriaticum, Silicea.

If the pain radiates below the ear: Natrum Phosphoricum, Silicea.

If the pain extends down into the eustachian tube: Silicea, Natrum Sulphuricum, Kali Sulphuricum, Natrum Muriaticum, Kali Muriaticum.

If the pain feels as if there is a plug or ball in the ear trying to push its way free: Natrum Sulphuricum.

For earaches with pain and itching combined: Kali Phosphoricum, Calcarea Phosphorica, Silicea, Natrum Muriaticum.

For earaches with pain and swelling combined: Calcarea Phosphorica, Kali Muriaticum, Silicea, Natrum Phosphoricum, Natrum Muriaticum, Ferrum Phosphoricum.

For swelling of the external ear: Kali Muriaticum, Ferrum Phosphoricum, Kali Sulphuricum.

For swelling of the internal ear: Kali Muriaticum, Kali Sulphuricum, Natrum Muriaticum, Calcarea Sulphurica, Ferrum Phosphoricum, Natrum Phosphoricum, Silicea.

If the external ear is red, hot, and swollen: Ferrum Phosphoricum.

If only one ear is red and swollen: Natrum Phosphoricum.

For swelling of the glands behind the jaw: Kali Muriaticum, Silicea, Calcarea Phosphorica.

For inflammation of the ear, in general: Ferrum Phosphoricum, Kali Muriaticum, Silicea, Magnesia Phosphorica, Calcarea Phosphorica, Calcarea Sulphurica, Kali Sulphuricum.

If the external ear is inflamed: Ferrum Phosphoricum, Kali Muriaticum, Silicea.

If the internal (middle) ear is inflamed: Ferrum Phosphoricum, Magnesia Phosphorica, Calcarea Phosphorica, Kali Muriaticum, Calcarea Sulphurica, Kali Sulphuricum.

If inflammation involves an offensive discharge from the ear: Kali Phosphoricum,

Silicea, Kali Sulphuricum, Calcarea Sulphurica, Calcarea Phosphorica, Ferrum Phosphoricum.

If discharge is bloody: Calcarea Sulphurica, Kali Phosphoricum.

If discharge is yellow: Kali Phosphoricum, Natrum Phosphoricum, Silicea, Kali Sulphuricum, Calcarea Sulphurica.

If discharge is thick and yellow: Silicea, Calcarea Sulphurica.

If discharge is watery and yellow: Kali Sulphuricum.

If discharge is bright golden yellow: Natrum Phosphoricum.

If discharge is brownish-yellow: Kali Sulphuricum, Kali Phosphoricum.

If discharge is greenish-yellow: Natrum Sulphuricum, Kali Sulphuricum.

If discharge is white: Kali Muriaticum.

If discharge is colorless, like raw egg white: Natrum Muriaticum, Calcarea Phosphorica.

If discharge is, in general, thick: Natrum Muriaticum, Calcarea Sulphurica, Natrum Sulphuricum.

If discharge is, in general, thin: Kali Sulphuricum, Silicea, Kali Phosphoricum.

If discharge is fluent: Natrum Muriaticum.

If discharge is constant or chronic: Kali Muriaticum.

If discharge brings no relief from pain: Ferrum Phosphoricum.

For a discharge of ear wax: Natrum Muriaticum.

For earaches and infections without or with very little discharge: Silicea, Natrum Sulphuricum, Calcarea Phosphorica.

For earaches and noises in the ears: Ferrum Phosphoricum, Natrum Muriaticum, Kali Phosphoricum, Natrum Sulphuricum, Kali Muriaticum.

For roaring in the ears: Natrum Muriaticum, Silicea, Calcarea Sulphurica.

For buzzing in the ears: Kali Phosphoricum.

For cracking in the ears: Ferrum Phosphoricum, Kali Phosphoricum, Kali Muriaticum, Natrum Muriaticum, Silicea.

If cracking occurs when chewing or blowing the nose: Natrum Muriaticum, Kali Muriaticum.

For whizzing in the ears: Ferrum Phosphoricum, Magnesia Phosphorica, Silicea.

For popping in the ears: Ferrum Phosphoricum, Silicea.

For ringing in the ears: Kali Phosphoricum, Ferrum Phosphoricum, Natrum Sulphuricum, Magnesia Phosphorica, Silicea.

If ringing is very loud, like the sound of church bells: Natrum Sulphuricum.

For humming sounds in the ears: Kali Phosphoricum, Natrum Muriaticum.

For a sound like running water in the ears: Ferrum Phosphoricum, Natrum Muriaticum.

If hearing is dulled or decreased by sounds in the ears: Silicea, Natrum Sulphuricum, Ferrum Phosphoricum, Kali Muriaticum, Calcarea Sulphurica, Kali Sulphuricum.

If hearing is increased despite sounds in the ears: Natrum Muriaticum, Kali Muriaticum.

If the patient has dulled or distorted hearing and yet is very sensitive to sound: Kali Phosphoricum, Magnesia Phosphorica, Silicea, Natrum Muriaticum, Kali Muriaticum.

If the patient is very sensitive to sounds inside his or her ears: Kali Phosphoricum, Silicea.

If the patient is being driven crazy by the sounds in his or her ears: Kali Phosphoricum.

If sound in the ears occurs when the patient is drifting off to sleep, awakening him: Kali Phosphoricum.

If the patient is very sensitive to external sounds: Magnesia Phosphorica, Kali Phosphoricum, Kali Muriaticum, Natrum Muriaticum.

If patient is startled by sounds: Kali Phosphoricum, Kali Muriaticum.

If the patient is very sensitive to the sound of the human voice or hears his or her own voice echoing in the affected ear: Magnesia Phosphorica.

If the patient is very sensitive to the sound of music: Natrum Muriaticum.

If the patient's ears are blocked and stuffed, then suddenly crack open with a sound that startles him: Silicea.

For earaches in which the ears feel stuffed up: Kali Muriaticum, Silicea.

For earaches that are worse in the morning: Natrum Sulphuricum, Natrum Muriaticum.

For earaches that are worse in the daytime in general: Natrum Muriaticum.

For earaches that are worse in the evening: Kali Sulphuricum, Natrum Sulphuricum.

For earaches that occur at bedtime: Ferrum Phosphoricum.

For earaches that are worse at night: Ferrum Phosphoricum, Natrum Sulphuricum.

For earaches that are relieved if the patient sticks his finger deep into the painful ear: Silicea.

For earaches in which there is the sensation that something is alive in the ear: Silicea.

For earaches in which there is a sensation of water sloshing in the ear: Natrum Muriaticum, Kali Muriaticum, Natrum Phosphoricum.

For earaches that occur during changes in the weather: Calcarea Phosphorica, Natrum Sulphuricum, Silicea.

For earaches that occur when the weather gets colder: Silicea.

For earaches that occur when the weather changes from dry to damp: Natrum Sulphuricum.

For earaches that occur after exposure to cold wind: Ferrum Phosphoricum, Natrum Muriaticum, Silicea.

For earaches that occur after patient gets cold and wet: Ferrum Phosphoricum.

For earaches in very young patients: Ferrum Phosphoricum, Kali Muriaticum, Calcarea Phosphorica, Silicea.

For earaches in elderly patients: Kali Phosphoricum, Silicea.

Measles

While less common than they used to be, measles are still among those diseases that can occur in childhood. Because of modern prevention, when measles do occur they present more of a threat now than they did in the past, when young children encountered the illness as part of the means by which they developed their adult immune systems.

There are really only five cell salts to consider in all cases of measles. One, Ferrum Phosphoricum, so dominates the ailment that it could, in and of itself, be considered a cure. The other remedies to consider along with Ferrum Phos are Kali Muriaticum, Calcarea Phosphorica, Kali Sulphuricum and Natrum Muriaticum.

Ferrum Phosphoricum

Ferrum Phosphoricum handles almost all the stages of measles. Use it for the first stage, with the onset of symptoms, including fever, and for all symptoms in the ear, eye, nose, and throat.

Note that in the early stages of the illness, if the fever is high, Ferrum Phos may be combined with Kali Muriaticum and both may be dissolved in water and given to the patient in sips until improvement begins. Often, you may not know what illness you are dealing with until the rash appears, and you can consider this to be a general upper respiratory ailment or flu. When rash appears, add Kali Sulphuricum into the remedy mixture.

Most often, Ferrum Phos will be used along with Kali Muriaticum, which almost always follows and deals with the aftereffects of the ailment, from diarrhea to the exhaustion and depletion that occurs after the illness has past. Kali Mur is given in almost all cases of measles to help restore the patient to full strength.

If Kali Muriaticum alone fails to restore the patient to full health, add Calcarea Phosphorica, after the symptoms of the disease have passed, to help strengthen the patient's system. Kali Mur and Calc Phos may be used in alternation or combination for this purpose.

Think of Natrum Muriaticum as a good second remedy as well, for cases in which thirst dominates, and in which the patient's eyes stream with tears. When the patient, weakened, wants to lie in bed and be left alone.

Think of Kali Sulphuricum for cases in which the rash associated with measles is suppressed. To help bring out the rash and speed healing, give Kali Sulph. Also give it if the rash appears and then disappears. Kali Sulph (or Natrum Muriaticum, for that matter) may be given along with Kali Mur in the second stage of the illness, after the initial fever has passed. Either will help strengthen the work of Kali Mur, if they are called for by the patient's symptoms. Calc Phos may be given after all other remedies have stopped, to bring the patient back to health.

Mumps

For treatment of mumps, we again turn to the combination of the two remedies that together help us with most conditions that involve fever and swollen glands: Ferrum Phosphoricum and Kali Muriaticum. In the case of mumps, the two remedies should be given together, instead of starting with Ferrum Phos and using Kali Mur as the follow-up remedy. Kali Mur is actually the more important of the two remedies for cases of mumps, and in many cases it will treat the condition on its own. But when fever is a part of the picture—and it is most of the time, to some degree or another—give Ferrum Phos as well. Dissolve a few tablets of both remedies in cool or warm water, as the patient desires, and allow him or her to sip the water every few minutes until improvement begins. Then slow the number of doses as improvement continues.

For cases in which salivation is an issue, when the patient has an excess of saliva that drips from their mouth, add Natrum Muriaticum into the mixture. Think of Natrum Muriaticum and add it immediately if male patients experience swelling of the testicles during mumps.

Give Calcarea Phosphorica once the mumps are over, as we often do following ailments that deplete the system. Calcarea Phosphorica, given as a follow-up after all other remedies are stopped, will help restore the patient to full strength. If the patient remains depleted even after Calc Phos has been given, give Silicea instead.

Chicken Pox

The one cell salt that is always used in the treatment of chicken pox is Ferrum Phosphoricum. Always use it at the first stage of the ailment, when fever is present. When the eruptions appear, in *all* cases, add Kali Muriaticum to the Ferrum Phosphoricum and then, from there, choose from among the following remedies the one that best matches the patient's individual symptoms: Calcarea Sulphurica, Natrum Muriaticum, Natrum Sulphuricum, Kali Sulphuricum, and Silicea.

Note that, once the chicken pox have passed, you should give the patient Calcarea Phosphorica as a final remedy to restore the patient to full strength.

Again, in all cases of chicken pox, combine or alternate Ferrum Phos and Kali Muriaticum as the eruptions begin to appear.

Kali Sulphuricum

If the eruptions are dry and scaly, give the patient Kali Sulphuricum. Look for an abundance of yellow scales on the skin. The skin itches wildly and burns as well.

Calcarea Sulphurica

If the eruptions have yellow scabs, consider Calcarea Sulphurica. The patient will likely feel chilled while the scabs appear. They may discharge blood-streaked yellow pus when they are scratched. The skin is dry, but the scabs are moist when touched or scratched.

Natrum Muriaticum

If the eruptions are watery, containing transparent fluid that may thicken to the consistency of raw egg white, give the patient Natrum Muriaticum. Think of Natrum Mur if the skin forms thin crusts that fall off easily and then reform again and again.

Natrum Sulphuricum

If the eruptions are warty, with a watery yellow pus or yellow scales, give Natrum Sulphuricum. If the skin is very sensitive and painful in addition to itchy, think of Natrum Sulph. Also, if the skin itches more when it is uncovered, think of Natrum Sulph.

Silicea

If the eruptions are extremely painful, consider Silicea. Consider it if swollen glands figure into the picture of the illness, if the eruptions have a coppery color, and if the eruptions ooze when scratched and are slow to heal. When the skin is very sensitive, when the patient suffers from itching and burning and harsh pain, the remedy to con-sider is Silicea.

Nosebleeds

There are several cell salts to consider when treating a nosebleed, or a patient with the chronic tendency toward nosebleeds. The major remedies are Ferrum Phosphoricum, Calcrea Phosphorica Calcarea Sulphurica, Kali Muriaticum, Natrum Muriaticum, Natrum Sulphuricum and Silicea. Often it will be the color and the quality of the blood or the frequency of nosebleeds that will indicate the remedy. The age of the patient will also be a factor.

Ferrum Phosphoricum

Ferrum Phosphoricum is especially indicated in nosebleeds in children. Think of this remedy first for all cases in which the blood is bright red. Think of this remedy espe-cially if the other symptoms common to the remedy are present: if the patient's face is red, dry, and hot; if fever is present; if the nosebleed is associated with the onset of a cold; if it is preceded by an itching or smarting in the nostrils, especially the right nos-tril. This is an excellent remedy to keep in mind for children who have frequent nose-bleeds, and who also are given to having frequent colds and/or ear infections. For nosebleeds in children age two to twelve. (Younger, think of Silicea if symptoms match; older, think of Natrum Muriaticum, as well as Ferrum Phos and Silicea.)

Calcarea Phosphorica

Calcarea Phosphorica is the remedy to think of for patients who get nosebleeds in the afternoon, or whose nosebleeds are preceded or accompanied by a sensation of cold on the tip of the nose. Think of this remedy for cases in which a headache over one or both eyes accompanies the nosebleed. For cases of chronic sinus congestion in which the nose bleeds after it is blown clear of crusts. When nosebleeds are part blood, part mucus. Note that Calc Phos is, as always, our best preventive remedy. For patients who are chronically given to nosebleeds, give Calc Phos following nosebleeds and dur-ing the time between nosebleeds to reduce this tendency and strengthen the patient's whole system.

Calcarea Sulphurica

This is a general remedy for simple acute nosebleeds. Think of Calcarea Sulphurica when only one side of the nose is affected. This is a remedy to consider for a nosebleed that occurs at the end of a cold, when the patient's nose has been discharging yellow mucus, when the edges of the nostrils are sore from sneezing and blowing.

Kali Muriaticum

Kali Muriaticum is the other general remedy for nosebleeds that occur as part of a cold, when the nose has been blown and irritated. Consider this remedy as the alternative to Calc Sulph for cases in which the nasal discharge was white before the nosebleed. (The Calc Sulph discharge will be yellow.) It is a remedy for simple, acute nosebleeds. This is also the best general remedy for chronic nosebleeds that occur periodically, every few days, every week or every month, without a known cause. This is our best general remedy for a chronic tendency toward nosebleeds.

Natrum Muriaticum

Think of Natrum Muriaticum especially for cases of nosebleed that occur when the patient coughs, and that are associated with allergies and hay fever. Think of this remedy for nosebleeds that occur when the patient stoops or bends forward, when it happens if the patient puts his or her head down, face forward. This is an important remedy, along with Natrum Sulphuricum, for female patients who get nosebleeds during menses. It should also be consider for patients—again females especially—who have a tendency toward nosebleeds during puberty and into middle age. For nosebleeds that are accompanied by headache, by sinus congestion, and that tend to occur during the day, especially in the morning. In stubborn cases in female patients, combine or alternate it with Natrum Sulphuricum to bring relief.

Natrum Sulphuricum

Natrum Sulphuricum is a remedy for nosebleeds that are specific to female patients who have nosebleeds during menses. For patients whose nosebleeds occur during a headache in which there is a pronounced sensation of weight in the head. As always, the need for Natrum Sulph suggests one or both of two things: that the complaint is chronic in nature, and that the complaint is aggravated by damp. Both are also true in the case of nosebleeds. This is not often a remedy for a simple acute nosebleed (think of Ferrum Phos or Calc Phos or Calc Sulph for those), but is a good remedy especially for female patients who are chronically given to nosebleeds. These patients will quite often need Natrum Sulph given in combination with Natrum Muriaticum to achieve relief.

Silicea

Silicea is the remedy of choice for chronic nosebleeds in very young and very old patients. Consider this remedy for infants with nosebleed. (Ferrum Phosphoricum may be given first, as it usually is the first remedy tried—but Silicea will follow Ferrum Phos very well in these cases and will bring about a successful result.) Consider this remedy

first for children under two years of age. Consider this remedy as well for all cases of elderly patients who have a tendency toward nosebleeds. For cases of nosebleeds in elderly
patients who are depleted, who are chilly, who want to be wrapped for warmth, who
want their heads covered. For cases in which the headache is accompanied by head
sweat or pain in the bones of the face. For cases of nosebleed in any patient suffering
from a chronic, debilitating disease, a wasting disease. For nosebleeds in which the tip
of the nose is bright red, in which the tip of the nose itches.

Specific Remedies for Nosebleed

For nosebleeds that are brought on by blowing the nose: Natrum Muriaticum, Calcarea Phosphorica, Kali Muriaticum, Kali Sulphuricum, Natrum Sulphuricum, Ferrum
Phosphoricum, Silicea.

For nosebleeds that are brought on by coughing: Natrum Muriaticum, Ferrum Phosphoricum, Silicea.

For nosebleeds in patients who are anemic: Calcarea Phosphorica, Ferrum Phosphoricum, Natrum Muriaticum.

For nosebleeds that occur during fever: Ferrum Phosphoricum.

For nosebleeds that occur during headache: Ferrum Phosphoricum, Natrum Muriaticum, Natrum Sulphuricum, Calcarea Phosphorica.

For nosebleeds that occur when washing the face: Kali Muriaticum.

For nosebleeds that occur when stooping or bending: Natrum Muriaticum.

For nosebleeds that occur periodically: Kali Muriaticum, Natrum Muriaticum,
Natrum Sulphuricum.

If nosebleeds occur monthly as part of a woman's menses: Natrum Sulphuricum,
Natrum Muriaticum.

For nosebleeds with bright red blood: Ferrum Phosphoricum.

For nosebleeds with watery blood that is hard to clot: Natrum Muriaticum.

For nosebleeds in which the blood tastes acrid: Silicea.

For nosebleeds in which the blood tastes salty: Natrum Muriaticum.

For nosebleeds during the day, especially in the morning: Natrum Muriaticum.

For nosebleeds in the very early morning: Natrum Sulphuricum, Natrum Muriaticum.

For nosebleeds in the afternoon: Calcarea Phosphorica.

For nosebleeds in the nighttime: Kali Muriaticum.

For nosebleeds in infants: Silicea, Ferrum Phosphoricum.

For nosebleeds in young children: Ferrum Phosphoricum.

For nosebleeds in adolescents: Natrum Muriaticum, Ferrum Phosphoricum, Silicea.

For nosebleeds in the elderly: Silicea, Ferrum Phosphoricum.

For patients with a predisposition to nosebleeds: Calcarea Phosphorica, Kali Muriaticum, Silicea, Ferrum Phosphoricum.

Toothaches

This general category considers acute toothache, as well as sensitivity in teeth and teething pains (see section below). The remedies for toothache are Ferrum Phosphoricum, Magnesia Phosphorica, Silicea, Kali Muriaticum, Kali Phosphoricum, Kali Sulphuricum, Natrum Muriaticum, Calcarea Phosphorica, and Calcarea Fluorica, which is our best general remedy for loss of enamel or for teeth with weak enamel.

Note that all the remedies listed here work best for toothache if you dissolve them in hot or cold water—whichever the patient desires—and have the patient sip it, holding it over the painful place for a few seconds before swallowing it. Repeat this as needed until relief begins, then give the remedy only as needed. The cell salts cannot cure a decayed tooth and a trip to the dentist will still be required. However, they can get you through a hard night until you can get to the dentist. Also, used preventively, the calcium-based remedies can help strengthen teeth against decay and loss of enamel, especially when given to young children or pregnant women.

Note that looking at the tongue is always a good idea when dealing with any toothache.

Ferrum Phosphoricum

Think of Ferrum Phosphoricum for sudden acute toothaches, especially those associated with a red, swollen, and inflamed gum; when the cheek on the affected side is swollen, red, and hot; when the root of the tooth is inflamed and the whole of the affected area is hot, worse from heat and better from cold. When the patient wants to put ice against his or her cheek to relieve the pain. When the patient wants to chew ice or eat ice cream for the pain. Think of this remedy first for sudden toothache that appears without warning, especially for sudden toothache at night.

Magnesia Phosphorica

Magnesia Phosphorica is an excellent remedy for acute toothache if it follows the usual modalities suggested by the use of this remedy: the pain will be shooting, it will travel along a nerve or shift suddenly from place to place, tooth to tooth, until the patient is not sure which tooth is affected; it will be worse from cold and better from heat, so the patient will want hot applications on the skin or hot liquids in the mouth to relieve pain; and the pain will be relieved by pressure (pressing the hot application hard against the cheek) and made worse by forcing the patient to try and sit still to avoid pain. Although the pain is made worse from any motion, the patient may be driven to pace the floor by the intensity of the pain, making it worse and making the patient ever more frantic. This is the remedy for the sudden toothache that comes in the night that may occur when the patient is brushing his teeth or getting into bed, that may occur from taking cold water into the mouth, that may occur in a tooth that is already filled. This is not an inflammatory toothache—there is no swelling and/or redness associated with it. The sudden, acute toothache will, therefore, usually call for a choice between Ferrum Phos (better from cold, worse from hot, with inflammation) or Mag Phos (better from warmth, worse from cold, without inflammation).

Silicea

Silicea is the remedy to think of for the case of a toothache that may be sudden or slow in coming on, that may be acute or chronic in nature, but has a keynote characteristic: it is improved neither by cold nor by heat. Think of this remedy first for all cases of abscessed teeth, for cases in which a toothache is preceded or accompanied by a sensation of cold feet. When a toothache comes on as the result of the patient getting his or her feet cold or wet. This can be a very deep-seated pain, one that suggests chronic issues with the teeth in general and with the hard tissues of the body—specifically with the teeth, nails, and bones. This is commonly a toothache that is much worse at night, in which the pain is dull in the day, intense at night. In which nothing can be done to relieve the pain.

Kali Muriaticum

Kali Muriaticum is the remedy to consider for all cases of toothache that involve swelling of the gums, cheek, and/or jaw that does not involve heat or inflammation. Look to the patient's tongue for the characteristic white or gray-white coating that suggests the need for Kali Mur.

Kali Phosphoricum

Think of Kali Phosphoricum immediately for all cases in which the patient is overwrought and emotionally very intense in times of tooth pain. Especially for the patient whose face is very pale and whose gums are red—the gums may bleed or may have a red threadlike line along them—during the toothache. This is the remedy for the patient whose toothache begins when he grinds his teeth or who grinds his teeth during the toothache. For the patient who wants attention, who becomes very demanding, but who cannot be comforted when in pain. Just as the Mag Phos patient can become very worked up and will walk the floor in pain, the Kali Phos patient may scream and cry, may flail about, or may want to be carried or held during pain. Like Mag Phos (which can be given in combination or alternation with Kali Phos if the symptoms suggest both remedies), this is a patient who may get a toothache in a filled tooth. The tooth-ache may also be in a tooth that has crumbled or is severely decayed.

Kali Sulphuricum

Kali Sulphuricum is a remedy for only one instance of toothache: if the pain comes on or is aggravated by the patient as a whole being becoming warm, if it is worse when the patient is in a warm, enclosed room. When the patient seeks the comfort of fresh air, wants to open a window or go outside to relieve the pain. The need for a cold compress suggests Ferrum Phosphoricum, the need to go outside into cold air suggests Kali Sulph. Along with toothache, think of this remedy first for chronic inflammation of the gums or chronic gum pain.

Natrum Muriaticum

Natrum Muriaticum is a good general remedy for toothaches that are not as intense as others might be (Silicea, Ferrum Phos, Kali Phos, Mag Phos), but are worse in the day. They are best indicated by looking at the patient's tongue and mouth. Think of this remedy for toothaches in which the patient's tongue is clean, or in which the tongue and mouth are filled with saliva, or in which the tongue is covered by a coating of transparent mucus. Think of this remedy immediately for cases in which tears involun-tarily run down the patient's face during the toothache. Toothaches tend to throb, and the gums tend to bleed easily.

Calcarea Phosphorica

The calcium-based remedies are good for general tooth pains and the pains associated with teething and pregnancy. Calcarea Phosphorica is excellent for toothache that occurs during pregnancy (it is a good remedy in general to use during pregnancy, to maintain good health in the mother while encouraging strength and the creation of strong bones and teeth in the fetus). It is an excellent general remedy for toothache in patients who are chronically predisposed to tooth decay and can be used preventively to help lessen future toothaches by lessening tooth decay. This remedy tends to have toothaches in the afternoon and in the early evening. The pain tends to be boring in nature. The gums will also be painful and will either be very pale or very bright red.

Calcarea Fluorica

Think of Calcarea Fluorica first and foremost for cases of sensitive teeth, teeth that are aggravated by chewing, by being touched by food. This is the remedy to consider if the teeth, in general, feel loose, have lost enamel, or have developed weak enamel. This is a general remedy for sensitive teeth, for strengthening teeth, just as Calc Phos is for preventing tooth decay. The two remedies may be used together in combination or alternation (give Calc Fluor first thing in the morning and Calc Phos one hour after each meal) to strengthen teeth and bones, and both are especially suited to pregnant women.

Calcarea Sulphurica

Calcarea Sulphurica is associated with toothaches that involve abscesses, especially when the abscess or ulcer is filled with yellow pus and blood. Along with Silicea, this is our great remedy for tooth pain from abscesses. Think of this remedy for cases of chronic gum disease, when the gums bleed every time the patient brushes his or her teeth. When the gums, especially the inside of the gums, is sore and swollen. For chronic tooth and gum pain that is accompanied by swelling of the cheek. For inflammation of the tooth, gum, and tongue, when the base of the tongue is coated yellow. The pain may travel down into the patient's throat.

Specific Remedies for Toothache

For a toothache that is better from cold: Ferrum Phosphoricum. Kali Sulphuricum, Natrum Sulphuricum.

For a toothache that is better from cold food or drink or applications: Ferrum Phosphoricum.

For a toothache that is better from cool or open air: Kali Sulphuricum.

For a toothache that is better from very cold air: Natrum Sulphuricum.

For a toothache that is worse from cold in any form: Magnesia Phosphorica.

For a toothache that is worse specifically from the patient's feet becoming cold or wet: Silicea.

For a toothache that is better from heat: Magnesia Phosphorica.

For a toothache that is worse from the patient becoming warm or when in a warm room: Kali Sulphuricum.

For a toothache that is better from holding water in the mouth: Ferrum Phosphoricum, Natrum Sulphuricum.

For a toothache that comes on after eating warm food: Ferrum Phosphoricum.

For a toothache with inflammation: Ferrum Phosphoricum, Natrum Sulphuricum, Calcarea Sulphurica.

If inflammation is acute: Ferrum Phosphoricum.

If inflammation is chronic: Natrum Sulphuricum, Calcarea Sulphurica.

For a toothache without inflammation: Magnesia Phosphorica, Kali Muriaticum.

For a toothache accompanied by the swelling of the cheek: Ferrum Phosphoricum, Kali Muriaticum, Calcarea Sulphurica.

If swollen cheek is hot and red: Ferrum Phosphoricum.

For a toothache that comes on from sensitive teeth, from having food of any sort touch the teeth: Calcarea Fluorica.

For a toothache with abscess or ulceration: Silicea, Calcarea Sulphurica.

For a toothache associated with badly decayed teeth: Kali Phosphoricum, Calcarea Phosphorica.

If the toothache is in a filled tooth: Kali Phosphoricum, Magnesia Phosphorica.

For a toothache associated with weak enamel or worn enamel: Calcarea Fluorica, Calcarea Phosphorica.

To help harden enamel: Calcarea Fluorica, Magnesia Phosphorica.

For toothache associated with loose teeth: Calcarea Fluorica, Calcarea Phosphorica, Magnesia Phosphorica, Silicea.

If pain is accompanied by a flow of tears or saliva: Natrum Muriaticum.

If the pain is accompanied by or alternates with a headache: Kali Phosphoricum.

For pain associated with a trip to the dentist: Magnesia Phosphorica, Natrum Muriaticum, Natrum Sulphuricum.

If dental pain is especially severe: Kali Phosphoricum.

If dental pain travels along a nerve or shifts from place to place: Magnesia Phosphorica.

If dental pain involves inflammation: Ferrum Phosphoricum, Kali Phosphoricum.

Teething Pain

When an infant is teething, the entire household can share his misery. But there are some very simple cell salt treatments that can help everyone get some sleep.

Calcarea Phosphorica

Calcarea Phosphorica is the general remedy for teething. Think of it whenever any trouble arises concerning teething. Consider it if the teeth are late in coming in. Give Calc Phos and Calcarea Fluorica together for cases of slow development or for teeth with weak enamel. But no matter what other remedy or remedies you give, always give Calc Phos to the infant who is teething. Think of it first for all cases in which the infant is fussy, restless, and upset during the pain, for the patient who squirms and screams while you try to comfort him. From there, let the symptoms guide you.

Specific Remedies for Teething

If the pain associated with teething is improved by placing a cool compress against the cheek: Ferrum Phosphoricum. As always, this is the remedy for any sort of inflammation. Give this remedy if the cheek or gums are inflamed, are red, ho,t and swollen.

If the pain associated with teething is improved by placing warm compress against the cheek: Magnesia Phosphorica. Again, this is perhaps our single most effective remedy for pain, especially for pain, like teething, that shoots, that runs along a nerve.

If there are any gastric problems, especially diarrhea, that are associated with teething: Natrum Phosphoricum.

If there is an increase in saliva or stool or both during teething: Natrum Muriaticum.

If the patient is exhausted and depleted during teething: Silicea. Silicea and Calc Phosphoricum should be used in alternation or combination for the infant who is slow to develop, underweight, and, in general, weak. Also, these two remedies work well for any infant at the point at which the teething pains have stopped. They are good general remedies to keep in mind for any child who struggles with his or her development, is underweight, or has a tendency toward illness, especially respiratory illness. (Note that, if that tendency is toward underdevelopment of bones and other hard tissues, use Calc Phos and Calcarea Fluorica.)

If the patient is out of control emotionally, if he or she is screaming and writhing and cannot be comforted and Ferrum Phos or Mag Phos has failed to work: Kali Phosphoricum should be added into the mix.

Headaches

In all honesty, headaches are hard to treat, especially acute headaches. Once they have begun, they are hard to dismiss without swallowing a pill. This has led many to throw in the towel and reach for the aspirin. But though the cell salts may not give immediate relief from any given headache, they are excellent remedies for those who suffer from chronic headaches. Taken for a period of time, they will lead to fewer and fewer headaches or to headaches that are milder and milder, until the patient realizes one day that he doesn't get them the way he used to. In these cases, the cell salts are remarkable remedies, as they offer a solution to a problem that allopathic medicine can only cover with a temporary analgesic.

The chief remedies for headaches are Natrum Muriaticum, Magnesia Phosphorica, Ferrum Phosphoricum, and Kali Phosphoricum. Other remedies for patients with headaches include Kali Muriaticum, Kali Sulphuricum, Natrum Phosphoricum, Natrum Sulphuricum, Calcarea Phosphorica, Calcarea Sulphurica, and Silicea.

Natrum Muriaticum

Natrum Muriaticum is our general remedy for patients with headaches, especially for patients who chronically have a predisposition toward having headaches. These can range from headaches that are dull, slightly achy, that lead the patient to want to lie down, to migraines that send the patient into his or her bed for a period of hours or days. For the classic "sick" headache in which the patient cannot bear light, sound, or human contact; in which the patient must withdraw from everything that he or she finds dear. Think of this for all headaches in the forehead that involve a sensation of weight or congestion in the frontal sinuses. For headaches that accompany constipation or that come monthly before a female patient's cycle (these headaches can also come monthly during or just after the flow). For headaches that chronically begin when the patient arises from bed in the early morning and grow worse as the sun rises over the horizon, worse through the morning, and that begin to improve as the sun sets. Headaches in which the patient's tongue is covered with transparent mucus, or in which the patient's tongue is perfectly clean but the mouth is filled with saliva. Headaches during which tears trail down the patient's face. Think of this remedy for the patient who has frequent headaches and for whom resting, even napping, only makes the headache worse. Think of this remedy for all headaches, acute or chronic. Chances are that, unless another remedy is specifically indicated, Natrum Mur will do some good.

Ferrum Phosphoricum

Ferrum Phosphoricum is one of two remedies that I can suggest for acute treatment of headaches. Think of this remedy for any headache that, very simply, is improved if the patient puts a cold compress on his or her head. Think of Ferrum Phos for any headache during which the patient's face is flushed and hot, especially if the patient's eyes are red and inflamed during headache pain. These are headaches that can come on from too much exposure to sun and heat (also, ironically, from too much exposure to cold, such as a headache after skiing on a sunny day). The headaches are bruising in character and the pain is made worse if this patient moves, especially if he moves his head forward or downward. Headaches in which the patient cannot bear any pressure against his head; cannot bear even to have his hair touched. Ferrum Phos headaches tend to be worse on the right side of the head, and often are located in a single spot on the head (that spot will be relieved by the application of ice). These headaches are congestive and inflammatory. Consider Ferrum Phos always for all headaches that occur during fever. Also consider Ferrum Phos as the first remedy for any headache that comes on after a mechanical injury to the head. Finally, think of this remedy for violent migraines that follow the indicating symptoms, especially if the headache causes the patient to vomit undigested food.

Magnesia Phosphorica

Magnesia Phosphorica is our other great remedy for acute headaches. Think of this remedy for headaches in which the pain is relieved by applications of heat and by pressure. When the patient pushes the compress hard against his head or even presses his head hard against a wall or pillow. As Mag Phos is a remedy for pain, it is an excellent general remedy for headaches if they follow the remedy's general pattern. Think of it especially for headaches in which the pain shifts around, and for headaches that come on suddenly and leave just as suddenly. Think of Mag Phos for all headaches in which the patient's vision is affected by the pain. When the patient sees shapes or sparks or flashes of color just before or during the headache. When the patient sees double during headache. When the patient cannot bear cold and the pain is worse from any contact with cold. When the pain is made worse by any motion, but is also worse if the patient lies down flat. When the pain drives the patient out of bed and forces him or her to walk the floor or to sit tall in a chair, staying as still as possible. Also think of this remedy for the patient who has chronic headaches, as long as they come in spells. Give Magnesia Phosphorica during headaches and Calcarea Phosphorica between headaches to act preventively.

Kali Phosphoricum

Think of Kali Phosphoricum for acute or chronic headaches in overly sensitive patients, in patients who are sensitive and overly reactive to everything in their environment: to light and noise, but also to emotion, to color, and to things that the patient finds ugly. Unlike most other remedies for pain, Kali Phos offers two symptoms that will often guide you to the remedy. First, the Kali Phos headache is improved if the patient moves about gently and gingerly. The Kali Phos may walk about slowly, sway or even dance while in pain, as it relieves the pain. Second, the Kali Phos is not made nauseous by the headache, as is the case with headaches that are relieved by most other remedies—quite the opposite, in fact. The Kali Phos may become hungry during the headache, may eat and find that the pain is relieved by eating. Often, the Kali Phos' headache pain will be accompanied by a sensation of total emptiness in his stomach and he will feel that he must eat. He will be driven to eat and should be allowed to do so. The Kali Phos headache is often accompanied by noises in the ear, especially by loud humming or buzzing sounds. It is almost always accompanied by or followed by a sensation of total exhaustion. The Kali Phos may stay up walking, moving about, and eating during the pain and then lie down following it, exhausted by the pain after the fact. Look at the patient's tongue as an indication of the remedy: the Kali Phos will have a tongue that is yellow, usually a rather dark-yellow, even brownish tongue, and will often have bad breath or body odor that accompanies the pain.

Kali Muriaticum

Always think of Kali Muriaticum if the patient vomits during the headache and if the patient vomits white mucus. Think of Kali Mur for the patient whose tongue is coated white or whitish-gray during the headache. This is a general remedy for those who suffer from headaches, most commonly for those who have frequent, sick headaches that are accompanied by nausea and by an inability to handle even the thought of food (Silicea will share this symptom). Look at the patient's face during the headache. If his or her face seems devoid of emotion but looks swollen, haggard, and pale, think of Kali Muriaticum.

Kali Sulphuricum

Kali Sulphuricum is not often indicated for headaches, but it is easy to recognize when it is called for. Think of Kali Sulph for headaches in which the patient cannot bear to be in a warm room or in an enclosed space. When the patient must open a window, or, more commonly, go outside for a walk to help him feel better. Think of this remedy when the headache comes on or grows worse in the early evening, when the patient walks off into the sunset to relieve himself of his headache pain.

Natrum Phosphoricum

Like the other sodium-based remedies, the headaches that respond to Natrum Phos tend to come on in the early morning. Either the patient will awaken with the headache or it will begin just as he or she gets up out of bed. These are headaches with the characteristics of congestion and throbbing. The patient will feel as if his or her head is too full, as if the pain is located deep within the skull, as if something is pressed up against the skull from within, pushing to get out. The headaches are commonly in the forehead or occiput, but can involve the entire head. Natrum Phos follows Ferrum Phosphoricum very well for congestive and inflammatory headaches when Ferrum Phos alone fails to cure. Look to the patient's tongue as an indicator of the remedy. Look for a creamy yellow-white coating on the tongue and in the back of the mouth.

Think of Natrum Phos as the remedy for patients who are lactose intolerant and who get headaches when they eat dairy.

Natrum Sulphuricum

Natrum Sulphuricum is the remedy to think of when headaches, especially chronic headaches, get really severe. Think of this remedy when motion brings agony. When the patient cannot even move his or her eyes without having terrible pain. When the patient cannot read anything during a headache. For headaches that are accompanied by a sensation of vertigo, when the room swims and spins during the headache. Like Natrum Mur and Natrum Phos, Natrum Sulph headaches tend to come on in the early morning. The patient will awaken with the headache, or, in this case, be awakened by it. Consider this remedy for all cases of chronic headache when a change in the weather from dry to damp brings on a headache. For headaches that come on as storms approach. For headaches that occur periodically, as part of a woman's monthly cycle, or that arrive every spring, or are especially worse during snow melt in the transition from winter to spring. For headaches that come on or are aggravated if the patient gets cold and wet. These are congestive headaches: the patient feels a rush of blood into the head, feels his pulse pounding in his head. The patient will feel the pain especially at the top of his head. These are headaches that, like Natrum Mur's, begin in the morning and last all day. They begin to improve at bedtime, as the patient lies down in bed at night. Like the other Natrums, Natrum Sulphuricum is improved by quiet, by being left alone. Look at the patient's tongue—the Natrum Sulph tongue is coated with a greenish coat. It can be greenish-yellow or greenish-gray, but look for the color green. This headache can lead to retching, to vomiting.

Calcarea Phosphorica

Calcarea Phosphorica is an excellent general remedy for headaches, whether acute or chronic. Like Natrum Muriaticum, the mere presence of a headache suggests the possible need for this remedy. Sometimes it is used most effectively for headaches in which there are no distinct symptoms. When you have no clear idea of a remedy to give, give Calc Phos. Think of this remedy in all cases of headaches in sensitive patients, especially in young patients. Think of this for patients who are affected deeply by change. For headaches that come on in spells, frequent for a time, during changes in weather or life situation. For headaches that come on in the child when the parents argue. For the child who has frequent headaches when his or her parents are getting a divorce. For the child who has headaches when he does not want to go to school, to speak in public, to do anything that threatens or frightens him. Think of this remedy for adult patients as well, who follow the same pattern of avoidance. The headaches associated with Calc Phos are not as severe as those of remedy types such as Natrum Sulphuricum or Magnesia

Phosphorica. They are headaches in restless people, who feel better from motion, worse from either heat or cold. The pain is also worse from pressure or touch. The patient does not want anything to touch or press against his or her head. Calc Phos headaches follow the same unique pattern of head symptoms that the remedy carries elsewhere: the patient's head will feel cold to the touch in the Calc Phos headache.

Calcarea Sulphurica

Calcarea Sulphurica is less commonly used for headaches than some of the other remedies, yet it has a unique niche. In general, this is a headache with nausea and with vertigo. It is a headache in which the patient's eyes go blank and seem to recede into the head. In which the pain starts in the forehead and radiates out from there to enclose the whole head. But think of this remedy especially for cases that are similar to the Calc Phos. Just as in the section on acne suggests, Calc Phos and Calc Sulph are companion remedies for young patients. Where the Calc Phos's eyes will shine when he or she has a headache, the Calc Sulph's will retreat; his or her being will pull in, while the Calc Phos's pushes out. So when you have a young patient who is suddenly having headaches, look at these two remedies and see which is the better match. Or consider the gender link, and think first of Calc Phos for young girls who are given to headaches, and Calc Sulph for young boys. This simple differentiation will not always hold up, but it will surprise you how often it does.

Silicea

Silicea headaches are almost always chronic and almost always linked to imperfect digestion. Silicea headaches may be the result of food allergies or environmental allergies or linked to chronic diseases of the digestion or to chronic wasting diseases, but they very seldom exist without a panoply of other symptoms and conditions also being present. Think of this remedy for cases of chronic headache in young or old patients, in patients with slim limbs, in patients who are chronically weak and chilly. For headaches that are linked to foot sweat or head sweat, that may be worse from foot sweat or from the patient's feet getting cold or wet. For headaches that may be improved or greatly aggravated by head sweat. For headaches in which the patient wants to wear a hat or wrap his head during the pain. Other than his head and/or feet, the patient's skin is totally dry. His complexion will look sickly during headache. In a more acute sphere, these are headaches that come on from overwork or over-study. For headaches in college students just before, during, or after finals. For headaches that accompany times of great stress or challenge, when the system is pushed past the level of what it can usually accomplish. This is also the remedy to think of (for all issues, not just headaches) for caregivers who put their own needs aside for the sake of the patient. Who do not look to their own needs in terms of food and rest for the sake of others, and who are weak, tired and in pain as a result. Silicea and Natrum Muriaticum together work very well for patients who are chronically given to headaches, especially if those headaches come to define their lives, causing them to retreat from the world into their room.

Specific Remedies for Headaches

For acute headaches: Ferrum Phosphoricum, Magnesia Phosphorica, Calcarea Phosphorica, Calcarea Sulphurica, Kali Phosphoricum, Natrum Muriaticum.

For chronic headaches: Natrum Muriaticum, Silicea, Calcarea Phosphorica, Calcarea Sulphuricum, Natrum Phosphoricum, Natrum Sulphuricum

If chronic headaches come in clustered in a specific period of time: Calcarea Phosphorica, Calcarea Sulphuricum.

If chronic headaches are also periodic: Natrum Sulphuricum, Magnesia Phosphorica.

If chronic headaches are better in the open air: Calcarea Sulphurica, Kali Sulphuricum.

If chronic headaches are linked to seasonal change: Natrum Sulphuricum.

If chronic headaches are linked to changes in the weather: Natrum Sulphuricum, Calcarea Phosphorica.

For headaches that are worse from cold: Magnesia Phosphorica, Calcarea Phosphorica.

For headaches that are worse in a cold room: Silicea, Natrum Muriaticum.

For headaches that are worse from warm: Ferrum Phosphoricum, Calcarea Phosphorica.

For headaches that are worse in a warm room: Kali Sulphuricum.

For headaches that are worse from sleeping: Natrum Muriaticum, Natrum Phosphoricum, Natrum Sulphuricum.

For headaches that are worse from lack of sleep: Kali Phosphoricum.

For headaches that are worse from motion: Ferrum Phosphoricum, Magnesia Phosphorica, Natrum Sulphuricum, Kali Sulphuricum.

For headaches that are worse from motion of the head: Ferrum Phosphoricum, Natrum Sulphuricum, Kali Sulphuricum.

For headaches that are worse even from the motion of the eyes: Natrum Sulphuricum.

For headaches that are worse from pressure against the head: Ferrum Phosphoricum, Calcarea Phosphorica.

For headaches that are better from pressure against the head: Magnesia Phosphorica, Silicea.

If the headache is better after a nosebleed: Kali Phosphoricum.

For headaches that are better from eating: Kali Phosphoricum, Natrum Phosphoricum.

For headaches that are worse from eating: Ferrum Phosphoricum, Natrum Sulphuricum, Natrum Muriaticum.

For headaches that are worse from light: Silicea, Kali Phosphoricum, Natrum Muriaticum, Natrum Sulphuricum, Natrum Phosphoricum.

For headaches that are worse from noise: Silicea, Ferrum Phosphoricum, Kali Phosphoricum.

For headaches that are better from soft, beautiful music: Kali Phosphoricum, Natrum Muriaticum.

For headaches with nausea: Silicea, Calcarea Sulphurica, Natrum Phosphoricum, Natrum Sulphuricum, Natrum Muriaticum, Ferrum Phosphoricum, Magnesia Phosphorica.

If nausea is accompanied by a sensation of chill: Magnesia Phosphorica, Silicea.

If nausea and hunger are combined: Kali Phosphoricum, Silicea.

For headaches with hunger: Kali Phosphoricum.

For headaches without hunger: Natrum Muriaticum, Magnesia Phosphorica, Ferrum Phosphoricum, Calcarea Phosphorica.

For headaches with vomiting: Natrum Muriaticum, Natrum Sulphuricum, Ferrum Phosphoricum, Natrum Phosphoricum, Kali Muriaticum, Calcarea Phosphorica.

If vomiting undigested food: Ferrum Phosphoricum, Natrum Phosphoricum.

If vomiting white mucus: Kali Muriaticum.

If vomiting yellow mucus: Natrum Phosphoricum.

If vomiting green mucus: Natrum Sulphuricum.

If vomiting water or clear mucus: Natrum Muriaticum, Calcarea Phosphorica.

For headaches with constipation: Natrum Muriaticum, Kali Muriaticum.

For headaches with diarrhea: Natrum Sulphuricum.

For headaches with flatulence: Calcarea Phosphorica.

For headaches with belching or hiccoughs: Magnesia Phosphorica.

For headaches with yawning: Kali Phosphoricum.

For headaches with red or inflamed eyes: Ferrum Phosphoricum.

For headaches during which tears run down the face: Natrum Muriaticum.

For headaches with changes in vision: Magnesia Phosphorica.

For headaches from reading: Silicea, Natrum Muriaticum, Natrum Sulphuricum.

For headaches from watching television: Calcarea Phosphorica.

For headaches with chills up and down the spine: Magnesia Phosphorica.

For headaches with chills in the feet: Silicea.

For headaches with a cool or chilly feeling in the head: Calcarea Phosphorica, Silicea.

For headaches in which the external head is cool to the touch: Calcarea Phosphorica.

For headaches in which the external face and head are hot to the touch: Ferrum Phosphoricum.

For headaches with dizziness or vertigo: Natrum Sulphuricum, Ferrum Phosphoricum, Silicea, Calcarea Sulphurica.

For headaches combined with a sensation of weight or heaviness: Natrum Muriaticum.

For headaches combined with a sense of sleepiness: Natrum Muriaticum.

For headaches combined with a sense of sleeplessness: Ferrum Phosphoricum, Kali Phosphoricum.

If the patient is exhausted, but still sleepless: Kali Phosphoricum.

For headaches accompanied by forgetfulness: Calcarea Phosphorica.

For headaches accompanied by irritability: Kali Phosphoricum.

For headaches accompanied by despondency: Kali Phosphoricum.

For headaches associated with menstruation: Natrum Sulphuricum, Natrum Muriaticum, Calcarea Sulphurica, Kali Phosphoricum, Ferrum Phosphoricum.

For headaches before or during menses: Calcarea Sulphurica, Ferrum Phosphoricum, Kali Phosphoricum, Natrum Muriaticum.

For headaches after menses: Natrum Muriaticum, Natrum Sulphuricum.

For headaches in the whole head: Calcarea Sulphurica, Natrum Phosphoricum, Natrum Sulphuricum, Ferrum Phosphoricum, Kali Phosphoricum.

For headaches in the forehead: Silicea, Natrum Muriaticum, Natrum Phosphoricum, Natrum Sulphuricum, Calcarea Sulphurica.

For headaches in the temples: Natrum Muriaticum, Natrum Phosphoricum.

For headaches in the back of the head: Natrum Sulphuricum, Natrum Phosphoricum, Kali Phosphoricum, Magnesia Phosphorica, Silicea.

For headaches at the top of the head: Natrum Sulphuricum, Ferrum Phosphoricum, Magnesia Phosphorica, Natrum Muriaticum.

For headaches in which the pain shifts: Magnesia Phosphorica, Kali Sulphuricum.

For headaches in which the pain extends into the spine: Magnesia Phosphorica.

For headaches in which the pain extends into the neck: Magnesia Phosphorica, Silicea.

For headaches that come on in the early morning, waking the patient: Natrum Sulphuricum.

For headaches that come on in the morning, when the patient awakens: Natrum Muriaticum, Natrum Phosphoricum, Natrum Sulphuricum.

For headaches that grow worse from early morning until noon: Natrum Muriaticum.

For headaches that are worse in daytime in general: Natrum Muriaticum.

For headaches that are worse or begin in the afternoon: Calcarea Phosphorica.

For headaches that are worse or begin in the evening: Kali Sulphuricum.

For headaches that are worse or begin late at night or in the early morning hours, waking the patient from sleep: Natrum Sulphuricum.

For headaches with bruising pain: Ferrum Phosphoricum, Kali Muriaticum, Natrum Muriaticum, Kali Phosphoricum, Calcarea Phosphorica.

For headaches with throbbing pain: Natrum Muriaticum.

For headaches with shooting pains: Magnesia Phosphorica, Natrum Muriaticum, Silicea.

For headaches with boring pain: Natrum Muriaticum, Magnesia Phosphorica, Ferrum Phosphoricum, Kali Phosphoricum, Kali Sulphuricum, Natrum Sulphuricum.

If the headache pain is as if a nail were being driven into the head: Natrum Muriaticum, Ferrum Phosphoricum, Magnesia Phosphorica.

For headaches with a hammering pain: Natrum Muriaticum.

For headaches with bursting pain: Natrum Phosphoricum, Natrum Sulphuricum, Kali Muriaticum, Kali Phosphoricum, Kali Sulphuricum, Silicea, Natrum Muriaticum, Calcarea Sulphurica.

For headaches with a dull, aching pain: Natrum Muriaticum, Calcarea Phosphorica, Kali Muriaticum, Kali Sulphuricum, Kali Phosphoricum, Silicea.

For migraines: Natrum Muriaticum, Ferrum Phosphoricum, Magnesia Phosphorica, Kali Phosphoricum, Natrum Phosphoricum, Natrum Sulphuricum, Silicea. Note that a migraine will usually take more than one remedy to relieve. Choose Natrum Muriaticum and either Ferrum Phos or Mag Phos, whichever is better indicated, and give the remedies as soon as possible, unless specific symptoms guide you to another remedy. Give Calcarea Phosphorica and/or Silicea following the migraine to restore strength and act preventively.

Insomnia

There are four major remedies for sleeplessness among the cell salts. They are Ferrum Phosphoricum, Magnesia Phosphorica, Kali Phosphoricum and Natrum Muriaticum. But other cell salts are used as well. Among these are Kali Muriaticum, Natrum Phosphoricum, Calcarea Phosphorica, and Calcarea Fluorica.

Ferrum Phosphoricum

Ferrum Phosphoricum is very interesting when it comes to sleep, as it seems to cause the opposite reaction to what the patient usually experiences. Therefore, look for it to be an excellent remedy, almost a sleeping pill, for those who chronically cannot sleep. It will knock them right out and works well as an acute remedy for chronic insomnia. It will also work well in cases of acute insomnia, most often when the insomnia is associated with a physical illness that includes inflammation and/or fever or as the aftereffect of excitement. But be aware that, when used in patients who usually sleep quite well, it may have the effect of making them sleepless. So use Ferrum Phos carefully at bedtime, since it may cause a sleepless night.

Magnesia Phosphorica

It is easy to know when to use Magnesia Phosphorica for sleeplessness. This is the remedy for the manic patient. For the patient who walks the floor in sleeplessness. Who cannot or will not stay in bed, but gets up to sit in a chair or to pace the floor the whole night through. These are patients in deep emotional turmoil or extreme upset. Who are too angry to sleep, too fearful of what will happen the next day. This is the sleeplessness caused by dread, by bitterness, and by terror. Think of this remedy after a patient has received bad news that causes sleeplessness. Think of this remedy when physical pain accompanies emotional distress on sleepless nights. Note that most often this is the remedy of an adult who cannot sleep. A child in the same emotional state may do better with Kali Phosphoricum, which is a more high-strung remedy type, as opposed to the intense Mag Phos. However, the two remedies work well together in combination or alternation for cases of insomnia.

Kali Phosphoricum

Kali Phosphoricum is our best general remedy and the first that should be considered and used for all cases of insomnia, acute or, especially, chronic, in which the patient has trouble getting to sleep. When the patient is overstimulated or becomes overstimulated very easily. When the television works him or her up, or when music, company, ideas, colors, foods stimulate patients into sleeplessness. (Think of this when caffeine keeps you awake) Think of this remedy for cases in which worry, especially worry over money, leads to sleeplessness. Think of this remedy when physical exercise results in sleeplessness. And think of this remedy for the patient who has to get up and urinate time and again during the night, resulting in a poor night's sleep. This is the first remedy to think of for all cases of disturbed sleep as well, when sleep is not refreshing, although the patient stays asleep. Think of this as well for all cases of sleepwalking. It can be helpful for cases in which the patient awakens suddenly from a nightmare and must be comforted in order to go back to sleep. The Kali Phos dreams of fire above all things, but also dreams of burglars, of ghosts, of monsters. Suffice it to say, this remedy is excellent for young patients who do not want to go to sleep and who awaken with night terrors.

Natrum Muriaticum

Natrum Muriaticum is the remedy for the insomniac who can get to sleep just fine, but who awakens in the night and cannot get back to sleep. Who awakens again and again at three or four in the morning, who stares at the ceiling before giving up and getting up. Think of this remedy for the person who, exhausted, gets up early, trudges through the day, goes to bed after dinner, falls into a deep exhausted sleep complete with snoring and with a flow of saliva to the pillow, and then awakens again for no apparent reason in the middle of the night. This is an excellent remedy for those who have chronic issues with staying asleep for the full night. It is an excellent remedy for middle-aged or older patients, especially post-menopausal women, who have chronic sleep issues. Think of it as well for restless sleepers who toss and turn in the night.

Kali Muriaticum

Kali Muriaticum is a good remedy for an acute occasion of insomnia, but it is more important as a remedy for the chronic case. Think of this remedy in the specific case of the patient who is a very light sleeper. Who can be awakened by any change in temperature, by any noise, by light, and who, once awakened, cannot go back to sleep. This is the remedy for those who awaken suddenly, quite sure that they have heard someone downstairs. These are restless sleepers, light sleepers, who keep the whole house from sleeping soundly.

Natrum Phosphoricum

Natrum Phosphoricum has a specific use. Think of Natrum Phos for cases in which the patient is physically too tired to sleep. In which the patient is exhausted beyond his or her endurance, but cannot go to sleep. It is an excellent acute remedy for sleeplessness. In its chronic use, think of this remedy for the patient who is kept awake by heartburn, by acidity.

Calcarea Phosphorica

Calcarea Phosphorica is an excellent general remedy for sleeplessness. For times in which the patient is tired, stretches, yawns, is all but asleep in his or her chair at the dinner table, but who is wide awake in bed by the time he or she makes it through the preparations for sleep. This remedy is excellent for those who chronically have trouble sleeping. For those who cannot sleep in times of change, who are kept awake by worry, by the feeling that "Something bad is about to happen." It is our best remedy for sleeplessness in the elderly. It is to older patients what Kali Phosphoricum is to young patients. It offers calm, centered sleep to those who cannot relax into it themselves.

Calcarea Fluorica

Calcarea Fluorica contrasts with Kali Phosphoricum, in that it also involves dreams. But where the Kali Phos is awakened from nightmares and is very upset, Calc Fluor patients have dreams that are noisy, vivid, colorful, but not nightmarish. Instead, these dreams are sweeping vistas that move them, and that then elude them after they awaken from them suddenly. Think of this remedy for those times when the patient awakens suddenly from a dream other than a nightmare and cannot get back to sleep. This is an excellent acute remedy for these occasions.

Appendix

The Simple Logic of Dr. Schuessler's Biochemic Theory

1. The human body contains twelve vital inorganic elements which are responsible for maintenance of normal cell-function.

2. When from some cause, one or more of these elements become deficient the normal cell-function or metabolism is disturbed and a condition arises known as disease.

3. By supplying to the system the lacking elements in the form of Schuessler Biochemic Remedies normal cell-function and health can be restored.

—J. B. CHAPMAN, M.D.,
DR. SCHUESSLER'S BIOCHEMISTRY

Resource Guide
to the Cell Salts

Because the number of books, Internet sites, and pharmacies that are dedicated to the cell salts are limited, it is important to try and gather together as much information as possible on the topic. Here, to my knowledge, are the best resources available on the biochemic remedies.

Books

As is common with books on homeopathy, many of those available today on the subject of the cell salts are reprints of earlier editions that were brought back into print by the Indian publishing house, B. Jain. As they are reprints, the dates of the edition may differ from mine because the date of a reprint is not always static (more copies of that same work may be printed again). So stay true to the title and the author when B. Jain is the publisher and you will be getting the right book.

Note also that different books offer different versions of the spelling of Schuessler's name and the name of his system of therapeutics. They are variously called cell salts, tissue salts, biochemic medicine, and biochemistry. All are the same thing, just as Schuessler and Schussler are the same man.

Finally, note that I have placed these books in what could loosely be called their order of importance, with the best books on the subject (in my opinion, at least) listed first, and some of the more entertaining but less useful works listed toward the bottom of the list.

The Twelve Tissue Remedies of Schussler, by William Boericke, M.D. and Willis A. Dewey, M.D., New Delhi, India: B. Jain Publishers, Ltd. (1987). This is the bible when it comes to the cell salts. Everyone who studies them or uses them owes a debt to Boericke and Dewey for this book. It offers a complete guide to each remedy as well as a repertory of the symptoms. Originally published back in 1914, this book has the same sense of completion and organization that Boericke offered in his *Pocket Manual of Homeopathic Materia Medica* for homeopathic remedies—a book that is still in common use today. If you are going to only get one book on the cell salts (excluding mine, of course), get this one.

Natural Healing with Cell Salts, by Skye Weintraub, N.D., Pleasant Grove, Utah: Woodland Publishing, Inc. (1999). This is an excellent little book. It runs in alphabetical order, which I always find a bit odd, so if you want to find a sore throat, you don't deal with a section on the throat or on upper respiratory conditions, but, instead, you look under "S." That works well as long as you and Weintraub agree on the way the condition should be worded. If you don't, you have to leaf through the book until you find what you are looking for. But my criticism over the structure of the book aside, it is a simple to understand, easy to use guide to the cell salts. The bulk of the book is a list of conditions and tips on how to use the cells salts to address them. What it lacks is a good materia medica of the cell salts (instead we get a couple of paragraphs on each and a page or two on how to use the remedies). At the end of the book are a couple of very brief case studies that seem to have been an afterthought.

The Biochemical Treatment of Disease, by W. H. Schuessler, M.D., New Delhi, India: B. Jain Publishers, Ltd. (2004). Now you would think this is the definitive book on the subject, as it is authored by the man who created the biochemic system of medicine. Instead it is a small book, under one hundred pages, that gives a scant few sentences on each remedy, a few quotes from Moleschott, and then lists conditions and gives tips on what remedy or remedies to give for each. This is not a particularly good book, nor is it a helpful one, in my opinion.

Schussler's Bio Chemic Pocket Guide with Repertory, by W. H. Schuessler, M.D., New Delhi, India: B. Jain Publishers, Ltd. (2004). No author is directly credited for this book, but the information in it seems to have been edited out of the *Biochemical Treatment of Disease* (see above), so Schuessler should get the credit. This is truly a pocket guide, very small, with the usual lack of information on the remedies and the appropriate way in which they are to be used. Instead, the book's seventy-five or so pages are dedicated to listing ailments and remedies, ailments and remedies. This is the sort of book that you get when the creator of a system has been dead for a long time and his works are in the public domain. Skip it.

Biochemic Tissue Salts: A Natural Way to Prevent and Cure Illness, by Andrew Stanway, M.B., M.R.C.P., Wellingborough, Northamptonshire, England: Thorsons Publishing Group (1982). This is a good little book. Long before the Internet came to be what it is today, Stanway somehow knew to structure his little book in the form of FAQs (the "frequently asked questions" that are listed on nearly every web page). His short chapters have titles like, "Where can I obtain the tissue salts?" and "Do people actually use them?" which I find particularly appealing. This is a little book that is crammed with solid, practical information. Should you come across it, it is worth a look.

Dr. Schuessler's Biochemistry: Twelve Biochemistry Remedies, A New Domestic Treatise, A Medical Book for Every Home, by J. B. Chapman, M.D., New Delhi, India: B. Jain Publishers Ltd. (2001). The title says it all. Actually, Chapman's book is one of the most respected on the topic of the cell salts and is quite good. He gives a very brief history of the salts, but does manage to work cell theory into it, and then gives brief sketches on the salts themselves, before giving an alphabetical listing of ailments and remedies. The best thing about this book is that it is based on Chapman's own work, and not on the pool of common knowledge on the salts, so some of the indicated remedies will be quite different from those in the other books available. If Chapman's methods work for you, it will be a valuable book to have. Note, however, that since this is a reprint of an older book, some of the language will be archaic to those who have not already studied homeopathy, so have an old medical dictionary nearby.

The Biochemic Handbook: How to Get Well and Keep Fit with Biochemic Tissue Salts, by J. B. Chapman, M.D. and Edward L. Perry, M.D., St. Louis, Missouri: Formur, Incorporated—Publishers, (1994). This is a reprint of the classic work *Biochemic Theory and Practice,* by the same authors, that was published by Luyties back in 1920. It is one of Chapman's best known works and contains the usual introduction to the remedies, the list of remedies, and a long list of ailments paired with suggested remedies.

Unique Combinations with Clinical Cases in Homeopathy and Biochemistry, Volumes 1 and 2, by R. L. Gupta, M.D., New Delhi, India: B. Jain Publishers, Ltd. (1996). What is extremely good about this book is that it takes its subject very seriously indeed. This is not a pocket manual or home guide. Instead, as the subhead suggests, is it a "Practitioner's Manual" that wastes no time giving basic information on the cell salts. Instead, it launches into in-depth case studies that will appeal to both serious students of homeopathy and biochemistry and medical professionals alike. The second volume is dedicated to a repertory of sorts that, while complete, offers nothing new in the way of information. Still, it is an excellent book to have at the ready and it will give those who want a deeper understanding of the cell salts a source of just that kind of information.

Repertory & Materia Medica of the Biochemic Remedies, by S. R. Phatak, M.D., New Delhi, India: B. Jain Publishers, Ltd. (1997). This is an updated version of the 1937 volume by Dr. S. R. Phatak, who one can only assume is the father of Dr. S. R. Phatak. The preface promises that the work has been reorganized into alphabetical order and, apparently, edited and fleshed out. The result is a handy volume that contains a good repertory that is structured like many modern homeopathic repertories, in alphabetical order, followed by a materia medica that is rather brief and to the point, all just as the title promises. While not the best book on the subject, it is certainly a worthy volume for those who want to have the full range of research available today.

Gems of Bio-Chemic Materia Medica, by J.D. Patil, M.D., New Delhi, India: B. Jain Publishers, Ltd. (1999). This is a practical, helpful look at the cell salts that is well thought out, well researched and organized very well to boot. Patil gives a really good background on biochemic medicine and solid information on how the minerals that become the cell salts function in the human body and what shifts in impact occur once potentization takes place. He looks at some of the families from which the remedies are made and at the remedies themselves, and concludes with a good glossary. This is a good reference work to have on your shelf.

Facial Diagnosis of Cell Salt Deficiencies: A User's Guide, by David R. Card, Prescott, Arizona: Hohm Press, (2005). I was most interested in the concept of this book and ordered a copy when I first heard about it. This is a large, oversized paperback that, while crammed with information on the cell salts (some of it is rather reminiscent of Carey's *Salts of Salvation*, as sections of that book on the individual remedies and astrological signs are lifted whole—this is not an act of deceit, by the way, as Carey encourages anyone to do just that), has a basic weakness, to me at least, which has to do with the reason for the book in the first place. Its purpose is to present color photographs that show just what the faces of individuals needing certain remedies would look like in terms of color, swelling, and so on. I thought this sounded great. The photos, however, were of little help, at least to me, because I could never see what it was that the author was indicating. In the end, I decided it is actually more helpful to simply describe in words what to look for and what you will find, especially when it comes to the tongue. By the way, I was also amazed that the author chose not to show the tongues of the different remedy types, as that might have actually photographed well and as this one part of the body is such a strong indicator of the different types. All told, while this book does have some good, solid information, it is a disappointment in terms of the photos.

Zodiac and the Salts of Salvation, by George Washington Carey and Inez Eudora Perry, York Beach, Maine: Samuel Weiser, Inc. (1932) may be the most famous book on the subject—or at least it was a few years back when the "New Age" was in its ascendancy. It is a book that combines astrology, poetry ("The Birth of the Author, 'The Saint George' of Biochemistry" by Edith F. A. U. Painton), and great gobs of arcane knowledge into something that sort of has to be seen to be believed. To clarify, I do not mean that as a recommendation, only a critique. This is an interesting book, to be sure, and it will appeal to those who wish such a synthesis of homeopathy and astrology (it has been attempted before with other remedies, in other books), but the fact that I am a Libra, according to this book, means that I need Natrum Phosphoricum. Would that it were that easy.

Homeopathic Cell Salt Remedies: A Simple Guide to Using Homeopathic Cell Salts, by Nigey Lennon and Lionel Rolfe, Garden City Park, New York: Square One Publications, (2004). This book really got me angry. It is a reprint of an older book, *Nature's 12 Magic Healers: The Amazing Secrets of Cell Salts,* which has had more than just a title change in this new edition. In the age of the reprint, when no book seems to ever go out of print, I guess it should not surprise or bother me, but the editors have taken the old book, which was published back in 1978 (thus the campy name) and tarted it up a bit with a new cover design and edited copy. They have drained it of all real homeopathic information in the hopes of making the book easy to follow and easy to use, and instead seem to want to make the cell salts into health and beauty aids. The original book, which I had happened upon at a book sale, was fun and an easy read. The new version is very much a pig with lipstick.

Harmony is the Healer: The Combined Handbook to Healing Flowers, Colour Therapy, Schussler Tissue-Salts, Emergency Homeopathy and Other Forms of Vibrational Medicine, By Indrid S. von Rohr, Rockport, Massachusetts: Element, Inc. (1992). This is just the book for you if you can't get enough vibrational medicine in your life, or if Carey's book on astrology and the cell salts fails to give you your full fix of the arcane. This book is a smattering of this and a dab of that. While it is a fun read, I can only hope that those who read it will not mix and match the remedies with the same abandon that they are written about.

Internet Sites

Although the cell salts merit mention on myriad Internet sites, the number of sites dedicated to them is surprisingly small. And, as with all other topics of study, the information available on the Internet swings wildly, in terms of quality.

Among the sites that I recommend for further study on the biochemic method are:

www.biochemics.info. This is the most complete and most thorough site I have found on the topic of the cell salts. It contains sections on Biochemics, Schuessler, and on related subjects ranging from the "Minerals of Life" to "The Funny Molecule." It is well worth a visit.

www.homeoinfo.com. While the site is by and large dedicated to the study of classical homeopathy, there are sections on both the cell salts and the Bach flower remedies. Choose the link for "Non classical topics" on the home page and then look under the rather interesting subheading of "Minimalists" for both offshoots of homeopathy.

www.hpathy.com/tissuesalts. Hpathy.com is one of the largest and most complete sites for all things homeopathic. Therefore it stands to reason that there is a nice sub-site link that deals with the tissue remedies. There is a good deal of information from books that have gone into the public domain and a discussion on the salts presented by site owner and noted Indian homeopath, Manish Bahtia.

www.elixirs.com. This is a commercial site, so its main purpose is to sell you cell salts, not to inform you about them. However, there is a list of FAQs on the cell salts that contains a good bit of basic information. The site (from which you can order your cell salts, if you like) also employs a counselor who is available to assist you in selecting the cell salts that are right for you.

Pharmacies

It's getting harder and harder to differentiate between the pharmacies and the Internet sites, as all the pharmacies that produce cell salts (and other homeopathic remedies) have an online presence. In the case of the cell salts, there are two homeopathic pharmacies that produce almost all the specific cell salt remedies and offer them in home kits, and such. Between these two pharmacies, I have a clear preference.

Luyties: Based in St. Louis, Missouri, this company has been in the business of making cell salts since 1853. They make a very good product and—this is important—they store their remedies in amber glass bottles, which I always prefer over remedies stored in plastic. For this reason, when offered a choice, I choose Luyties' remedies. They can be ordered by phone at 1 (800) Homeopathy, or online by going to www.1-800homeo pathy.com. This is a site that offers many different forms of homeopathic remedies, single remedies, and combinations, and sells a very inexpensive travel kit of cell salts which stores easily in any home medicine chest. Although they do not at this point sell my books, I still recommend them highly.

Hyland's Homeopathic: Based in Los Angeles, California, Hyland's has been making cell salts since 1903. This company offers an excellent product as well, although their pellets are chalkier than those made by Luyties, and for that reason you will sometimes have trouble getting children to take them. Also, they store their remedies in white plastic bottles, which, in my opinion, make them more likely to lose potency over time. They, too, have their own Internet site at www.hylands.com. This is a big site, from which you can order any homeopathic remedies, as well as cell salts. They also sell kits. They can be reached by phone at 1 (800) 624-9659.

Index

About the Author

Vinton McCabe is the author of seven books on the subject of health and healing. Most notably, he is the author of several books on the subject of homeopathy, published by Basic Health Publications. These include the two companion volumes to *The Healing Echo*, *The Healing Enigma* (2006) and *The Healing Bouquet* (2007), as well as *Household Homeopathy* (2005). McCabe also wrote *Homeopathy, Healing & You* (1998) and *Practical Homeopathy* (2000), both published by St. Martin's Press. He is also the co-author, with Dr. Marc Grossman, of *Greater Vision*, a book on natural vision improvement, which was published in 2002 by Keats Publishing.

He has studied homeopathy for the past three decades, and served as a homeopathic educator for fifteen of those years. He also served as the president of the Connecticut Homeopathic Association from the establishment of that non-profit organization in 1985 until his move to rural Connecticut in the year 2000. As the chief educator for that organization, he has been responsible for training thousands of laypeople and medical professionals alike in the basics of homeopathic philosophy and in the proper uses of homeopathic remedies.

In addition, McCabe has served on the faculty of both the Open Center of Manhattan and the Wainwright House of Rye, New York as a homeopathic educator. He has taught homeopathy at the Learning Annex, the Omega Institute, the New York Botanical Garden, and the Seminar Center in Manhattan, and has served as a member of the Board of Directors for the Hudson Valley School for Classical Homeopathy, for whom he developed educational materials. He has traveled throughout the United States, teaching courses in homeopathic philosophy and the uses of homeopathic and Bach flower remedies.

McCabe has worked with medical professionals, including acupuncturists, naturopaths, and chiropractors, as a homeopathic consultant. In addition, he is a trained vision therapist, and practiced vision therapy for seven years (1993–2000) at the Rye Learning Center in Rye, New York.

Aside from his work in vision therapy and homeopathy, Vinton McCabe has won awards for his journalism, as well as for poetry and theatrical writing. He is a published novelist. He was awarded an individual artist grant by the Connecticut Commission on the Arts for the creation of his first full-length drama, "Appassionata." In 1990, he was given the Dewar's Young Artist award in poetry.

Vinton McCabe has also worked as a producer, a writer, and a host in both television and radio. He was producer and host of the PBS series *Artsweek*, and creator and executive producer of *Healthplan*, an award-winning healthcare special produced by Connecticut Public Television. On radio, he has acted as a film and theater critic and hosted his own daily talk show.

As a print journalist, Vinton McCabe has done features work for many weekly and daily papers, as well as monthly publications, including *New England Monthly*, *The Stamford Advocate*, and *The New York Times*.

THE HEALING ENIGMA
DEMYSTIFYING HOMEOPATHY
Vinton McCabe

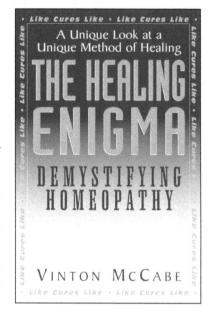

In his twenty-five years as a homeopathic educator, Vinton McCabe has taught thousands of medical professionals and laypersons alike both the philosophy and practice of homeopathic medicine. And through his books on the subject, he has reached many more, giving his readers both the tenets of homeopathy as put forth originally by Samuel Hahnermann more than two hundred years ago and his own unique viewpoint on the subject of homeopathic healing.

In *The Healing Enigma: Demystifying Homeopathy*, McCabe makes use of his full experience in homeopathy to give a fully rounded assessment of the principles of homeopathy and the manner in which it is practiced today. Throughout a text that combines a passionate argument for a mode of healing that is "rapid, gentle, and permanent" in its action, with personal insights and unexpected humor, readers will not only learn what constitutes classical homeopathy and the possibility for healing that it represents for their own lives, but they will also be challenged to consider that the reality of the healing process fundamentally differs from the allopathic concept of curing disease.

Where other books on the subject of homeopathy are limited in their scope to readers who are interested in the mechanics of its practice and the oversimplified selection of remedies, *The Healing Enigma* speaks as much to the practitioners and patients of traditional "allopathic" medicine as it does to those already in the alternative camp. While the "enigma" of the title speaks most directly to the practice of homeopathy, the underlying mystery has to do with the nature of healing itself and the methods that can be used to encourage the healing process.

240 pages • 6 x 9 Paperback • ISBN: 978-1-59120-071-0

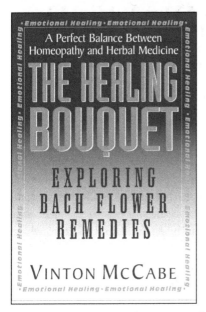

THE HEALING BOUQUET

EXPLORING BACH FLOWER REMEDIES

Vinton McCabe

Many books on the Bach Flower Remedies are written by nutritionists, herbalists, and practitioners of traditional Western or allopathic medicine. *The Healing Bouquet* has been written by Vinton McCabe, the author of seven books on the subject of homeopathy, health, and healing. In this companion volume to *The Healing Enigma*, McCabe places the Bach Flower Remedies within their natural context—that of homeopathic medicine.

As the author comments, "We have to remember that Edward Bach was an allopathic doctor—and a highly successful one—who, after reading the writings of Samuel Hahnemann, began to incorporate homeopathic philosophy in his practice of medicine. His evolution as a physician ultimately led him to close his medical practice in order to dedicate the last part of his life to the creation of a new pharmacy of healing tools, which today we call the Bach Flower Remedies. Given his background as both an allopath and a homeopath, the remedies he created are totally unique. They represent the perfect balancing point between homeopathic and herbal medicine."

In *The Healing Bouquet*, Vinton McCabe fully explores the history of the Bach remedies, as well as the philosophy behind their appropriate use. He also explains Bach's own philosophy of healing, one that stresses the need for emotional healing and the role that it plays in physical health. More importantly, he gives in-depth portraits of the guiding symptoms for each of Bach's thirty-eight remedies, portraits created with insight, humor, and an understanding of human emotions and behaviors that will allow readers to identify themselves and those who are part of their lives within these pages.

464 pages • 6 x 9 Paperback • ISBN: 978-1-59120-072-7

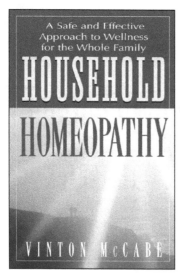

HOUSEHOLD HOMEOPATHY

A Safe and Effective Approach to Wellness for the Whole Family

VINTON McCABE

Homeopathy is an alternative medical practice that treats a health condition by administering minute doses of a remedy that would produce symptoms of that condition in a healthy person. Homeopathy is the full expression of holistic medicine, one that sees all people as whole beings in body, mind, and spirit, in whom all symptoms must then be both interconnected and interrelated. As a specific form of medical treatment, homeopathy dates back to just over 200 years ago, but the underlying principles of homeopathy go back to the time of Hippocrates.

Those who wish to gain a practical understanding of homeopathy know that study and dedication are required. This book makes the subject of homeopathy as down to earth and as practical as it can be and provides readers with plenty of food for thought. It discusses the most common homeopathic remedies—such as Arnica, Hypericum, Calendula, Aconite, and many others—and how they can be used safely and effectively. Household Homeopathy teaches readers how to promote healing in themselves and their loved ones—in their own homes. It covers how to handle remedies, how to select them, and how to use them wisely.

From short-term solutions to long-term fixes, the homeopathic approach to wellness can benefit sufferers of virtually every common health condition—from headaches and sore throats to digestive ailments and motion sickness. There will be no need to turn to potentially harmful medications to relieve everyday health complaints. This also means fewer trips to the doctor and reduced medical expenses. Armed with the information in this book and the will to fully understand homeopathic treatments, readers will be able to take control of their well-being and that of their loved ones safely and effectively.

400 pages • 6 x 9 Paperback • ISBN: 978-1-59120-070-3

CPSIA information can be obtained
at www.ICGtesting.com
Printed in the USA
JSHW021459260121
11202JS00004B/141